Health Services

Policy and Systems for Therapists

Third Edition

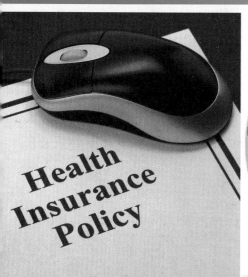
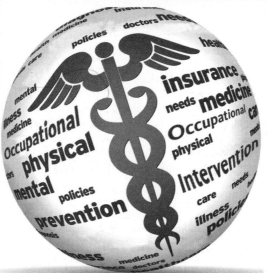
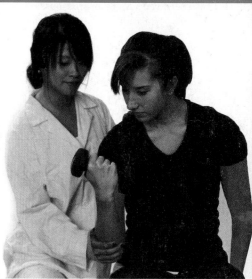

Robert W. Sandstrom PhD, PT
Department of Physical Therapy
Center for Health Policy and Ethics

Helene L. Lohman OTD, OTR/L, FAOTA
Department of Occupational Therapy

James D. Bramble PhD, MPH
Department of Pharmacy Sciences
Center for Health Services Research and Patient Safety

School of Pharmacy and Health Professions
Creighton University
Omaha, Nebraska

Publisher: Julie Levin Alexander
Publisher's Assistant: Regina Bruno
Editor-in-Chief: Marlene McHugh Pratt
Executive Editor: John Goucher
Editorial Program Manager: Monica Moosang
Editorial Assistant: Erica Viviani
Director of Marketing: David Gesell
Executive Marketing Manager: Katrin Beacom
Marketing Coordinator: Alicia Wozniak
Marketing Specialist: Michael Sirinides
Production Project Manager: Patricia Gutierrez
Senior Operations Supervisor: Nancy Maneri-Miller
Project Management Team Lead: Cynthia Zonneveld

Creative Director: Jayne Conte
Cover Designer: Bruce Kenselaar
Text Designer: Mary Siener
Cover Art: aceshot1/Shutterstock, Inc. & kbuntu/Fotolia
Chapter Opener Art: DrHitch/Fotolia
Media Director: Amy Peltier
Lead Media Project Manager: Lorena Cerisano
Full-Service Project Management: Anandakrishnan Natarajan
Composition: Integra Software Services, Ltd.
Printer/Binder: Edwards Brothers Malloy State St
Cover Printer: Lehigh-Phoenix Color/Hagerstown
Text Font: Times Ten LT Std, 10/12

Credits and acknowledgments borrowed from other sources and reproduced, with permission, in this textbook appear on the appropriate page within text.

Notice: The author and the publisher of this volume have taken care that the information and technical recommendations contained herein are based on research and expert consultation, and are accurate and compatible with the standards generally accepted at the time of publication. Nevertheless, as new information becomes available, changes in clinical and technical practices become necessary. The reader is advised to carefully consult manufacturers' instructions and information material for all supplies and equipment before use, and to consult with a health care professional as necessary. This advice is especially important when using new supplies or equipment for clinical purposes. The authors and publisher disclaim all responsibility for any liability, loss, injury, or damage incurred as a consequence, directly or in directly, of the use and application of any of the contents of this volume.

Many of the designations by manufacturers and sellers to distinguish their products are claimed as trademarks. Where those designations appear in this book, and the publisher was aware of a trademark claim, the designations have been printed in initial caps or all caps.

Library of Congress Cataloging-in-Publication Data

Sandstrom, Robert W.
    Health services : policy and systems for therapists / Robert W. Sandstrom, Helene L. Lohman, James D. Bramble.—3rd edition.
      p. cm
    Includes bibliographical references and index.
    ISBN-13: 978-0-13-311061-6 (alk. paper)
    ISBN-10: 0-13-311061-3 (alk. paper)
    I. Lohman, Helene, author.   II. Bramble, James D., author.   III. Title.
    [DNLM: 1. Health Services Accessibility—organization & administration—United States.   2. Health Policy—United States.
    3. Occupational Therapy—organization & administration—United States.   4. Physical Therapy Specialty—organization & administration—United States. W 76]
    RA395.A3
    362.1068—dc23
                                                                                                                2013010757

10 9 8 7 6 5 4 3 2 1

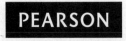

ISBN 10:   0-13-311061-3
ISBN 13: 978-0-13-311061-6

Contents

Preface to the Third Edition

Since the second edition was published in 2008, health policy has significantly changed.

The enactment of the Patient Protection and Affordable Care Act of 2010 (PPACA) in March 2010 (followed by its legal affirmation by the United States Supreme Court in June 2012 and a political re-affirmation by the reelection of President Obama in November 2012) is the largest regulatory overhaul of the United States health care system since the enactment of Medicare and Medicaid in 1965. The effects of the PPACA will be played out over several years, if not decades. In the years to come, this law is sure to affect the practice of all health care providers, including occupational therapists and physical therapists. In addition, a number of changes have occurred to other important public policies affecting therapist practice, for instance, in Medicare. Cumulatively, these developments have prompted this new edition of our textbook.

The central purpose of the book remains unchanged from the first edition published in 2003. We have striven to produce a comprehensive introduction to the policies and systems where occupational therapists, physical therapists, and therapist assistants find their work and provide their care. In doing so, we have made several changes in response to the users and reviewers of the book. We are very grateful to those persons who gave their time, expertise, and constructive criticism to help us improve this edition. The changes are as follows:

- The book has been increased from twelve to thirteen chapters. In this edition, we created a new chapter on global and population health. The global health content provides an international perspective on the health care systems of several industrialized nations. We have moved the public health content into this chapter and emphasized its relationship to population health. We view population health as a growing area of importance for occupational therapists and physical therapists in our evolving health care system.
- The advocacy chapter has moved from the end of the book to a position after the principles of health and public policy chapters. We believe that public policy advocacy skills need to have a stronger emphasis in occupational therapist and physical therapist entry-level curricula. We hope that this change will help students develop stronger policy analysis and advocacy skills by placing this content closer to the content that explains principles of policy. We encourage the use of the advocacy skills material to understand the reimbursement policy and systems chapters that follow this chapter.
- We welcome two new contributors (Creighton colleagues) to this edition of the textbook. Anna Domina OTD and Katherine Young OTD wrote a new chapter on special education and the mental health care systems. We are grateful for their participation and believe this chapter offers a significant, positive contribution to this edition. We also thank Yolanda Griffiths OTD for her assistance with this chapter.
- Several of the chapters on reimbursement policy (Chapters 6–9) had significant updates to reflect the statutory changes from the PPACA. As a result, we moved the content on casualty insurance, workers' compensation, and long-term care insurance to the private insurance chapter (Chapter 7). The Medicare chapter was rewritten to better explain the reimbursement strategies to their different benefits.
- All chapters have had content and emphasis updates and revisions that reflect changes in policy and the health care system since the second edition. We have tried to emphasize application to therapy practice.
- Key terms for each chapter are updated and defined in the Glossary. We have tried to be sensitive to the appropriate use of "patient" and "client" terminology when writing the narrative.

Increasingly, the challenge has been to make the book a comprehensive introduction to health policy and the health care system experienced by physical therapists and occupational therapists without making it too specific or overwhelming in detail. This has been challenging with all of the regulatory changes of the past few years and in recognition that many students have had little, if any, public policy or business background prior to encountering this content. There are outside resources that instructors will include that are not in this textbook and we recognize that there are portions of the book that will be excluded for one or more reasons. Given that a number of changes due to the PPACA have not yet occurred or are not widespread (e.g., health insurance exchanges or accountable care organizations), we expect that other resources will be accessed by instructors to provide students an appropriate education in these policy areas. Even as we conclude this edition, the Congress and president are considering Medicare and Medicaid reforms that may affect the content presented in this edition. For these still-to-be-determined changes, we have done our best to introduce concepts so as developments do occur the student will be able to recognize and understand the new policy or system landscape. We hope that we have been successful in meeting our primary goal to provide a strong foundation for a health services course in the therapy disciplines, apart from the traditional administration or management course. We offer this textbook as a tool to assist students and instructors in this endeavor.

We recognize and thank Mark Cohen, John Goucher, and the people of Pearson Education for their ongoing support of this project. A special thanks to Melissa Kerian and Anandakrishnan Natarajan for their patience, expert guidance, and editorial work as we have completed this edition. To our families, we offer our deepest thanks and love for their partnership with us on this book.

R.W.S.
H. L. L.
J.D.B.
Omaha, Nebraska

Reviewers

Rhea Cohn, PT, DPT
George Washington University
Washington, DC

Gail Fisher, MPA, OTR/L, FAOTA
University of Illinois at Chicago
Chicago, Illinois

Dory Marken, PhD
Eastern Kentucky University
Richmond, Kentucky

M. Beth Merryman, PhD, OTR/L
Towson University
Towson, Maryland

Rupal Patel, PT, MS
Texas Woman's University
Houston, Texas

Theodore Peterson, OTR, ATP, DrOT
Idaho State University
Pocatello, Idaho

Douglas Simmons, OTR/L, PhD
University of New Hampshire
Durham, New Hampshire

Laurie Walsh, JD, PT
Daemen College
Amherst, New York

Debbie Waltermire, MHS, OTR/L
Elizabethtown College
Elizabethtown, Pennsylvania

Public Policy and Therapists

CHAPTER OBJECTIVES

At the conclusion of this chapter, the reader will be able to:

1. Explain the interaction between policy, systems, and everyday practice in occupational therapy and physical therapy.

2. Define power and describe how policy is used to create and distribute power in a society.

3. Compare and contrast the uses of private policy and public policy as a method to effect social change.

4. Discuss the experience of disablement using the medical disablement, social disability, and universalism models.

5. Differentiate medical care and human services systems as components of the health care system for persons with disabilities.

KEY WORDS

Biomedical Model
Disablement
Distributive Justice
Dualism
Health Services
Marginalization
Social Disability
Universalism

CASE EXAMPLE ··

Susan is a 22-year-old single woman who works full time in a low-wage job as a hotel housekeeper. Her employer does not offer health insurance to employees. Susan does not qualify for any public insurance program. Susan is among the 46 million Americans without health insurance. She does not have a regular health care provider.

Susan lives with her grandmother, Sarah, who is age 70. Sarah worked for many years at a local factory and has been retired for the last five years. She receives a small pension and a Social Security payment each month. Sarah has health insurance through the Medicare program. Her low monthly income qualifies her to receive assistance from the Medicaid program for her Medicare deductibles. This benefit is important since last year Sarah had surgery and was hospitalized. Sarah did not pay for any out-of-pocket costs for her surgery.

Susan's mother, Ann, was injured in a motor vehicle accident three years ago and is unable to find work in her community. Since then, she has lost her job and has spent most of her life savings on medical expenses and monthly bills. She is waiting for a decision on her application for permanent disability status from Social Security. This would permit her to qualify for health insurance through Medicare and a disability benefit. She would like to work, but she has had difficulty finding vocational training options in her small community to help her learn new skills.

Case Example Question:

1. What are reasons for the differences in access to health care for Susan, Ann, and Sarah?

Introduction

Policies and systems are established to improve the lives of people and the overall community. This book is about an important and complex set of policies and systems in the United States: **health services**. Health services include the organization, financing, and operational delivery of medical care and certain human services to persons who experience disease, illness, injury, and **disablement**. We are most interested in the health services that affect disablement because this book is intended for physical therapists and occupational therapists. Specifically, we are going to explore the policies that support and direct therapy care as well as the systems that organize these services. It is our intent that as you become better informed about health services, you will become a better advocate for your patients and profession in order to improve existing policies and systems.

This chapter will introduce broad concepts regarding the development and implementation of health services affecting both occupational therapy and physical therapy. While our two professions are different, we are often similarly affected by policy. The next two chapters will introduce and explore the three foundational principles of health care policy: access, cost, and quality. Chapter 4 discusses public policies designed to address social disablement (i.e., marginalization and discrimination against persons experiencing disability). In Chapter 5, we present information about advocacy or how you can understand and potentially change the policies that we are going to discuss in this book. As you will learn, these policies have profound effects on the financing and organization of health care, including therapy services. First, we begin in this chapter by discussing the social structures that generate the policy and systems affecting therapists and persons with disabling conditions. Second, we will discuss different theoretical models of disablement and how they can explain different policies and systems.

We begin this chapter by introducing and discussing the issue of power as it affects health services. Specifically, we will discuss how power is distributed in American society through two policy-creating mechanisms: government (public) and private enterprise. Next, we will study different viewpoints about what it means to experience disablement. One's perspective on disablement affects the type of policy that is created and how its effectiveness is evaluated. Third, we will integrate the concepts of a medical care system and human services system into our discussion. All of these systems affect the organization of health services for persons who are experiencing temporary or permanent disablement. We will conclude the chapter with a historical review of the development of the U.S. health care system in the 20th century and discuss the future of health care delivery in the 21st century.

Policy and Power

On March 23, 2010, President Obama signed the Patient Protection and Affordable Care Act of 2010 (PPACA). This executive action culminated a year of congressional deliberation and debate about the structure and function of the U.S. health care system. The PPACA achieved reform of the private insurance and public insurance programs and incentivizes changes in the U.S. health care system when prior attempts at reform (e.g., President Truman's and President Clinton's initiatives to create a national health care system) had failed. The success of the PPACA, in light of the failures of prior national leaders to achieve health care reform, illustrates the interplay between history, policy, and power. These reforms matter to occupational therapists, physical therapists, and the patients that seek our services. As we will discuss in this book, access to health care is affected by insurance status and cost. Policy incentives create social and economic forces that affect the ability of therapists to create or expand therapy practices.

The lack of uniformity in health services in the United States can be traced to our system of policy **dualism** (see Table 1-1). Both the government and private enterprise are involved in the financing, organization, and delivery of health services, including occupational and physical therapy. While the PPACA changed the market for health insurance in the United States, its effects were controversial, primarily because it affected the balance of power between these two social forces. The sources of power for these two forms of health services policy-making are the core documents of our republic and the dominant economic system, free market capitalism. Physical and occupational therapy services are shaped by each source of power.

As noted in Table 1-1, health services originate from two sources of *power* in the United States: public and private. The allocation of resources and the organizational ability of government and the free enterprise system create the foundation for health services in the United States. As we will discuss in later chapters, government uses its taxing and regulatory authority to create access to medical and rehabilitation services, and, in some cases, to provide them to persons in need. Health services are also large economic enterprises (see Chapter 2). Both not-for-profit and for-profit enterprises have privately invested in the delivery and financing of health care, including therapy services. The generation of profit from this investment creates economic power that influences the health services system. The tension and interplay between private policy and public policy affecting health services are dynamic and political.

Table 1-1 Dualism and American Health Services Policy

	Government	Free Enterprise
Source of power	Constitution	Capitalistic markets
Role	Financing	Financing
	Regulation	Organization and delivery
	Organization and delivery	

While policy is often affected by government decisions and economic investment, effective and fair health services policy must consider those who are powerless. The lives of many persons who experience disablement are characterized by poverty, unemployment, lack of adequate housing and transportation, impaired access to medical care services, and barriers to equal social and economic opportunity in the broader society. Policies reflect the distribution of power in the decision-making process and the values and ethics of the broader society. Just policy considers the life and circumstances of the powerless and creates opportunities for empowerment and advancement for all persons in the society (Banja and DeJong 2000; Purtilo 1995).

In summary, policies are expressions of power that allocate and organize resources to address identified needs in a society. As we will discuss later, systems are established that respond to policy decisions. Just policies affirm the human rights of those who are powerless and provide a pathway for advancement. In the next section, we will discuss in more detail the sources of power that drive health services: government and private enterprise, as well as moral/ethical principles.

Sources of Power

Government

In the United States, the power of the government is established in the Constitution and other core documents. The United States was founded in a revolt against the authority of central government, based on the idea of promoting individual liberty. In general, the American democratic republic is a system of limited and distributed government. The American system distributes power among three branches: executive, legislative, and judicial. Government authority is further divided between the national government and the states. Laws enacted by legislative bodies require executive approval and are reviewable by the courts. All of these decisions are reported, analyzed, and commented upon by a free press to the governed citizenry. American citizens have a right to address their government, and public policymakers are held responsible for their decisions by election on a regular basis. As a result, government power is expected to be used cautiously, for understood reasons, and only when necessary.

When it does act, government power is coercive (Weiner and Vining 1992). Government has the power to unilaterally ascertain, restrict, permit, or direct resources of private individuals and organizations. Through the establishment and enforcement of laws and regulations, government can force behavior change on individuals and organizations that may not agree with the policy or that would not implement the same policy on their own. We also need to recognize the important role of government in establishing the "playing field" for private enterprise. Laws are government policies that establish private property and regulate markets that help to create the conditions that allow competition and the efficient, effective allocation of economic resources, including health services. When and under what circumstances can government use this power?

We can summarize two reasons for government action: failure of the private market to work as expected and a consensus among the governed populace for government action (Weiner and Vining 1992). In certain circumstances, private markets are perceived to be ineffective in meeting individual or community needs. For example, government provides the resources and ensures that roads and bridges are available to meet the transportation needs of society. It is accepted that it would be ineffective for each individual or community to privately organize and maintain a system of roads and bridges that permit people to work, shop, trade, or use recreational resources. It is a government responsibility to perform this responsibility. Government action is also expected to address concerns raised by the will of the people. For example, the Americans with Disabilities Act of 1990 (see Chapter 4) was enacted to improve the civil rights of all Americans with disabilities and reflected the social consciousness that this was the "right thing to do." It would be very difficult, if not impossible, for civil rights to be achieved in all communities unless government power was used.

POLITICAL PROCESS   The will of the people is exercised through the political process at all levels of government. Chapter 5 will introduce you to the principles and application of advocacy related to the political process. It is useful now, however, to discuss the

Table 1-2 Political Perspectives on the Role of Government in Health Care

	Libertarian	Egalitarian
Source of responsibility	Individual	Society
Health care	Earned reward	Prerequisite for work
Treatment of poor	Private charity	Government programs

Source: Based on Long, M.J. Social Values and the Medical Care System. In *The Medical Care System: A Conceptual Model.* Health Administration Press, Ann Arbor, 1994, p. 23–40.

political process as it relates to the distribution of power. It is within the political process that priorities are determined and actions taken or not taken by government to address societal concerns.

Political power derives from electoral activity, position, and the power of persuasion. Elections determine the representatives who will make decisions regarding policy. Elections reflect a perspective on the proper role of government in solving societal issues, (e.g., health care problems). In Table 1-2, two contrasting political perspectives on the role of government are presented. A libertarian perspective views the primacy of the individual and freedom from government intervention as important. Health care is viewed as an earned reward for work, and persons who have difficulty receiving health care are best served by private charity. In contrast, egalitarian philosophy emphasizes the society (its rules, attitudes, and barriers) as the source of societal problems. Government action is encouraged from this perspective to improve overall freedom. Health care is looked upon as a prerequisite for work and government programs as the solution to improve the health care system. While not presented in this table, Long (1994) also discussed a *utilitarian* perspective on health care that emphasizes the greatest good for the greatest number of people. This viewpoint is the foundation for many public health initiatives (see Chapter 13) that improve health by ensuring clean water or proper vaccinations against communicable disease. Elections determine a dominant perspective; although, in our political debates, it is common to hear views that blend both perspectives. Policymakers have decision-making power by virtue of their position, whether elected or appointed by an elected official. Persuasion is commonly demonstrated by the influence of interest groups, which is expressed through lobbying on legislative matters. This system is carried over to regulators who develop regulations concerning medical care policy.

Active Learning Exercise

Reflect upon your personal political philosophy. Would you describe yourself as a libertarian or egalitarian or somewhere in between? Think about the issue of providing mandatory, national health insurance for all Americans. To what extent does the social issue affirm or change your perspective?

Private Enterprise

Private enterprise creates power by the investment of capital and the organizational ability of individuals and institutions that create systems each day to exchange economic resources in a marketplace. The American system of capitalism provides opportunities for individual success and allows unsuccessful enterprises to fail. In this economic system, private enterprises accept the risk of failure, create strategy, innovate, and implement services that meet the needs of consumers. People who successfully do this have a proprietary advantage, a form of economic power. This proprietary advantage creates business activity, initiates competition, allocates economic resources efficiently, and creates wealth.

Decisions that meet the demands of the marketplace in an efficient manner result in rewards to the owner of the resources, that is, a profit. Profits are used to pay creditors, create new investment, and provide for the personal well-being of the owners (Helfert 1997). Profits create economic power. Investment and the incentive to invest provide the economic resources to build hospitals and clinics, hire therapists, educate the next generation of providers, and deliver critical medical care services to the ill or injured.

The generation of economic resources also finances the government. Individuals and businesses pay taxes that support governmental action. While government and private sources of power are different, we must recognize that they are symbiotic and, at times, complementary. This relationship fuels the reality of interest group politics, the necessary advocacy of specialized, private groups for governmental action, and political action committees, groups that privately finance the candidates for government office who support their perspectives. The American Physical Therapy Association (APTA) and the American Occupational Therapy Association (AOTA) have long recognized this reality at all levels of government and expend considerable time and resources to involve members in the political process.

Ethics and Values

Complex societies, like the United States, are always changing. Changing economic conditions, emergence of new threats to the public health or welfare, and developing technologies alter the lives of persons. These changes often mean that existing social structures or policies are inadequate for the present or emerging circumstances. For a society to be well ordered and functioning to permit maximum quality of life for its citizens, the policies or social contracts of persons within the society must be just. The principal focus of ethics is often on individual duty and responsibility as a professional to one's patient. However, social policy also reflects ethical values. The key concept for thinking about and determining the ethics of social policy is **distributive justice**. One of the purposes of this book is to help you understand health policy and be able to reflect upon the rules, regulations, and systems that you work in, so that you can understand their effect on your practice and advocate for a more just society. In Chapter 5, we will explain the specific skills to be an effective advocate. In this section, we are going to think about ethical principles from three important philosophers about social policy in their worlds: Aristotle, John Rawls, and Michael Long. From their ideas and reflections, we can ascertain some principles upon which to think about the fairness and equity of the world in which we live and work.

For policy to be just, Aristotle (as summarized by Denier [2007], pp. 18–19) stated that social goods should be shared in a community "as far as it complies with the principle of equality of geommetrical proportion. This means that justice demands to *treat equals equally and unequals unequally*". Aristotle understood that distributive justice requires policy whose outcome or effect is not equivalent for all persons. As described by Denier, the dilemma is that a definition or standard of the meaning of "equals" or "unequals" is often difficult to determine. She describes four Aristotelian criteria or descriptors of persons that could be used to evaluate the distributive justice implications of social policy in this paradigm: personal needs, contributions to the society, status, and assignment by merit. Aristotle believed that assignment by merit was the best justification for unequal distribution of social goods. While there is no consensus understanding of ethical social policy, Aristotelian theory establishes the ethical framework for a social response that is customizable to the attributes and needs of individual persons. How does this framework support the ethics of social policy for persons with disabilities or in need of therapy services?

As we have already indicated, many people experience disenfranchisement from the mainstream of society. Socioeconomic disadvantage, discrimination, and isolation from opportunities affect the lives of people who are "different" from the majority in the community. Persons with disabilities have historically experienced these circumstances (Banja 1997). Policies that affect everyone, including the powerless, should be fair and equitable. Laws and private policies reflect the basic values and ethics of the society and must be considered along with economic power and government authority in any debate on health services. John Rawls was a very influential 20th-century American philosopher on the subject of social justice, social policy, and social institutions. In *A Theory for Justice* (1999), Rawls identifies two principles for creating or determining just social policies and institutions:

1. Each person has an equal right to a fully adequate scheme of basic liberties that is compatible with a similar scheme of liberties for all (Equal Liberty Principle).
2. Social and economic inequalities are to satisfy two conditions. First, they must be attached to officers and positions open to all under conditions of fair equality of opportunity, and, second, they must be to the greatest benefit of the least-advantaged members of society (Difference Principle).

In Rawls's perspective, the first principle should be the first priority, and the Difference Principle has secondary priority. Both principles have priority over other considerations, for instance, welfare or efficiency in determining the ethics of social policy. Rawls did not specifically identify health care, but he did identify wealth and income as basic liberties in his first principle. "Rawlsian" theory is useful because it clarifies and expands upon Aristotle's ideas about the justice of inequalities in a society. Just social policies and structures permit all persons to have access to social goods based on equality of opportunity, and the "greatest benefit" is given to persons who are disadvantaged or marginalized.

Long (1994) describes four values that form the ethical base for health policy in the United States: freedom, equality, rewards, and treatment of the poor. Table 1-3 outlines the four principles and provides an example of a contemporary health services policy issue that is an application of the principles developed by Long. Freedom is a social construct that describes our relationship to one another and our ability to make and act upon individual decisions. Related to the ethical principle of autonomy, the ability to make choices about health care and have access to services are examples of policy matters related to the principle of freedom. Should people have the freedom to choose their health care provider without limitations from a managed care plan? Related to the ethical principle of beneficence, the principle of equality defines the sharing and disbursement of rewards and responsibilities in society. Who is entitled to receive health care services? How will health care services be distributed to people? The large number of Americans without health care insurance (prior to the PPACA) demonstrated that we do not have a system that guarantees equal access to health care (see Chapter 2).

The principle of rewards addresses this question: Is health care a basic right, or is it payment for contributions to the greater social good? Our core government documents do not define health care as a basic right of citizenship. A universal, national health insurance plan for all Americans has not been enacted. However, we have some laws (e.g., a right to emergency care) that create a legal expectation that all persons are eligible for a level of health care. Finally, according to Long (1994), health care policy must address the issue of the powerless and the poor. Treatment of the poor is an issue of social justice. A civil and just society will have policies and systems that provide for the care and treatment of all people, not only the economically advantaged or socially elite. Government intervention in health care has often been predicated on meeting the needs of historically disadvantaged groups (see Chapters 7 and 8).

Table 1-3 Ethical Considerations of Health Services Policy

Ethical Principle	Contemporary Issue
1. Freedom	Medicare therapy cap
2. Equality	Uninsured Americans
3. Rewards	Universal or employment-based health insurance
4. Treatment of the poor	Medicaid program changes

Based on M. Long, *The Medical Care System: A Conceptual Model* (1994).

In summary, health services are affected by competing and complementary sources of power in society: government and private enterprise. To be workable, social policy, including health care policy, must be perceived as meeting moral and ethical values in the society. This is a dynamic and changing situation that is created by multiple stakeholders making decisions each day. The PPACA of 2010 changed the social structure of health care in the United States in an attempt to improve access and reduce the number of persons without health insurance. Health care in the United States is political, and the decisions made in private enterprises and government affect the experience of disablement for millions of Americans. Let us now turn our attention to the experience of disablement and discuss how changing perspectives on this issue have affected the development of health services for persons with disabilities.

Experience of Disablement

The special interest of this book is how policy and systems affect people with disabilities and the people who care for them. Physical therapy and occupational therapy exist as professions to serve a societal need to treat people with disabilities. The incidence and prevalence of temporary and permanent disablement create a human and social need for assistance, new opportunities for independence, and community.

The experience of disablement creates foundational paradigms for the understanding of what needs to be done and the organization of rehabilitation health services. Disablement is experienced as a biomedical problem, an economic challenge, and a socio-political issue. Disablement is a major social problem. The size and prevalence of disablement mean that solutions require the involvement of major social institutions.

Disablement is common to the human experience and has existed throughout human history. It is only in the last 150 years, however, as Western society has industrialized, that formal attempts have been made to define disablement and to develop a major, organized, social response beyond the family unit. In the United States, a fundamental principle for defining and determining this social response is the individual's ability or inability to work (Alston 1997; Kennedy and Minkler 1998). The inability of a person to work jeopardizes the ability of the person and family unit to be self-sustaining. As a result, a broader social response is needed to provide the individual and family unit with support. At odds with this idea is the societal expectation that everyone capable of self-support and work will do so. Society can ill afford a policy that provides generous benefits to individuals and family units that are capable of working for self-support.

Ability to work as an establishing principle for defining disablement creates three new questions for policymakers: Who can work or not work? What types of services are needed by people who cannot work? What can society afford to provide to those who are unable to support themselves and their social unit? The first two questions have been addressed to medical care providers. The third question is a matter of continuing contention within and between private and public policymakers.

Answers to these questions are affected by the prevailing definition of the disablement experience. The basic characteristics of three major perspectives of disablement are summarized in Table 1-4. Historically, the **biomedical model** has been the dominant model of thinking about disablement in the United States. The social disability model has arisen in complement to and, in some cases, opposition to the biomedical model. Universalism challenges the notion that disablement is a special or separate policy issue. All three models affect the organization and delivery of therapy services to persons with disability in the United States.

Biomedical Model

In order to determine eligibility for benefits, policymakers have turned to health care providers to determine the type and extent of disablement. Since the late 19th century, medical doctors have been granted power to determine and certify who is disabled and who, within the guidelines of the policy, can receive benefits. This policy decision resulted in the "medicalization" of disablement (Craddock 1996a; Williams 1991). As the scientific rationale for medical practice grew exponentially in the 20th century, disablement became increasingly viewed as a biomedical problem.

Table 1-4 **Disablement Models**

	Medical Rehabilitation	Social Disability	Universalism
Source of disablement	Person	Social attitudes and policies	Both
Experience of disablement	Structure and function of body	Discrimination and isolation	All persons have potential
Response	Medical care	Human services	Integrated system

The focus of the biomedical model is to explain the patient's experience by understanding the source of the problem in terms of basic science and cellular pathology. This perspective emphasizes the role of the physician. The expansion of science and the acceptance of the biomedical model fostered a sophisticated and expensive medical care system with an emphasis on the identification and cure of pathology. Disablement was understood as a problem of medical pathology.

The biomedical model has limits, however, in its ability to explain disablement. Disablement is not "curable." Disablement often begins at the point where medical practice has limited effectiveness to eliminate disease or reverse injury. The manifestations of the pathology are not acute. Instead, they are usually chronic. A definition of disablement and the ultimate determination of success in treating disablement go beyond the terms used in treating acute illness, that is, morbidity and mortality. By the mid-1960s and thereafter, with the emergence of the Nagi model (Nagi 1965), new biomedical models emerged to explain the experience of disablement.

These models of "medical disablement" broaden our understanding of the manifestations of disease and injury. Impairments, functional limitations, and disability defined the organ/tissue, whole person, and societal role effects of chronic illness and disablement (Brandt and Pope 1997). The philosophy of medical disablement supports policies that develop systems to address these concerns. Physical therapy and occupational therapy services that improve function and address pain, weakness, contracture, and similar problems, can be defined as "medically necessary" and, therefore, are reimbursed through medical care insurance. This policy supports the provision of necessary services for those who are recovering from recent or recurring illness or injury.

The definition of "medical necessity" also limits independent therapist action and direct access to therapy services by the public. Many insurance plans, including public plans, require physician certification of therapy services in order for persons with disablement to access therapy care. We will discuss these issues in depth in Chapters 6–9. The medicalization of therapy services has also organized complex systems that employ therapists within the medical care system, typically dominated by physicians. We will explore this system in detail in Chapters 10 and 11. In summary, the medicalization of disablement has made it possible for many people to receive therapy services funded through medical care insurance. The dominance of the medical model, however, has also limited direct access to rehabilitation therapy care for persons with medically stable disabling conditions. While providing many employment opportunities, the medical rehabilitation model also constrains the distribution of therapists to the medical care system.

While the medical disablement model broadens the understanding of disablement to include more than pathology, the focus of the disablement experience remains on the individual. This conceptualization reinforces the importance of the patient-provider relationship to the exclusion of broader societal influences on the experience of disablement. As a result, some theorists reject the biomedical model as an inadequate explanation of disablement. Since medicine has limits to its effectiveness in treating chronic and disabling conditions, they argue, improvements in lifestyle and the barriers that affect people with disabling conditions must be addressed by different mechanisms.

Social Disability Model

Social disability thinking has developed as "a dynamic social phenomenon that has as much to do with cultural norms and socioeconomic status as it is due to the individual's physiologic condition" (Kennedy and Minkler 1998). Social disability theory can be traced to the responses of people with chronic disease and illness to the limits of the biomedical model in explaining their experience and to the American civil rights movement of the 1960s (Craddock 1996b). The social disability movement has instigated the development and study of disability as a culture and has caused the rethinking of the policy response to disablement.

From the perspective of social disability theory, medical disablement models are ineffective in explaining the situation of people who are physiologically stable but have ongoing disablement, social, and human services needs. Social disability theorists argue that the focus of medical disablement models on the person as the source of disability reinforces three negative stereotypes (Kennedy and Minkler 1998; Williams 1991). First, there is an excessive reliance on the health care provider as a source of solutions for disablement. Second, the biomedical model emphasizes a continual need for the person with a disabling condition to assume a "sick role" in order to receive services. Finally, the understanding of the disablement experience from a pathophysiologic perspective ignores other powerful social influences. From the social disability perspective, the source of disablement is not the pathophysiologic condition of the person but the sociopolitical environment.

Rather than originating as a pathologic event, disablement is created as the result of a social process of **marginalization** of persons with disabilities by the larger society and its policies. Marginalization of the disabled results in stigmatization by others (Williams 1991; Zola 1989). The inability to work weakens the economic power of people with disabilities, and, as a result, their political voice weakens. Those who are not disabled begin to view the expensive and special services required for full social participation by people with disabilities as a drain on other pressing social needs. Persons with disabilities are then forced to compete for limited social resources but experience barriers in their attempts to do so. In summary, one social disability theorist writes that disability "becomes a problem when it causes a person to consume rather than produce economic surplus" (Kennedy and Minkler 1998). From this perspective, disablement is not found in the person with physical or mental impairments. Disablement is created by a pattern of social and economic discrimination by the majority of the population against one group through a mechanism of isolation and exclusion.

The effect of the social disability model on policy has led to the enactment of numerous civil rights laws over the last 25 years that address discrimination against persons with disabilities. Policies have also been enacted to support a human services system that empowers persons with disabilities to live more full and productive lives in the community. For example, the Rehabilitation Act of 1973 created Centers for Independent Living and state vocational rehabilitation programs that provide services to address the issues of community integration and socioeconomic discrimination. We will cover many of these programs and laws in Chapter 4.

It is important to note that the medical rehabilitation system and the human services system are distinct from one another. Although both serve persons with disabilities, there is little formal integration and varying levels of coordination of policies and services between them. As we have discussed, their philosophical foundations, policy histories, and organizations are quite different. The problem of division, experienced in both theory and practice, is addressed by the concept of **universalism**.

Universalism

The historical development of disablement policy in the United States has created two separate systems. The medical rehabilitation system is organized using the biomedical model, focusing on the person as the source of disablement and directing interventions, including therapy services, at improving the quality of life from this perspective. The human services system is based on a social disablement model that identifies the policies and attitudes of the society as the source of disablement. Services that empower the person with disability through expanded civil rights, access to employment, improved housing, and transportation are provided by organizations supported by policies that address social disablement.

Both of these models and systems emphasize the experience of separation and difference for persons with disability. Universalism attempts to explain disablement not as a condition that affects a few individuals who require specialized medical or human services but rather as a situation to be recognized by the entire population at risk for disablement (Zola 1989). All of us live in a temporary state of nondisablement. The universalism philosophy advocates that most people will be affected by disability at some point during the aging process. As a result, policies should be developed to integrate all persons and to educate the population about living with a disability. Universalism addresses the fundamental problem of the marginalization of those with disabling conditions, whether on biomedical, social, economic, or political terms.

Universalism attempts to bridge the gap between the biomedical and social disability models. Integrated and coordinated policy that addresses the biologic, social, economic, and political reality of disablement is needed to truly address the experience of disablement. Ideally, an integration of medical and human services would be of the greatest benefit for persons who are experiencing disablement (Leutz 1999; Leutz, Greenlick, and Capitman 1994; Rothman 2010). There are few current examples of this form of pragmatic policy and systems development for persons with disabling conditions in the United States.

Internationally, there has been progress in conceptualizing the experience of disablement from a perspective that integrates both medical and social disablement models (Hurst 2003; Vrkljan 2005). The implementation of the International Classification of Functioning, Disability and Health (ICF) is an important development for therapists to understand and utilize when assessing patient status, effectiveness of treatment, and population health. The ICF was introduced in 2001 as a revision of the 1980 World Health Organization International Classification of Impairments, Disability and Handicap (ICIDH). The ICF describes "how people live with their health condition" (WHO 2013). The ICF assesses body structure and function, activities and participation, and contextual factors, that is, the environment and personal factors (Jette 2006). Body structure and function, activities, and participation are similar to the previously described conditions of impairments, disabilities, and handicap in the ICIDH (similar also to the medical model we discussed earlier). Environmental conditions include social variables (e.g., attitudes and services), systems, and policies as they affect persons with disabilities. The ICF has been operationalized in several of these domains and is progressing towards a useful measure of both medical and social disablement.

Active Learning Exercise

Visit the WHO ICF website and learn more about the ICF (http://www.who.int/classifications /icf/en/) Reflect upon a patient/client you have worked with and describe their disablement status using the ICF model.

Therapists and The Health Care System

The practice of occupational therapy and physical therapy has been shaped and transformed by the models of conceptualizing disability and the sociopolitical process that defines the priorities of the society and the health care resources needed to address these priorities (see Table 1-5). Today, it is difficult to comprehend the state of health care delivery at the beginning of the 20th century. At that time, health care was a small, unregulated, and privately funded enterprise. The number of health care providers was relatively small and lacked uniform educational standards. Competing philosophies of treatment (e.g., allopaths vs. homeopaths) applied care in a largely unregulated and unscientific environment. Limited technologies were available to diagnose or treat disease. Acute illness (e.g., infectious disease) was the predominant problem. Most care was provided in private homes or for the poor, in substandard hospitals designed to quarantine illness. A small public health structure existed in only a few urban areas. Disablement was not a major health care issue, and the social response was limited primarily to families.

Table 1-5 Development of U.S. Health Care in the 20th Century

	1900	1950	2000	➤2010
Philosophy of care	Competing philosophies/ little science	Dominance of allopaths/rise of bioscientific model	Increasing interdependence/ increased emphasis on understanding the sociology and economics of health care	Interdependent systems
Funding	Private pay	Private pay/ small insurance industry	Large insurance programs/ small private pay	Large insurance programs/ small private pay/ providers share risk
Primary location of care	Home	Hospital	Outpatient settings	Integrated systems, e.g., accountable care organizations or medical homes
Role of government	None	State regulation	Federal insurance programs	Large federal insurance programs
Concept of disablement	No social response	Medical problem	Medical and social response	Medical and social response
Status of OT and PT	Nonexistent	Rationalized within organizations; dominated by medicine	Growth of private practice; work in acute and postacute care environments	Strong demand for services; need to integrate into emerging systems
Primary societal health policy objective	Standardize and improve quality	Improve access to care	Restrain growth in cost	Restrain growth in cost; improve access to care

The first half of the 20th century witnessed the development of a private health care system dominated by allopathic medicine. Other providers, (e.g., homeopaths, naturopaths, and chiropractors) were marginalized. This development was supported by the growth of a bioscientific understanding of disease, standardization of educational qualifications of providers, the emergence of new technologies, the establishment of environments to support these technologies (i.e., the hospital), and strong political activity, especially at the statehouse level. Private health insurance emerged in midcentury as a way to provide an inexpensive benefit to workers. Private pay, however, dominated the financing of health care. Both physical therapy and occupational therapy were established in the health care system during this period but came to be dominated by medicine and rationalized within hospital organizations.

The second half of the 20th century saw significant changes, especially in the financing of health care. The enactment of Medicare/Medicaid in 1965 and the development of managed care in the late 1980s into the 1990s marked the entrance of both government and corporations into the operations of health care delivery. Both of these programs greatly increased the amount of money available to fund health care but, as concerns about the high cost of health care rose, increased the power of these entities in determining how and where this money is spent. This led to an expansion in the size and scope of the health care system followed by a reorganization and reintegration of health care services. Health care was no longer provided in hospitals but in a number of settings in the "post acute" environment. Chronic diseases, many associated with the modern lifestyle, emerged as dominant problems. Occupational therapy and physical therapy grew with the health care system and emerging problems. A private practice emerged in both professions during the latter half of the century. To varying degrees, therapists achieved freedom from the dominant position of allopathic medicine, although medicine retains an influential position in relation to both professions. Health care has become increasingly a federal political issue; although, the country has rejected several attempts at national health insurance or a national health care system.

What about the 21ˢᵗ century? The first decade of the century was characterized by continuing growth in health care and concern about health care costs, especially as they affect the federal government budget. The PPACA is the most significant reform of the health insurance industry since Medicare and Medicaid. While expected to decrease costs to the federal government versus the status quo, the PPACA primarily addressed lack of access to health insurance (see Chapter 6). However, PPACA reforms also advanced system changes (i.e., the development of patient-centered medical homes and accountable care organizations) (see Chapter 10). If these new systems develop as planned, physical therapists and occupational therapists will be challenged to meet new opportunities not as solo practitioners but rather in concert with other professionals in integrated models of care (Johnson and Abrams 2005; Kigin, Rodgers and Wolf 2010).

As can be noted from this review, both occupational therapy and physical therapy have grown and adapted as occupations with the changes in the health care system. The future of both professions, especially their autonomy, will be affected by these social forces and the continuing/emerging needs of the society (Domholdt 2007; Sandstrom 2007). In this book, we are going to introduce the structure of the policies and systems where therapists do their work. Coupled with an appreciation for the historical context of this work, the book should give the reader an viewpoint to the future opportunities and challenges facing the professions and their work.

Conclusion

In this chapter, we have introduced the principles that affect the creation of policy and systems to deliver rehabilitation services to people with disabilities as well as the practice of occupational therapy and physical therapy. Policy is about distributing power to maintain the status quo or to effect needed social change. The power to develop health services policy has two sources: government and private enterprise. Health services policy has social, economic, and ethical effects. Just policy distributes health care in an equitable and fair manner with special concern for persons who are disadvantaged. Policy development and implementation is a political process. Much of the remainder of this book will discuss the effects of policy decisions made in both private and public forums.

Health services policy that addresses disablement has developed in response to the dominant perspective that has defined the disabling experience. The medical model focuses on the person as the source of disablement.

Important in determining eligibility for medical and social benefits (see Chapters 6–9), this model has reinforced the development of an acute and postacute health care system (Chapters 10 and 11). The social disability model finds the source of disablement in the community and society. This model has fostered the development of a community and educationally-based system of services for persons with disability that is explored in Chapter 12. Finally, we will focus on global and population health perspectives in Chapter 13.

Access, cost, and quality are three foundational principles that drive all health policy, including policies that affect occupational therapy and physical therapy. An ideal system would maximize access to high-quality health care at a reasonable cost. In the next chapter, we will review the successes and challenges for U.S. health services policymakers as they attempt to achieve two of these objectives: access and cost.

Chapter Review Questions

1. Define the relationship between power and policy.

2. What are the sources of power in the policymaking process?

3. Who is involved in policy formation, and how is policy formed?

4. Identify the uses and limitations of private policy and public policy in meeting social need and effecting social change.

5. Describe the principles that can be used to evaluate the distributive justice of health policy.

6. How does "ability to work" affect policy toward persons with disabilities?

7. Compare and contrast the characteristics of the biomedical and medical disablement models.

8. Define the source of disablement according to the social disability model.

9. What is universalism?

10. How have perspectives on the experience of disablement affected the development of system responses to disablement?

Chapter Discussion Questions

1. Some people advocate for government action to improve health care. Others believe that private market solutions are the better choice for increasing access to quality and affordable health care for more Americans. What are the pros and cons of each of these philosophies on health services policy?

2. Compare and contrast the positions of the social disability and medical disability models of disablement. Which of these models do you believe is most effective in meeting the needs of persons with disability? Why?

3. Rawls describes two complementary and competing principles for just social policy: equal liberty and preferential benefits to the disadvantaged. Do you agree with his theory? Discuss its strengths and weaknesses.

4. Physical therapy practices primarily within the model of medical disablement. Occupational therapy also practices within the context of social disability. How does the orientation of each profession affect the type of services provided?

References

Alston, R. J. 1997. Disability and health care reform: Principles, practices, and politics. *J Rehabil* 63(3): 15–19.

Banja, J. D. 1997. Values, function, and managed care: An ethical analysis. *J Head Trauma Rehabil* 12(1): 60–70.

Banja, J. D., and G. DeJong. 2000. The rehabilitation marketplace: Economics, values, and proposals for reform. *Arch Phys Med Rehabil* 81: 233–39.

Brandt, E.N., and A.M. Pope, eds. 1997. *Enabling America: Assessing the role of rehabilitation science and engineering.* Washington DC: National Academy Press.

Craddock, J. 1996a. Responses of the occupational therapy profession to the perspective of the disability movement. Part 1. *Br J Occup Ther* 59(1): 17–21.

_____. 1996b. Responses of the occupational therapy profession to the perspective of the disability movement. Part 2. *Br J Occup Ther* 59(2): 73–78.

Denier, Y. 2007. *Efficiency, justice and care.* Dordrecht: Springer.

Domholdt, B. 2007. The meanings of autonomy for physical therapy. Invited commentary. *Phys Ther* 87(1): 106–08.

Helfert, E. 1997. *Techniques of financial analysis: A modern approach.* 9th ed. Chicago: Irwin Press.

Hurst, R. 2003. The international disability rights movement and the ICF. *Disabil Rehabil* 25(11–12): 572–76.

Jette, A. 2006. Toward a common language towards function, disability, and health. *Phys Ther* 86(5): 726–34.

Johnson, M., and S.L. Abrams. 2005. Historical perspectives of autonomy within the medical profession: Considerations for 21st century physical therapy practice. *J Orthop Sports Phys Ther* 35: 628–36.

Kennedy, J., and M. Minkler. 1998. Disability theory and public policy: Implications for critical gerontology. *Int J Health Law* 28(4): 757–76.

Kigin, C.M., M.M. Rodgers, and S.L. Wolf. 2010. The Physical Therapy and Society Summit (PASS) meeting: Observations and opportunities. *Phys Ther* 90: 1555–67.

Leutz, W. 1999. Five laws for integrating medical and social services: Lessons from the United States and the United Kingdom. *Milbank Q* 77(1): 77–110.

_____, M. R. Greenlick, and J. Capitman. 1994. Integrating acute and long-term care. *Health Affairs* 13(4): 59–74.

Long, M. J. 1994. *The medical care system: A conceptual model.* Ann Arbor MI: AUPHA Press.

Nagi, S. Z. 1965. Some conceptual issues in disability and rehabilitation. In M. B. Sussman, ed., *Sociology and rehabilitation* (110–113). Washington DC: American Sociological Association.

Purtilo, R. 1995. Revisiting the basics of professional life. *PT Magazine* 3: 81–82.

Rawl, J. 1999. *A Theory of justice* (rev. ed.). Cambridge MA: Belknap Press of Harvard University. pp. 52–76.

Rothman, J.C. 2010. The challenge of disability and access: Reconceptualizing the role of the medical model. *J Soc Work Disabil Rehabil* 9: 194–222.

Sandstrom, R. 2007. The meanings of autonomy for physical therapy. *Phys Ther* 87(1): 98–105.

Vrkljan, B. 2005. Dispelling the disability stereotype: Embracing a universalistic perspective on disablement. *Can J Occup Ther* 72(1): 57–59.

Weiner, D.L., and A.R. Vining. 1992. *Policy analysis: Concepts and practices.* Englewood Cliffs NJ: Prentice Hall.

Williams, G.H. 1991. Disablement and the ideological crisis in health care. *Soc Sci Med* 32(4): 517–24.

World Health Organization (WHO). 2013. International Classification of Functioning, Disability and Health. Retrieved from http://www.who.int/classifications/icf/en/

Zola, I. 1989. Toward the necessary universalizing of a disability policy. *Milbank Q* 67 (suppl 2, pt. 2): 401–28.

2

Access and Cost of Health Care

CHAPTER OBJECTIVES

At the conclusion of this chapter, the reader will be able to:

1. Distinguish the different components that define access to health care services.

2. Describe the role of health care insurance with regard to accessing health care services and a person's health status.

3. Explain the relationship of health care insurance, access to health care services, and a person's health status.

4. Discuss the major components of health care revenue and expenditures in the United States.

5. Explain the economic, demographic, and systems reasons for the growth in health care costs.

6. Discuss the effects of different payment mechanisms on health care costs.

7. Explain the concept of direct access to therapy services.

KEY WORDS

Acceptability
Access
Accessibility
Accommodation
Affordability
Availability
Capitation
Case Rate
Cost-containment
Direct Access
Expenses
Fee for Service
Global budgeting
Gross Domestic Product
Markets
Predisposing Factors
Revenue
Uninsured

CASE EXAMPLE ··

Joe had worked for several years as a supervisor in a manufacturing plant before losing his job to the restructuring of the plant. Now out of a job, he decided to return to school to get a degree. So Joe started to work part time and enrolled as a full-time student at the local community college. His goal was to become a physical therapist assistant. Up to this time, Joe regularly visited his physician. Due to lack of health insurance and having a lower-paying, part-time job, physician visits were put on hold. Joe felt he had to make this decision since out-of-pocket insurance was too expensive. Having been relatively healthy, making this decision did not seem unwise.

During this time Joe developed what he thought was a hang nail on his left index finger. Joe noticed that his finger had become red and swollen. At first, he treated the finger by soaking the nail in disinfectant. Joe was concerned so he went to his physician. At that time, Joe was informed that the nail would need to be surgically removed. The procedure would cost $200, and he would need to bring that in cash since he did not have insurance. But without insurance and without the cash, he did not return. After several months of continuing to feel sick and his finger not healing, Joe went to the area's free health clinic.

By this time, gangrene was present, and the infection was present in the bone (i.e., osteomyelitis). All of this was the result of undiagnosed and untreated diabetes.

This is a typical story about how the lack of health insurance and the high cost of health care combine to delay diagnosis. Additionally, when treatment is sought, it is often incomplete since the follow-up care needed is too costly. In the example above, we should note that the neuropathy and circulatory complications indicate that Joe probably had been diabetic for more than two years. It was not until exhaustion and gangrene developed that medical treatment came into play. However, diagnosing and treating diabetes early can help avoid or delay complications; thus, highlighting the importance regular visits and medical screenings (Sered and Fernandopulle 2005).

Case Example Questions/Discussion:

1. Describe Joe's access to health care services and how his care was impacted by his access.

2. Discuss what activities could have been done better to improve the care services Joe received.

Author's note: This story was summarized from S. Sered and R. Fernandopulle (2005). *Profiles of the Uninsured: Uninsured Americans Tell Their Stories.* The complete article as well as additional stories can be found at http://www.cmwf.org/General/General_show .htm?doc_id=256036

Introduction

In Chapter 1, we introduced broad themes and theories that describe the goals of the health care system and how policy is developed and changes over time. In this chapter, we get more specific about how to think about the system you will work in and to evaluate health policy. The "three-legged stool" of health care policy in the United States is **access**, cost, and quality. These three major constructs are commonly used in describing and evaluating the health care system (Barton 1999). A set of relatively simple questions can illustrate the importance that each of these constructs has in our discussion of health care services. For example, when an individual is in need of medical attention, is the needed care for complete recovery both available and accessible in a timely manner? Does the person receive the necessary referrals for medical care from the appropriate provider? Is the health care provided appropriately? Are the desired outcomes achieved? How much will the health care cost? How will the provider be paid, and who will pay for the health care received? The current chapter focuses on issues surrounding both the access to, and the cost of, health care services. Quality will be addressed in the Chapter 3.

Access to Health Care Services

The conversation about access to the health care system often is centered on the presence or absence of health insurance. While a lack of health insurance is the largest barrier to access, it is not the only barrier that individuals face as they enter the health care system. Unlike the situation in much of the industrialized world, access to health care in the United States is not a guaranteed right (Fuchs 1993). Thus, a person's ability to access needed health care services is a perennial issue for health care providers and policymakers. There are many different dimensions worthy of consideration in conceptualizing access to health care services. For example, Penchansky and Thomas's (1981) conceptualization of access that examines the fit between the characteristics of the health care system and the expectations of patients is presented in Table 2-1. Penchansky and Thomas examine this fit along five dimensions: **availability**, **accessibility**, **accommodation**, **acceptability**, and **affordability**.

Availability

Availability refers to the relationship between the amount and type of services provided by health care workers and the amount and type of services required by the population in need. The goal is to have the best possible match between the services provided and those needed. For example, a community with a large elderly population should have more geriatric services than a community with a younger demographic.

Accessibility

Another barrier to utilizing health care services is accessibility, such as geographic factors; thus, the second dimension examines the accessibility of health care services. Accessibility describes the relationship between the location and supply of health care providers and services (e.g., therapy clinics) and the location and transportation resources of the population (i.e., potential patients). Health services tend to be located in population centers that are large enough to support them. People living outside of these centers, such as sparsely populated rural areas, may not have access to the full range of health care

Table 2-1 Penchansky and Thomas's Access Factors

Availability—the amount and type of services provided related to the population's need.
Accessibility—the location and supply of health care services related to the population's location and transportation resources.
Accommodation—the organization and appropriateness of health care services, as well as the population's ability to use those services.
Acceptability—the attitude between health care providers and the population towards one another.
Affordability—the price of health care services related to the population's ability to pay.

Source: Penchansky and Thomas Access Factors in The Concept of Access: Definition and Relationship to Consumer Satisfaction. *Medical Care* 19, 2(1981):127–40. Used by permission.

services, regardless of their ability to afford those services. People who must travel great distances to reach the care that is needed may postpone or go without needed medical services. Practically, this means that though services are available, they are not accessible to the individuals in need. Rural communities across the country are some of the most at risk in having less than ideal access to health care services. Even in urban areas, there are barriers to the accessibility of health services, including human-made barriers (e.g., freeway patterns) and natural barriers (e.g., rivers).

Accommodation

The third dimension, accommodation, addresses three related issues: (1) the manner in which health care providers, services, and facilities are organized; (2) the population's ability to use these providers, services, and facilities; and (3) the population's opinion of the appropriateness of the providers, services, and facilities. Accommodation is affected by temporal factors that can create barriers which may keep care-seekers from accessing health care providers and services. Among these barriers are, for example, the potential mismatch between the schedules of providers and patients that results from inflexible working hours, the ability to attain childcare, or a host of other factors. These issues need to be considered when organizing health care services so that they are "accommodating" to potential patients.

Acceptability

The fourth dimension, acceptability, examines the attitudes and perceptions that health service providers and the population have toward one another. For example, cultural differences, including language barriers, differing values on health, or conflicting customs or beliefs, may exist. All of these differences may prevent an individual from reaping the full benefits of available health care services, even though the care may be available, accessible, accommodating, and affordable.

Affordability

The final dimension, affordability, is concerned with the price of health care services or the ability of the population to pay. Financial access to health care services is closely tied to health insurance and the ability to obtain insurance coverage. (Health insurance is addressed more fully in Chapters 6–9.) However, as has been discussed, health insurance coverage or one's ability to afford medical care is not the only factor to consider in examining access to health care services. Health insurance, by itself, does not guarantee access to care; for example, the necessary health care provider or therapy clinic may not be available where the patient lives (see the discussion on structure of the health care system in Chapter 3). Additionally, patients may need a referral from a primary care physician to seek specialized services (e.g., physical therapy or occupational therapy).

As Penchansky and Thomas's conceptualization demonstrates, there are many factors that may affect the ability to access health care services. All of these dimensions (i.e., availability, accessibility, accommodation, acceptability, and affordability), along with the predisposing factors of potential patients (e.g., age, sex, and occupation), need to be considered to fully understand the degree of access that defined populations have to health care services. **Predisposing factors** are individual characteristics that indicate a "propensity to use" health care (Andersen and Newman 2005). Women, persons with prior illnesses, elderly persons, and children are well known to more commonly access health care. Policymakers and health care practitioners must account for the many dimensions of access as they plan for the delivery of health care. However, it is difficult to determine which barrier is most important. Each person may have his or her own unique barriers to overcome; thus, the most problematic barrier to receiving care varies across individuals.

Though barriers vary across individuals, as a whole, our country's biggest access-related problem is the affordability of health care services (Vistnes and Zuvekas 1999). Adequate health insurance is essential to overcome the affordability barrier and gain access to appropriate and timely medical care. Though health insurance, as has been argued, is only one of the dimensions of access, it is an important part of the financing and delivery of health care services in this country; the next section takes a closer look at this barrier.

Access and Health Insurance

One key factor in making health care services accessible is health insurance coverage. The affordability of health care services is one of the greatest barriers we face as a nation with regard to access to the health care system (Stoddard, St. Peter, and Newacheck 1994). It is one of the main reasons that almost every presidential administration has introduced some sort of health care reform. Improvement of access to, and the affordability of, health care services was a major policy objective addressed by the Patient Protection and Affordable Care Act of 2010 (PPACA). We will be discussing a number of policy changes enacted by this law that affects the health insurance marketplace in Chapter 6.

Financial access to health care services is assured mostly by means of securing some form of health care insurance. Over the years, health insurance has provided the means for individuals to access the health care system and for health care providers to collect payment for services rendered. For most Americans under 65 years old, health insurance is obtained through their employer or the employer of a family member (Clemans-Cope, Garrett, and Hoffman 2006). In 2005, 62 percent of non-elderly Americans (those below 65 years old) belonged to employer-based health plans (Fronstin 2007). While the majority of non-elderly persons are covered through private insurance, Medicare provides coverage for people over 65, and Medicaid pays for services for those eligible to receive funds from the Temporary Assistance to Needy Families or the Supplemental Security Income program (SSI). While the specifics of health insurance plans are discussed in later chapters, the focus of this section is on the large problem of the uninsured and how it relates to accessing health care services.

Characteristics of the Uninsured

Over the last decade, the number of individuals without health insurance has steadily increased over time (see Figure 2-1). However, in 2011, the U.S. Census Bureau reported that those without health insurance dropped by 1.3 million from the previous year (Collins, Davis and Garber 2012).

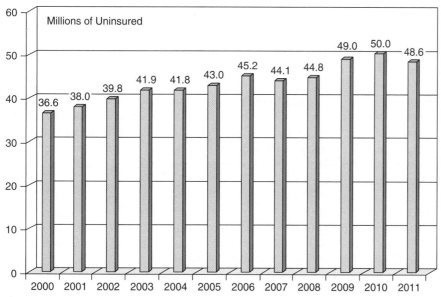

FIGURE 2-1 The Number of Non-Elderly Uninsured (in Millions)

Source: Income, Poverty, and Health Insurance Converge in the United States: 2011. United States Census Bureau, September 2012.

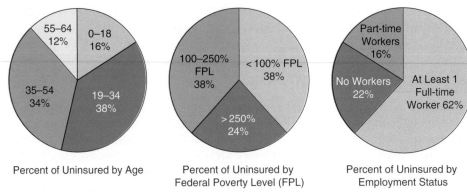

FIGURE 2-2   Characteristics of the Uninsured, 2010

Source: "The Uninsured: A Primer - Data Tables", (#7451-08), The Henry J. Kaiser Family Foundation, October 2012.

This information was reprinted with permission from the Henry J. Kaiser Family Foundation. The Kaiser Family Foundation, a leader in health policy analysis, health journalism, and communication, is dedicated to filling the need for trusted, independent information on the major health issues facing our nation and its people. The Foundation is a nonprofit private operating foundation, based in Menlo Park, California.

While the ranks of the uninsured continue to be high, the demographics and factors that place people at risk for being uninsured go relatively unchanged. The Kaiser Commission on Medicaid and the Uninsured (KCMU) reported a number of factors that contribute to the risk of being uninsured (KCMU 2012):

- Adults more than children are likely to be uninsured (see Figure 2-2). Low income children qualify for Medicaid or SCHIP (see Chapter 9), but adults only qualify for Medicaid if they are disabled, pregnant, or have dependent children. This situation was addressed by the Medicaid expansion provisions of the PPACA.
- Minorities are more likely to be uninsured than white Americans. Disparities in the number of uninsured are not solely tied to income.
- The poor and the near-poor are at the greatest risk of being uninsured (see Figure 2-2). This is due, in large part, to the high cost of health insurance. Of the nation's uninsured, two-thirds of them are classified as poor or near-poor. The PPACA aims to provide subsidies to the poor and near-poor to improve affordability of insurance.
- Most uninsured work (see Figure 2-2). Four out of five uninsured come from working families.

Health Status of the Uninsured

Discussions of health care reform are often centered on the attainment of a sense of equity with regard to the delivery and accessibility of health care services (Seiden 1994). Whether or not a person has health insurance makes a difference when and where they get the medical care they need. Currently, a lack of insurance coverage results in large discrepancies between the health care services available to the insured and the **uninsured**. The amount and type of health care services that people who are uninsured can afford and obtain are severely limited. The consequences of having limited access to needed health care services can be severe.

One reason that the uninsured do not get timely needed care is the lack of a regular place to receive care. As shown in Figure 2-3, over 50 percent of non-elderly uninsured do not have a regular place to go for advice or consultation (KCMU 2012). The lack of a regular provider is likely the main reason that those without health insurance are three times more likely to report problems with getting needed medical care. Other reasons for not getting needed care include the cost associated with that care. High costs may prohibit those without insurance from filling needed prescriptions as part of a physician's care plan (see Figure 2-3). The postponement of seeking care can have catastrophic consequences. For example, Braveman, Schaaf, Egerter, Bennett, and Schecter (1994) found that uninsured patients with appendicitis were more likely to have their appendix rupture due to delaying surgical intervention than were insured patients. More recent studies

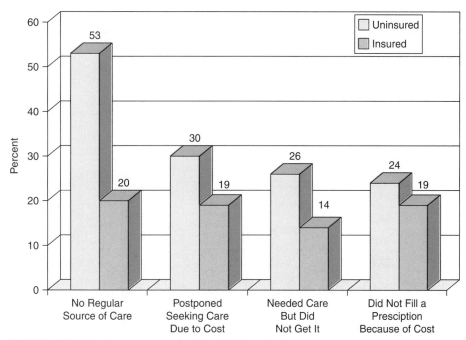

FIGURE 2-3 Barriers to Accessing Health Care Services

Source: "Summary of New Health Reform Law", (#8061), The Henry J. Kaiser Foundation, April 2011.

This information was reprinted with permission from the Henry J. Kaiser Family Foundation. The Kaiser Family Foundation, a leader in health policy analysis, health journalism, and communication, is dedicated to filling the need for trusted, independent information on the major health issues facing our nation and its people. The Foundation is a nonprofit private operating foundation, based in Menlo Park, California.

continue to support this conclusion. As reported by Davidoff and Kenney (2005) nearly half of the non-elderly uninsured have some type of chronic condition. In addition to postponing needed care, the uninsured are less likely to receive timely preventive care that may have an impact on their health status (Franks, Clancey, and Gold 1993). The KCMU reports (2006) that those with insurance are significantly more likely to have had recent mammograms and colon and cervical cancer screenings. Consequently, uninsured individuals with cancer are diagnosed in later stages of disease, which usually results in poorer outcomes, including dying earlier than those with insurance (Ayanian et al. 2000; Institute of Medicine 2003). This is just one example of how the lack of health insurance adversely affects the health of individuals, at least in part, because of inadequate access to health care services.

The Working Uninsured

So why are there so many uninsured, and why has the number of uninsured continued to increase over the years? There are multiple factors to consider in examining the increasing trend of uninsured persons. Two of these factors are the declining trend of employer-based insurance benefits and the rising premium costs for those who have insurance through their employer, as well as for those who buy health insurance individually.

Health insurance in the United States has historically been tied to employment (Kuttner 1999), but recently most of the uninsured in the United States are in working families. A 2012 Kaiser report on the uninsured indicates that more than three-quarters of the uninsured are in working families. There are many reasons that there are working uninsured, including a reduction in employer-sponsored insurance. Many of the reasons can be tied to one of the following two issues: 1) the high cost of health care services resulting insurance premiums, and 2) increases in employees' contributions to their health benefits (Cunningham, Aritga, and Schwartz 2008).

Employers, especially smaller employers, are sensitive to changes in health care premiums. With the continued growth rate of health insurance premiums, many employers either do not offer health benefits or have trouble affording their share of the health insurance premium. This results in greater financial burdens being placed on the patient/consumer. Employees must cover more and more of the health insurance premium. As shown in Figures 2-4 and 2-5, from 2001 to 2011, the burden has nearly doubled for both single and family coverage.

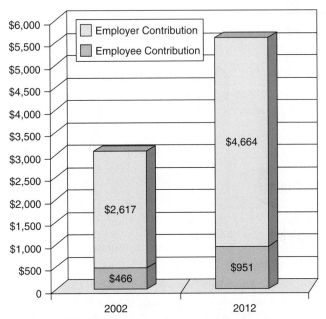

FIGURE 2-4   Employer and Worker Premium Costs for Individual Coverage

Source: "Medicaid Benefits: Online Database - Benefits by Service: Physical Therapy Services (October 2010)", The Henry J. Kaiser Family Foundation.

This information was reprinted with permission from the Henry J. Kaiser Family Foundation. The Kaiser Family Foundation, a leader in health policy analysis, health journalism, and communication, is dedicated to filling the need for trusted, independent information on the major health issues facing our nation and its people. The Foundation is a nonprofit private operating foundation, based in Menlo Park, California.

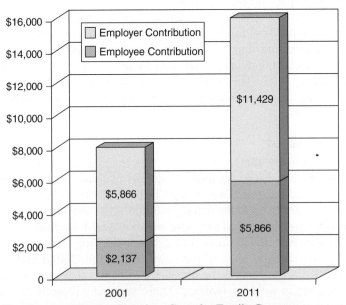

FIGURE 2-5   Employer and Worker Premium Costs for Family Coverage

Source: "Medicaid Benefits: Online Database - Benefits by Service: Physical Therapy Services (October 2010)", The Henry J. Kaiser Family Foundation

This information was reprinted with permission from the Henry J. Kaiser Family Foundation. The Kaiser Family Foundation, a leader in health policy analysis, health journalism, and communication, is dedicated to filling the need for trusted, independent information on the major health issues facing our nation and its people. The Foundation is a nonprofit private operating foundation, based in Menlo Park, California.

As can be seen, access to health insurance and health care services have been long-standing policy weaknesses of the U.S. health care system. In Chapter 13, we will discuss health systems in other industrialized nations where access to health care has been addressed quite differently. A major goal of the PPACA is to address this situation primarily by a combination of reform of the private insurance marketplace, an individual mandate to purchase health insurance, limits on the ability of private insurers to deny insurance coverage, and an expansion of the Medicaid program. Given that many of these reforms have not been fully implemented, it is unclear about the effect of these changes on access to care.

Cost of Health Care Services

This section will introduce concepts that help us understand why the cost of health care is such an important issue and will summarize health care financing in the United States, including an overview of health care expenditures, where the money comes from, and where it goes. After exploring the sources of **revenues** and **expenses**, we discuss the possible reasons for the unprecedented growth in health care spending, the role of government, and **cost-containment** mechanisms that have developed to slow the growth of health care spending here in the United States and internationally. Since affordability of health care is a major impediment to access, it is important to understand where the money comes from and how or where the United States spends money for health care.

With both private and public resources developing a multitude of health care programs and health plans, the financing of medical care in the United States is very complex. The percentage of gross domestic product spent on health care represents millions of dollars in revenue for many businesses and industries. Thus, the provision of health care services is big business. According to the data from the U.S. Centers for Medicare and Medicaid as reported in the Census Bureau's 2012 Statistical Abstract (U.S. Census Bureau 2012), total health care expenditures reached nearly $2.49 trillion, representing 17.6 percent of the U.S. **gross domestic product** (GDP). Of this amount, over $2.08 trillion represent personal health care expenditures, a per-capita level of $7,578. These expenditure data support an earlier statement by the Center for Medicare and Medicaid Services (CMS) that projected health care expenditures will reach $4 trillion by 2015 (Borger et al. 2006).

Health Care Financing: Where It Comes From

As shown in Figure 2-6, in 2009, 47.4 percent of personal health care expenditures were funded by private sources (e.g., private health insurance and out-of-pocket costs), while public sources such as Medicare and Medicaid funded 39.1 percent of national health care spending (U.S. Census Bureau, 2012).

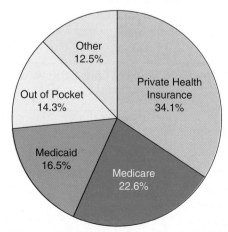

FIGURE 2-6   Personal Health Care Expenditures by Source of Funds

Source: U.S. Census Bureau.

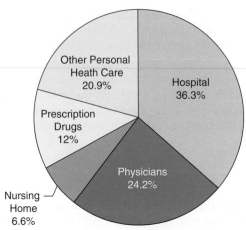

FIGURE 2-7   Personal Health Care Expenditures by Type of Expense

Source: U.S. Census Bureau.

Americans spent $801.2 billion for private health care insurance in 2009, representing an increase of 8.6 percent over the previous year (U.S. Census Bureau 2012). This data also reports that Medicare spending for health care in 2009 grew to $502.3 billion, an increase of 11.6 percent over the previous year. Medicaid spending also rose from the preceding year to $373.9 billion, an increase from 2008 of 8.9 percent.

Health Care Financing: Where It Goes

Figure 2-7 shows where health care expenditures went in 2009. Hospital care is the largest single component of personal health care spending, representing 36.3 percent of personal health care expenditures. The next-largest component of expenditures is physician services, which account for 24.2 percent of the national expenditures. The remaining expenditures break down as follows: 12 percent for prescription drugs, 6.6 percent for nursing home care, and 20.9 percent for other health care expenditures, which included visits to nonphysician providers, medical supplies, and other health services (U.S. Census Bureau, 2012). Of the two largest health care expenditures, hospitals accounted for $759.1 billion in 2009 and physicians $505.9 billion, which translated to a growth of 5.1 and 3.9 percent over 2009.

The Growth of Health Care Expenditures

As noted earlier, the health care expenditure in the United States is significant, and it has had almost uninterrupted growth over the past few decades and continues to represent a larger portion of the GDP. This is important since rising health care costs place pressure on other societal needs and priorities (e.g., education or infrastructure). Health care costs have been cited as a major reason for rising government expenditures and budget challenges. As stated earlier, it is estimated that health care expenditures will rise to over $4 trillion by 2015. Reasons influencing this growth in expenditures include a complex interaction of economic factors, demographic changes, and system factors (see Table 2-2).

Table 2-2 Reasons for Growth in Medical Care Expenditures

A. Economic
   1. Inflation
   2. Market structure
   3. Insurance

B. Demographic change

C. System
   1. Provider behavior
   2. Technology

Economic factors relating to the growth in health care spending include inflation, market structure, and insurance. Most experts would agree that, of all the potential reasons, inflation (both general and for medical care) is the major driving force behind the increases in health care expenditures. Health care **markets** are unique and different from other economic markets, such as commodity markets (Folland, Goodman, and Stano 1997). "Perfect" markets balance supply and demand at a price that is competitively determined by buyers and sellers in a marketplace. The marketplace has many informed buyers and sellers who know what they are buying and selling. Buyers and sellers are free to enter and exit the market as conditions warrant. Perfect markets create competition that allows for the production of goods and services at an affordable price. Health care markets differ from perfect markets in many ways. Access to health care services is not uniform; thus, price is not always competitively determined, but rather is regulated and fixed. Consumers are often at an information disadvantage in making health care purchasing decisions; therefore, it is difficult for consumers to evaluate their purchases. Part of this disadvantage for consumers is that when seeking health care services they are often ill or injured and not in a position to wait for care, negotiate, or seek better prices. Another disadvantage is that prices are almost never known prior to treatment, so consumers are not able to make informed choices. Fee-for-service payments encourage not only increase in medical prices, but an increase in the quantity of services, especially high-priced tests that may add only minimal value to the patient's care (Emanuel et al. 2012). Providers are often prevented by regulation, licensure, and tradition from entering high-cost markets in order to offer a comparable service at a lower cost. Finally, health care insurance has a unique effect on health care markets.

The role of health insurance is a major contributor to the growth in health care expenditures (Fuchs 1990; Peden and Freeland 1995). The protective role of health care insurance has acted to insulate consumers from the true costs of their health care purchases. Because of this, some observers cite the market failure of health care insurance as a major cause of expenditure growth. In sum, inflation, market structure, and health insurance have prevented the forces of competition from working to restrain the growth of health care costs.

Demographic effects also play a role. The elderly population (i.e., those over 64) continues to grow very rapidly. For example, 36.8 million persons in 2005 were 65 or over, an increase of 3.2 million, or 9.4 percent, from 1994 (U.S. Department of Health and Human Services 2007). The elderly population, due to the increase in the incidence of sickness with age, accounts for a large portion of health care expenditures. Indeed, persons 65 and over have many more contacts with their health care provider. For example, the National Center for Health Statistics (2006) shows that elderly males have one-and-a-half to two times as many physician office or hospital outpatient visits than those 55 to 64 years old, and the gap between younger cohorts is even greater. As the post–World War II "baby boom" generation retires, we must prepare ourselves for the influence of an aging population on both the higher cost and utilization of health care services.

System factors also affect growth in health care costs, including administrative bureaucracy, provider behaviors, the lack of a well-coordinated care system that may lead to unsafe duplicative or conflicting care plans, and the American affinity for high-technology health care (Davis et al. 2007). For example, Davis et al. point out that the complexities associated with duplicative, uncoordinated requirements and administrative costs for providers lead to high overall administrative costs, including the proportion of insurance premiums that are used to cover those costs. Indeed, according to the Commonwealth Fund National Scorecard (2006) on U.S. Health System Performance, the United States spends a higher percentage than any other country, and almost three times as much as Canada, on health administration and insurance.

Inefficiency is not only a result of complex administrative systems, but also a product of provider behavior. Some of the abuse is a result of physicians practicing "defensive medicine" in order to protect themselves from costly legal actions. The practice of defensive medicine is an expenditure-increasing activity, and some analysts believe that major savings would be produced if it could be stopped (Emanuel et al. 2012; Mello, Chandra, Gawande, and Studdert 2010), while others report that malpractice reform would save only a small fraction of the total health care expenditures (Thomas, Ziller, and Thayer 2010). As we will discuss shortly, incentives in payment mechanisms also have powerful effects on provider utilization of health care services and overall costs. Finally, the American fascination with high-technology health care has resulted in the identification and treatment of more disorders (Sultz and Young 1999). The costs of delivering this technology are associated with higher overall costs to the system.

Payment Mechanisms

Efforts to contain health care costs have led to various payment mechanisms designed to control health care spending. The intent of these payment mechanisms is to slow the growth of health care expenditures. This section briefly explains the various payment mechanisms for health care providers and the incentives that each of these mechanisms has created. Specifically, four major payment structures are discussed in this section: (1) **fee-for-service**, (2) **case-based**, (3) **capitation**, and (4) **global budgeting**. All four of these payment systems are currently used in the U.S. health care system (Reinhardt 1993). You will read about applications of these mechanisms in Chapters 6–9. Their basic features are summarized in Table 2-3.

After World War II, the growth in availability of health insurance and the introduction of Medicare and Medicaid created a formal payment system for health care providers. At this time, the health care industry was much smaller and relatively inexpensive. While hospitals were paid either on a per-day or a per-stay basis, the primary payment mechanism for physicians was known as fee-for-service (FFS). This approach entailed charging the patient a separate fee for each service or procedure provided by the provider (e.g., therapist or physician). If the patient had health care insurance, the insurer paid the fee either in full or at least in part. Some of the FFS charges depended on the physician's specialty and geographic region. Thus, variation existed in the charges for certain services across physicians. For this reason, some payers began to institute a more uniform payment system that was still fee-for-service, but based on usual, customary, and reasonable charges for a given area. As occupational therapy and physical therapy services grew with the overall system, a similar payment structure was utilized.

With few limits on utilization, this payment mechanism created an incentive for providers to add additional days of care or tests. For example, physicians added a test that would have results that were interesting but not essential. Similarly, hospitals were inclined to keep a patient an extra day "just to be sure" it was safe and the patient was ready to leave the hospital. Occupational therapy and physical therapy services were viewed as an extension of medical care and thus had similar incentives. In this payment system, the patient (or insurer) bears all of the financial risk of predicting how much to pay while the provider has no risk at stake. In cases when patients have health insurance, FFS drives up expenditures. Patients are not fiscally responsible because their insurance is handling all payment claims. Providers have no incentive to limit procedures or avoid unnecessary care. Several observers have cited the inflationary effect of this type of payment structure (Reinhardt 1994).

Table 2-3 Characteristics/Incentives of Payment Mechanisms

Payment Mechanism	Characteristics	Incentive on Risk/Costs
Fee-for-service	Provider paid for each procedure rendered	Highest utilization/costs All risk borne by payer
Case-based rate	Provider paid for each episode of care	Shared risk with payer
Capitation	Provider paid flat rate	All risk borne by provider
Global budgeting	Flat, all-inclusive budget	Known, capped costs

As the shortcomings of the fee-for-service payment mechanism were exposed, alternative payment structures began to emerge. One of these changes was the enactment by Medicare in 1983 of a change from a fee-for-service payment system for hospitals to case-based payment. This reimbursement system shifted payment from a retrospective reimbursement system to a prospective payment system (see Chapter 8). Reimbursement in this mechanism was predetermined primarily on the basis of the patient's diagnosis. This diagnostic-related group (DRG) payment system provided one payment for all services relating to a given diagnosis, instead of paying separately for all the different services used in treating the patient. The DRG payment schedule included adjustments based on the teaching status of the hospital, its geographic location, and outlier cases (i.e., patients whose treatments significantly exceeded the norm in cost). The incentive created by DRG payments was for hospitals to use resources more efficiently and avoid unnecessary procedures in treating patients. Today, prospective payment systems are a major part of financing health care services in the public and private sectors. Essentially, prospective payment systems put providers on a budget with regard to how they use resources to care for their patients. As we will see in Chapter 8, case-based payment is very commonly experienced by therapists providing care in institutional settings (e.g., hospitals, nursing homes, and home health agencies).

The third payment mechanism, the flat fee per patient per month, a feature of some types of health maintenance organizations, is a form of managed care (see Chapter 7). This payment mechanism is known commonly as capitation and pays a monthly fee for each patient enrolled in their practice. If the cost of treating a patient is less than the capitation rate, greater profits are realized; however, if a patient's care is more than the monthly capitation rate, the health care provider loses money. This system creates an incentive for the provider to keep the patient well to avoid costly care and thus keep most of the capitation as profit. The incentives in a capitated payment system are opposite of those in a fee-for-service environment. In addition, the financial risk to the provider of greater utilization of service than anticipated is also much higher. The concern of the prospective and capitated payment systems is that if the fee schedule or payment is set too low, it may have a negative incentive on care such that insufficient services are provided thus having a negative impact on patient care.

Global budgeting, the fourth payment mechanism, is used primarily for hospitals, especially in Canada. Provinces provide a predetermined amount to a hospital to cover all of its operational expenses. In the United States, the Indian Health Service (see Chapter 9) uses a global budgeting mechanism.

Access and Cost: A Therapist Perspective

Even when an individual has adequate health care insurance, access to health care practitioners may be limited. Historically, physicians have controlled access to physical and occupational therapy services. As will be discussed in Chapters 6 and 7, many insurers require that the insured see a primary care doctor before visiting a specialist, including physical and occupational therapists. The primary care physician acts as a gatekeeper who must refer patients to more specialized care.

In states throughout the United States, both physical and occupational therapists are working from a legislative standpoint to improve **direct access** to their services. Thus, patients would be able to bypass their primary care physician and go directly to a therapist for evaluation and treatment. Direct access to therapy services takes various forms. In some states, there are no requirements for physician referral for evaluation or treatment. In other states, a patient may receive an evaluation without physician referral but the therapist must receive a physician order for treatment. In other states, a time limit (e.g., 30 days) is imposed on direct access to treatment. Any patient contact over 30 days requires a physician evaluation. A fourth form of direct access is to limit it to certain environments (e.g., educational environments). Various combinations of these forms of direct access are present in the states. Physical therapists are licensed in all states. Currently, 47 states permit some form of direct access to physical therapy (APTA 2013). Occupational therapists are regulated in all states; regulation varies from licensure (the strictest form) to title protection (the weakest form). Thirty-seven states have no physician referral requirements for occupational therapy (Smith 2000). Nine states permit an evaluation but no treatment without physician referral. Four states permit evaluation and treatment in nonmedical settings or educational settings only.

EFFECTS OF DIRECT ACCESS ON THERAPY PRACTICE   The research evidence indicates that 9–12 percent of a U.S. physical therapist's practice may be by direct access. These studies are dated but provide some insight into the extent of direct access to physical therapy. In a study of 1,580 patients with low back pain treated by 208 health care providers in North Carolina, Mielenz et al. (1997) reported that 12.6 percent of the patients received physical therapy through direct access. Additionally, one-third of responding physical therapists in Massachusetts used direct access, which accounted for 8.8 percent of their practice (Crout, Tweedie, and Miller 1998). In an early study of direct access to physical therapy, Domholdt and Durchholz (1992) reported that 45 percent of physical therapists utilized direct access, which accounted for 10.3 percent of their practice. McCallum and DiAngelis (2012) reported that one in three Ohio therapists in their sample utilized direct access and that direct access accounted for 6–10 percent of their patients. A report by Snow, Shamus, and Hill (2001) found that three in four persons would go to a physical therapist by direct access but two in three persons had no knowledge of their ability to do so. Internationally, utilization of direct access is higher. Leemrijse, Swinkels, and Veenhof (2008) found that 28 percent of physical therapy patients in the Netherlands came by direct access.

More recent work has focused on the clinical decision-making ability of physical therapists related to direct access. Jette et al. (2006) found that physical therapists made correct decisions 87 percent of the time for musculoskeletal conditions, 88 percent of the time for noncritical medical conditions, and 79 percent of the time for critical medical conditions. Correct decision-making percentages were higher for physical therapists who were certified orthopedic specialists. Childs et al. (2005) found that experienced physical therapists had better knowledge than medical students, physician interns, and medical residents in managing musculoskeletal conditions. Physical therapists in military settings have been found to have the requisite knowledge to be effective in a direct access environment (Childs et al. 2007).

A common argument against direct access to physical therapy services alleges that it is unsafe and the cost and usage of therapy services both increase when there is no physician referral or control over utilization. The evidence demonstrates that direct access to physical therapy does not increase and can lower cost or utilization rates vs. physician-referred therapy (Mitchell and deLissovy 1997; Pendergast et al. 2011). Sandstrom (2007) found no difference in physical therapist malpractice in states that permitted direct access vs. states where it was prohibited. Moore et al. (2005) found that military personnel being treated through direct access were at "minimal risk for gross negligent care." Boissonault and Ross (2012) report "numerous examples of physical therapists using effective multifactorial screening strategies for referred and direct-access patients, leading to timely referrals to physicians"(p.446). Deyle (2006) summarizes the evidence and concludes that "the risk from either diagnosis or intervention from a physical therapist is extraordinarily low, with the possibility of substantial benefit"(p.633).

Conclusion

In this chapter, we have explored and discussed access and cost issues facing the U.S. health care system and will discuss quality in the next chapter. These three principles, access, cost, and quality, form the foundation for effective health policy. Simultaneous achievement of an optimal state for all three principles is very difficult but is the goal of policymakers. The Patient Protection and Affordable Care Act of 2010 will certainly change the landscape of access to affordability of health care services in the coming years. This Act promotes coverage by expanding Medicaid programs as well as providing premium subsidies to make health insurance more affordable. As noted in this chapter, however, access to health care comprises many different facets, and we will have to wait to determine the real impact of the Affordable Care Act. As the country and the therapy professions move forward, the use of these three principles will be an effective method to evaluate the effect of health care reform on the population's health.

Chapter Review Questions

1. Recall the three foundational policy principles that define health policy.

2. Define predisposing factors, need factors, and enabling factors.

3. Define each of Penchansky and Thomas's five dimensions of access.

4. What is the relationship between health insurance and access to health care services?

5. Define the characteristics of the uninsured.

6. Describe the effect of direct access to therapy services on the cost and quality of health care.

7. Identify and describe the basic sources of funding for the U.S. health care system.

8. Identify and describe the major expenditures for U.S. health care.

9. Identify major causes for growth in U.S. health care expenditures.

10. Review the major mechanisms for physical therapist and occupational therapist payment: fee for service, case rate, and capitation.

Chapter Discussion Questions

1. The development of a marketing plan for a therapy practice will benefit from a consideration of the principles of access. Discuss how you could use Penchansky and Thomas's model of access to determine whether to open a therapy practice.

2. Discuss how the unique American policy decision to support both private and public health insurance affects access to health care.

3. Is direct access to occupational and physical therapy essential? Do you think it will increase access for the population? Explain your answer.

4. The United States is the only major industrialized democracy without a system of national health care insurance. How would the development and implementation of national health care insurance in the United States affect the cost of health care?

5. It is estimated that more costs of health care may be transferred to the consumer from the employer/government in the form of higher premiums, deductibles, and co-payments. What would the effect of these changes be on the growth of the costs of health care? On occupational therapists and physical therapists?

6. Discuss the incentives of fee-for-service and capitated payment systems on the cost of health care. How do these systems promote or inhibit access to care?

7. Americans spend more money on specialized, high-technology medical care than people in other countries. This decision may affect the availability of resources for other worthwhile social goals (e.g., education, transportation). What effect do you believe this policy decision may have on persons with disabilities or with other forms of medically stable, chronic diseases?

References

American Physical Therapy Association (APTA). 2012. Direct access to physical therapy services: Overview. http://www.apta.org/StateIssues/DirectAccess/Overview/ (accessed April 10, 2013).

Andersen, R., and J.F. Newman. 2005. Societal and individual determinants of medical care utilization in the United States. *Milbank Q* 83. Online-only. doi: 10.1111/j.1468-0009.2005.00428.x (accessed December 7, 2012).

Ayanian, J.Z., J.S. Weissman, E.C. Schneider, J.A. Ginsburg, and A.M. Zaslavsky. 2000. Unmet health needs of uninsured adults in the United States. *JAMA* 284(16): 2061–69.

Barton, P.B. 1999. *Understanding the U. S. health services system.* Chicago: Health Administration Press.

Boissonault, W.G., and M.D. Ross. 2012. Physical therapists referring patients to physicians: A review of case reports and series. *J Orthop Sports Phys Ther* 42(5): 446–54.

Borger, C., S. Smith, C. Truffer, S. Keeehan, A. Sisko, J. Poisal, and M.E. Clemens. 2006. Health spending projections through 2015: Changes on the horizon. *Health Affairs* 25(2), Web exclusive, 61–73.

Braveman, P., V.M. Schaaf, S. Egerter, T. Bennett, and W. Schecter. 1994. Insurance-related differences in the risk of ruptured appendix. *N Engl J Med* 331(7): 444–49.

Childs, J.D., J.M. Whitman, P.S. Sizer, M.L. Pugia, T.W. Flynn, and A. Delitto. 2005. A description of physical therapists' knowledge in managing musculoskeletal conditions. *BMC Musculoskelet Disord* 6: 32.

Childs J.D., J.M. Whitman, M.L. Pugia, P.S. Sizer Jr., T.W. Flynn, and A. Delitto. 2007. Knowledge in managing musculoskeletal conditions and educational preparation of physical therapists in the uniformed services. *Mil Med* 172(4): 440–45.

Clemans-Cope L., B. Garrett, and C. Hoffman. 2006. Changes in employees' health insurance coverage, 2001–2005. Kaiser Commission on Medicaid and the Uninsured, Issue Paper (Report #7570).

Collins, S.R., K. Davis, and T. Garber. 2012. 1.3 million Fewer People were uninsured in 2011. *The Commonwealth Fund Blog.* http://www.commonwealthfund.org/Blog/2012/Sep/Fewer-People-Were-Uninsured-in-2011.aspx (accessed December 7, 2012).

Commonwealth Fund National Scorecard. 2006. *The Commonwealth Fund Commission on a high performance health system, why not the best? Results from a national scorecard on U.S. health system performance.* The Commonwealth Fund.

Crout, K.L., J.H. Tweedie, and D.J. Miller. 1998. Physical therapists' opinions and practice regarding direct access. *Phys Ther* 78(1): 52–61.

Cunningham P., S. Aritga, and K. Schwartz. 2008. The fraying link between work and health insurance: Trends in employer-sponsored insurance for employees, 2000-2007. Kaiser Commission on Medicaid and the Uninsured (Report #7840).

Davidoff, A., and G. Kenney. 2005. Uninsured Americans with chronic health conditions: Key findings from the national health interview survey. The Urban Institute and the University of Maryland. http://www.urban.org/publications/411161.html (accessed May 2005).

Davis, K., C. Schoen, S. Guterman, T. Shih, S.C. Schoenbaum, and W. Ilana. 2007. Slowing the growth of U.S. health care expenditures: What are the options? The Commonwealth Fund. http://www.cmf.org/publications/publications_show.htm?doc_id=449510 (accessed June 2007).

Deyle, G.D. 2006. Direct access physical therapy and diagnostic responsibility: The risk to benefit ratio. *J Orthop Sports Phys Ther* 36(9): 632–34.

Domholdt, E., and A.G. Durchholz. 1992. Direct access use by experienced therapists in states with direct access. *Phys Ther* (8): 569–74.

Emanuel E., N. Tanden, S. Altman, et al. 2012. A systematic approach to containing health care spending. *N Engl J Med* 370(10): 949–54.

Folland, S., A.C. Goodman, and M. Stano. 1997. *The economics of health and health care.* 2nd ed. Upper Saddle River NJ: Prentice Hall.

Franks, P., C.M. Clancey, and M.R. Gold. 1993. Health insurance and mortality. *JAMA* 270(6): 737–41.

Fronstin, P. 2007. *Employment-based health benefits: Access and coverage, 1988–2005.* Washington DC: Employment Benefit Research Institute (Issue brief no. 303).

Fuchs, V. 1990. The health sector's share of the gross national product. *Science* 247(4942): 534–38.

_____ 1993. National health insurance revisited. In J.K. Iglehart, ed., *Debating health care reform: A primer from Health Affairs* (81–91). Bethesda MD: Project Hope.

Institute of Medicine. 2003. *Hidden costs, value lost: Uninsurance in America.* Washington DC: The National Academies Press.

Jette, D.U., K. Ardleigh, K. Chandler, and L. McShea. 2006. Decision-making ability of physical therapists: Physical therapy intervention or medical referral. *Phys Ther* 86(12): 1619–29.

KCMU. 2012. The uninsured: A primer. Kaiser Commission on Medicaid and the Uninsured Report. www.kff.org

Kuttner, R. 1999. The American health care system: Health insurance coverage. *N Engl J Med* 340(2): 163–68.

Leemrijse, C.J., I.C.S. Swinkels, and C. Veenhof. 2008. Direct access to physical therapy in the Netherlands: Results from the first year in community-based physical therapy. *Phys Ther* 88(8): 926–46.

McCallum, C.A., and T. DiAngelis. 2012 Direct access: Factors that affect physical therapist practice in the state of Ohio. *Phys Ther* 92(5): 688–706.

Mello, M.M., A. Chandra, A.A. Gawande, and D.M. Studdert. 2010. National cost of the medical liability system. *Health Affairs* 29(9): 1569–77.

Mielenz, T.J., T.S. Carey, D.A. Dyrek, B.A. Harris, J.M. Garrett, and J.D. Darter. 1997. Physical therapy utilization by patients with acute low back pain. *Phys Ther* (10): 1040–51.

Mitchell, J.M. and G. deLissovy. 1997. A comparison of resource use and cost in direct access versus physician referral episodes of physical therapy. *Phys Ther* 77(1): 10–18.

Moore J.H., D.J. McMillian, M.D. Rosenthal, and M.D. Weishaar. 2005. Risk determination for patients with direct access to physical therapy in military health care facilities. *J Orthop Sports Phys Ther* 35(10): 674–78.

National Center for Health Statistics. 2006. *Characteristics on trends in the health of Americans.* Hyattsville MD.

Peden, E.A., and M.S. Freeland. 1995. A historical analysis of medical spending growth, 1960–1993. *Health Affairs* 14(2): 235–47.

Penchansky, R., and J.W. Thomas. 1981. The concept of access: Definition and relationship to consumer satisfaction. *Med Care* 19(2): 127–140.

Pendergast, J., S.A. Kliethermes, J.K. Freburger, and P.A.Duffy. 2011. A comparison of health care use for physician-referred and self-referred episodes of outpatient physical therapy. *Health Serv Res* 47(2): 633–54.

Reinhardt, U.E. 1993. Reorganizing the financial flows in American health care. *Health Affairs* 12:172–93.

_____.1994. Planning the nation's workforce: Let the market in. *Inquiry* 31(3): 250–63.

Sandstrom, R. 2007. Malpractice by physical therapists: Descriptive analysis of reports in the National Practitioner Data Bank Public Use Data File, 1991–2004. *J Allied Health* 36(4): 201–08.

Seiden, D.J. 1994. Health care ethics. In A.R. Kovner, ed., *Health care delivery in the United States* (486–531). New York: Springer.

Sered, S., and R. Fernandopulle. 2005. *Profiles of the uninsured: Uninsured Americans tell their stories.* http://www.cmwf.org /General/General_show.htm?doc_id=256036 (accessed June 2007).

Smith, K. 2000. Direct access important to profession's future. http://www.aota.org/Pubs/OTP/Columns /CapitalBriefing/2000/cb-052200.aspx (accessed July 10, 2007).

Snow, B.L., E. Shamus, and C. Hill. 2001. Physical therapy as primary health care: Public perceptions. *J Allied Health* 30(1): 35–38.

Stoddard, J.J., R.F. St. Peter, and P.W. Newacheck. 1994. Health insurance status and ambulatory care for children. *N Engl J Med* 330(20): 1421–25

Sultz, H.A., and K.M. Young. 1999. *Health care USA: Understanding its organization and delivery,* 2d ed. Gaithersburg MD: Aspen Publishers.

Thomas, J.W., E.C. Ziller, and D.A. Thayer. 2010. Low costs of defensive medicine, small savings for tort reform. *Health Affairs* 29(9): 1578–84.

U.S. Census Bureau. 2012. The 2012 Statistical Abstract: The National Data Book. http://www.census.gov/compendia /statab/cats/health_nutrition/health_expenditures.html# (accessed July 2012).

U.S. Department of Health and Human Services. 2007. A statistical profile of older Americans aged 65+. U.S. Department of Health and Human Services, Administration on Aging. http://www.aoa.gov/PRESS/fact /pdf/Attachment_1304.pdf.

Vistnes, J.P., and S.H. Zuvekas. 1999. *Health insurance status of the civilian noninstitutionalized population: 1997.* MEPS Reseach Findings No. 8. AHRQ Pub. No. 99–0030. Rockville MD: Agency for Health Care Research and Quality.

3

Quality of Health Care

CHAPTER OBJECTIVES

At the conclusion of this chapter, the reader will be able to:

1 Compare and contrast the population- and personal-based conceptualizations of health care quality.

2 Describe the following basic components of a quality health care system:
   a. Adequate structure
   b. Effective processes
   c. Evidence-based practice
   d. Satisfactory outcomes

3 Review the mechanisms and provide examples of measuring and reporting on the quality of the health care system, using:
   a. Peer review
   b. Accreditation
   c. Report cards

4 Discuss the legal foundations for quality in the health care system:
   a. Professional regulation
   b. Patient rights
   c. Medical negligence

5 Identify future developments to improve health care system quality and address health disparities.

KEY WORDS

Acceptable
Accreditation
Clinical Practice
   Guideline
Effectiveness
Efficacy
Efficiency
Equitable
Evidence-based
   Practice
Health Disparities
Informed Consent
Interpersonal
   Excellence
Legitimate
Medical Negligence
Outcomes
Optimal
Patient Privacy
Pay for Performance
Peer Review
Process
Professional Regulation
Scope of Practice
Structure
Technical Excellence
Utilization Review

CASE EXAMPLE ··

Sue is a busy manager of a hospital-based physical therapy department. She learned today that the hospital's accreditation body will be visiting next year. She needs to develop quality improvement processes to meet the accrediting body's expectations. To do so, she focuses on the most common processes in her department and creates outcome measures that demonstrate the high quality of care provided by her therapists. She develops a tracking mechanism and goals for response times for patient referrals. She uses an outcome measuring survey to determine the functional status of her patients upon admission and discharge. Her staff finds the feedback useful to their care planning and implementation processes.

Case Example Question:

1. Explain how staff therapists can use quality improvement information to improve their care processes. Why would it be important to do so?

Introduction

In Chapter 2, we explored two of the three legs of the policy "stool": access and cost. In this chapter, we will introduce and discuss the third principle of health policy: quality. Quality is an important principle since it describes the effectiveness of a health care intervention or service. It is also the principle that is most directly under the control and responsibility of a health care provider (e.g., a physical or occupational therapist). While a description of quality may seem straightforward on its face, a definition of quality can be surprisingly complex.

People and society want access to, and are willing to pay only for, a high-quality health care system. In this section, we will explore the meaning of quality health care. Recent studies have pointed out serious deficiencies in the health care system, such as the high rate of medical error (Institute of Medicine 1999). Depending on one's perspective, Americans either are receiving the highest-quality health care in the world or are not getting an adequate return on quality from the most expensive health care system in the world. We will also discuss the basic components of a quality health care system: structure, process, and outcomes. We will introduce methods to measure the quality of each of these components. Finally, we will review the basic foundation of quality: the legal rights of patients to be protected and informed when interacting with the health care system.

Perspectives on Health Care Quality

There are two fundamental paradigms with which to analyze the quality of health care services in the United States: one is personal based and the other population based. Each of these perspectives is influenced by the structure of the current system, contemporary social expectations, and legal mandates to ensure quality health care. The personal-based perspective focuses on the patient–provider relationship and the organization, delivery, and outcome of the services patients receive. It is the perspective used most commonly by physical therapists, occupational therapists, and other providers. The population-based perspective analyzes health care quality by examining the experiences and health status of populations and subgroups. The roots of the population-based perspective of health care quality can be traced to the universalism philosophy. A definition of quality from this perspective includes not only medical care, but also socioeconomic status and the community environment. Increasingly, policymakers are using a population health perspective to design health policy. Table 3-1 compares and contrasts the population- and personal-based concepts of quality.

Table 3-1 Population-Based vs. Personal-Based Concepts of Health Care Quality

	Population-based	Personal-based
Theoretical model	Public health	Medical
Key components	Quality of life/health status Function Satisfaction	Patient–provider interaction Structure, process, outcome Satisfaction
How to measure?	Survey, interview Community-based	Peer review, accreditation Within the health care system

For patients with chronic diseases and disabilities, the quality of their health entails much more than medical care. The population-based quality perspective is increasingly being used to understand the quality of life of persons with disabilities living in community environments. A plethora of measures of quality of life for persons experiencing disablement exist, including both general and disability-specific measures of health status. General measures of health status—(e.g., the Medical Outcomes Study SF-36; Ware and Sherbourne 1992)—can compare the health status of a person experiencing disablement with that of the age-matched general population. Disease-specific measures (e.g., the Arthritis Impact Measurement Scales 2) are often more sensitive and specific to health status in these specific populations, but have limited ability to define quality of life in comparison to that of the general population. As we will discuss later, these measures also provide a method for assessing the outcomes of physical therapy and occupational therapy and demonstrating the effectiveness of the care involved.

A personal-based perspective is common to the administration and practice of physical therapy or occupational therapy services. The Institute of Medicine (1999) defines quality of health care as "the degree to which health services for individuals and populations increase the likelihood of desired health outcomes and are consistent with current professional knowledge" (p.211). In contrast to population-based perspectives, this definition focuses on services: how they are delivered and what their result is. In 1990, Avedis Donabedian postulated several key concepts or terms that define quality of health care. **Efficacy** and **effectiveness** define quality within the patient-therapist relationship. Effectiveness is the best care provided under ordinary, everyday circumstances. Efficacy is the best care provided under ideal circumstances. Effectiveness is the definition that is the usual expectation for day-to-day clinical performance by therapists (e.g., in utilization review or an evaluation of a medical negligence claim). However, other Donabedian conceptualizations are increasingly important to policymakers as the quality of health care is evaluated based on its effects on a population. Care that is **efficient**, **legitimate** or **optimal** relates to the cost-benefit ratio of therapy services. The relationship of cost to the amount of improvement defines the efficiency of care with the ideal cost-benefit ratio being the definition of optimal therapy services. As we introduced in Chapter 2 and will further explore in Chapters 6-9, increasing the out-of-pocket expenses for therapy services is a policy incentive for patients to be more efficient consumers. Legitimate health care is optimal health care that meets societal expectations (see the Medicare definition of "skilled" therapy services in Chapter 8). Health care quality can also be defined to be **acceptable** or **equitable**. Acceptable care is available, accessible, and accommodating to the needs of patients (see Chapter 2). Equitable care meets societal expectations for fairness and justice (see Chapter 1 and the health disparities section later in this chapter). These definitions are increasingly important today as policymakers work to control costs (see pay for performance later in this chapter) and focus on the health of populations (see also Chapter 13).

These perspectives on quality health care are affected and reinforced by the legal mandates to assure high-quality health care services. The basis for governmental actions is the expectation that providers have a responsibility to provide the best care for the patients they serve. It is important to understand the legal requirements for health care quality as the "floor," or minimum societal expectation, for health care quality. Legal mandates focus on public safety. For example, the tort system of law provides a legal recourse for people to address medical errors. Provider-caused medical errors and negligent practices are harms that are remediated in the courts. Licensure and other forms of regulation ensure a base level of provider capability to serve the public and protect it from harmful practices. The law also establishes fundamental rights for patients in their interactions with the system.

Structure, Process, and Outcomes: Three Dimensions of Quality

In 1966, Avedis Donabedian put forth a template that is widely accepted today as the basis for understanding the framework of quality in the health care system. This template has three components: **structure, process,** and **outcomes**. Structure comprises the permanent features of the health care system—hospitals and the various health care providers. Process is the method of delivery of care. Outcomes are the results of the health care encounter. Over the years, the definition and measurement of quality have developed steadily from an initial focus on structure, to how health care is delivered (process), to outcomes. Today, outcomes (e.g., medical error rates and functional outcomes) are very important to the examination of the quality of health care in America. In the last few years, the federal government and nongovernmental accrediting agencies (see Accreditation section) have made outcomes data publicly available (see Report Cards section). Let us first consider each of the three components of health care quality separately. The basic features of structure, process, and outcome are displayed in Table 3-2.

STRUCTURE   Structure is the basic foundation or infrastructure of the health care system. It comprises the services and the organization of the health care system and, as such, is closely related to the health policy principle of access. A quality system has to have the physical and human resources with which to deliver services at locations that can be accessed by the public it serves. If a location or region lacks the facilities or the types of providers to provide appropriate care, it is defined as "medically underserved"; in other words, it lacks a proper structure to meet the needs of the population it serves. The Health Resources Services Administration maintains a database of health professional shortage areas and provides grant funding to alleviate structural problems of this kind. Health care systems with these problems are typically in rural areas or poor districts of urban areas. Besides impaired access, regulation of providers, whether they be therapists or long-term care facilities, is the basis for the determination of adequate structural quality.

Active Learning Exercise

Visit the Health Resources Services Administration, Bureau of Health Professions Data Warehouse at its website: http://hpsafind.hrsa.gov/. Look up your home county. Is it a Health Professional Shortage Area or Medically Underserved Area?

Table 3-2 Features of Structure, Process, and Outcome

	Structure.	Process	Outcome
Key components	Physical facilities Human resources	Technical excellence Interpersonal excellence	Results
How measured?	Access to care Professional regulation	Standards Peer review	Survey Interview

PROCESS   Process is the method by which health care is delivered. It has two components: **technical excellence** and **interpersonal excellence** (Donabedian 1988). Interpersonal excellence is the caring aspect of health care and is typically measured by patient satisfaction survey. Technical excellence comprises the ability of the health care provider to make informed decisions, as well as the skill of the health care provider to improve the patient's situation. In essence, a quality health care intervention should shorten the length of time of a disabling condition, reduce its severity, or both. The measurement of technical excellence requires the utilization of accepted intervention protocols and a mechanism of review to determine the appropriateness of the actual intervention. For example, occupational therapy and physical therapy are routinely utilized in the postoperative treatment protocols for total joint arthroplasties. Therapy services are provide technical excellence in the process of the care of these patients.

For the last decade, the emphasis in health care quality is on **evidence-based practice**, defined as the "integration of the best research evidence with clinical experience and patient values" (Sackett, Strauss, and Richardson 2000, p.1). The goal of this emphasis is for clinicians to ascertain, interpret, and utilize the best evidence in making treatment decisions. A number of studies of occupational and physical therapists indicate that therapists recognize the importance of evidence-based practice and are working to implement evidence-based practice into their work. In an early study, Dysart and Tomlin (2002) found that lack of time, high costs, weak research analysis skills, and a higher value placement on experience versus research limited the incorporation of evidence-based practice into the work of occupational therapists. Similarly, access to evidence, problems with interpreting evidence, other "organizational barriers," negative attitudes towards research, and lack of education limited the implementation of evidence-based practice for physical therapists (Bridges, Bierema, and Valentine 2007; Maher, Sherrington, Elkins, Herbert, and Moseley 2004; Salbach, Jaglal, Korner-Bitensky, Rappolt, and Davis 2007). It has been demonstrated that the desire for learning, the highest degree held, and practicality were positively associated with use of evidence-based practice (Bridges, Bierema, and Valentine 2007; McCluskey and Lovarini 2005). Bennett, McKenna, Hoffmann, Tooth, McCluskey, and Strong (2007) found that a discipline-specific online database improved the ability of occupational therapists to access evidence. Recently, Crowell, Tragord, Taylor, and Deyle (2012) have advocated short "critically appraised topics" as a successful method to integrate evidence-based practice into the busy schedules of therapists.

OUTCOMES   Outcomes are the results of the patient's care and an important measure of the quality of the health care system. They are typically measured by examining the health status of the person or, in the case of a person with a disability, the status of disablement. Generic health status measures are commonly used to measure quality of life. A variety of disease-specific measures are available to assess health status for specific populations. Both types of measures are used to measure outcomes. As accountability for system performance has increased, the measurement and reporting of outcomes has become more important.

Generic health status assessment is one type of patient outcomes measurement. Tools have been designed to measure health status, quality of life, and global health outcomes. Generic health status surveys are especially valuable when a clinician wants to monitor the health status of an individual or a population. These surveys typically measure overall health status across physical, psychological, and social domains to provide a more complete picture of health. Another advantage to certain generic health status measures is norm referencing and, in some cases, age-matched referencing. This feature allows a comparison of results with the average health of the population. The Medical Outcome Study–Short Form (SF-36), developed by Ware and Sherbourne (1992), is a well-known global health status measure. The SF-36 is a quick norm-referenced survey of eight domains of physical, social, emotional, and mental health status. It is widely used as a measure of outcomes for many types of medical pathologies.

Many diseases have outcome measures to assess health status and patient outcomes for persons who experience those diseases. These measures are advantageous in that they assess specific features of the condition and are usually more sensitive to detecting an improvement or a change in condition than a generic health status survey is. An example of a disease-specific outcome measure is the Arthritis Impact Measurement Scales 2, which measures the health status of persons with arthritis in physical, emotional, and social domains (Meenan, Gertman, and Mason 1980).

Improved functioning and a lowered need for external-care assistance is a critical outcome in the care of persons with temporary or permanent disablements. Contemporary outcomes measurement in rehabilitation settings includes patient-reported measures of health status, a report on interpersonal excellence, clinical measures of disablement, and a descriptive report of all patients served by a provider (Dobrzykowski 1997). A number of outcome measurement and reporting systems have been developed in the last 20 years.

The Focus on Therapeutic Outcomes (FOTO) tool, a commercially available outcomes management system, measures disablement in outpatient orthopedic settings (FOTO 2012). Studies of the FOTO database have demonstrated the effectiveness of outpatient orthopedic rehabilitation procedures (Amato, Dobrzykowski, and Nance 1997; Dobrzykowski and Nance 1997). In 2006, APTA introduced the Outpatient Physical Therapy Improvement in Movement Assessment Log (OPTIMAL) as an outcome reporting system for outpatient settings (Guccione et al. 2005). In medical rehabilitation, the Uniform Data System for Medical Rehabilitation (1997) and its outcome measurement tool, the Functional Independence Measure (FIM™) (and its pediatric version WeeFIM™), is the standard for functional-limitations outcomes assessment.

REPORT CARDS Report cards are intended to increase consumer awareness of the quality of the health care they are purchasing and receiving. Werner and Asch (2005) stated that the intent of report cards is to promote the preferential selection of good physicians and to motivate physicians to compete on quality. Wicks and Meyer (1999) identify five features of a useful report card system for quality reporting: interested consumers, understandable report cards, a focus on outcomes and high-priority quality areas, utilization of accurate measures, and a reward system to encourage provider accountability based on the results of the report card. The adoption by Medicare of the use of report cards to inform the public of the quality of hospitals, nursing homes, and home health agencies has increased attention on provider report cards. Occupational and physical therapists are currently being paid a bonus fee for providing outpatient quality data on their services. In the near future, this reporting will become mandatory. Public report cards have been associated with reduced mortality rates for cardiac surgery (Epstein 2006). Their overall effect, however, has been modest, with some reports of greater usage when patients are dissatisfied with or changing health plans (Braun, Kind, Fowles, and Suarez 2002; Schultz, Thiede-Call, Feldman, and Christianson 2001).

Active Learning Exercise

Visit the Medicare consumer website at http://www.medicare.gov/HomeHealthCompare/search.aspx. Enter in the zip code for your area and choose one or more agencies that offer therapy services. Compare the quality of occupational therapy or physical therapy services for the chosen home health agencies by selecting the quality of patient care and patient survey results tabs. How useful did you find this information? Would it influence your purchasing decision?

UTILIZATION REVIEW **Utilization review** is a process in which insurance representatives review medical records of treatment for appropriateness of care (Lenz 2008). **Clinical pathways** are written guides that apply evidence to practice and plan care for clinical conditions. There is no one definition for clinical pathways; however, a recent Cochrane Review (Rotter et al. 2010) suggests that clinical pathways should be multidisciplinary, provide guidelines or evidence, detail the intervention approach, have timeframes or criteria for progression, and help standardize care. In addition to insurers, utilization review is commonly performed by institutional providers (e.g., hospitals) (see Chapter 8). Failure of the process to meet these standards of appropriateness of care or outcomes can result in the denial of payment or transfer of the patient to a more appropriate level of care (see Chapter 11). At the level of institutions, quality of care is assured by accreditation.

ACCREDITATION   **Accreditation** is the primary method by which institutional providers measure their structure, process, and outcomes against consensus quality standards. Most individual providers—e.g., private therapy clinics—are not accredited. Payer review of provider documentation is the dominant method for determining the quality of individual practitioner performance. Accreditation is a voluntary process performed by a nongovernmental organization by which an institutional provider allows a focused survey of its organization and operations using the accrediting body's standards. If the institution meets the accrediting body's standards, it receives a public proclamation of its quality until the next accreditation is required. We will discuss three major accreditation organizations that are of interest to occupational therapists and physical therapists: the Joint Commission on the Accreditation of Health Care Organizations, the Commission on the Accreditation of Rehabilitation Facilities, and the National Committee on Quality Assurance.

JOINT COMMISSION   The Joint Commission on the Accreditation of Healthcare Organizations (JCAHO) is the oldest accrediting body of health care organizations in the United States (JCAHO 2007). Originally established in 1951 to accredit hospitals, JCAHO now accredits a full array of health care organizations, including skilled nursing facilities, home health agencies, and behavioral health organizations. JCAHO has developed performance standards for the structure, organization, and processes of the institutions it accredits. Surveys are conducted by teams of JCAHO employees who conduct on-site reviews and interview key leaders and workers. JCAHO uses the ORYX program to demonstrate an outcomes management system. JCAHO maintains an online report card of its accredited organizations at http://www.qualitycheck.org.

Active Learning Exercise

Visit http://www.qualitycheck.org and search for a hospital in your hometown. How useful is the information to help you understand the quality of care in this facility?

A major initiative of JCAHO has been the development and assessment of provider performance related to patient safety and quality improvement. In November 1999, the Institute of Medicine released *To Err Is Human: Building a Safer Health System*, a major report on the quality of health care in the United States. This report found that up to 98,000 deaths annually in the United States could be attributed to medical error. The report attributed more deaths to medical error than to highway accidents, breast cancer, or AIDS. Falls have been identified as one of the most common forms of adverse events experienced by elderly patients (Rothschild, Bates, and Leape 2000; Thomas and Brennan 2000). Most of these errors were attributed to the design of the health care system and not to individual provider practices (Casarett and Helms 1999; Leape 1997). Mu, Lohman, and Scheirton (2006) found that most errors committed by occupational therapists were related to interventions, especially treatments or supervision of patients.

In 2001, the Institute of Medicine released *Crossing the Quality Chasm: A New Health System for the 21st Century*. This report advocates a redesign of the health care system to bolster the clinical information infrastructure, encourages the use of evidence-based practice by clinicians, and calls for the inclusion of clinical quality indicators, as well as cost-efficiency measures in determining the system's functioning. In response, JCAHO has implemented the National Patient Safety Goal initiative to focus attention on quality and safety improvement in the health care system. Goals have been established for many of the care settings in the health care system (e.g., hospitals, ambulatory care, home health agencies, long-term care facilities, laboratories, and behavioral health providers) (The Joint Commission 2012).

Active Learning Exercise

Go to the Joint Commission website on the National Patient Safety Goals and learn more about the priorities to make the U.S. health care system safer this year: http://www.jointcommission.org/standards_information/npsgs.Abx1spx.

The Commission on the Accreditation of Rehabilitation Facilities (CARF) was created in the late 1960s to perform institutional quality-review assessment for organizations that serve persons with disabilities (CARF 2000). CARF accredits a wide variety of institutions, community-based providers, and organizations that serve persons with physical and behavioral disabilities. Like JCAHO, CARF utilizes performance standards to determine quality, but unlike JCAHO, it utilizes part-time surveyors recruited from the clinical fields to conduct the surveys. The CARF accreditation process emphasizes patients' rights and a provider commitment to quality improvement.

The National Committee on Quality Assurance (NCQA) was formed in the 1990s by business, labor, and the insurance industry as a body to accredit quality in health plans—specifically, forms of managed care (NCQA 2007). NCQA assesses health plans in regard to access and service, provider qualifications, wellness and prevention activities, and care for people who have chronic diseases and illnesses. NCQA utilizes a focused survey of health plans to make its accreditation decisions.

LEGAL ISSUES AND QUALITY   For certain health care quality and safety issues, the government has set mandatory minimum standards for medical care and has established mechanisms to enforce these standards. These issues include **professional regulation, patient privacy,** and **medical negligence**.

Government regulation of professional practice is intended to assure a basic level of safety and competence in providing services, including occupational therapy and physical therapy. The National Board for Certification in Occupational Therapy is the certification body for occupational therapists (NBCOT 2007). The Federation of State Boards of Physical Therapy is the organization of regulatory boards for physical therapists. Schmitt and Shimberg (1996) have identified three purposes for professional regulation: protection from unethical provider activities, public assurance of the basic competence of a practitioner to provide safe and effective care, and providing the public with a procedure for the discipline of a professional who performs unsafe or incompetent acts. Licensure laws vary from state to state. A typical licensure law codifies the scope of practice, educational qualifications, testing requirements, and disciplinary procedures for a professional. A **scope of practice** defines the procedures or limits on the types of procedures a professional can perform. Regulations promulgated from a licensing board or agency will further define the scope of practice. Scope of practice statutes and regulations vary from state to state. A model state practice act for physical therapy has been presented by the Federation of State Boards of Physical Therapy (see www.fsbpt.org for more information). A model practice act for occupational therapy has been developed by the American Occupational Therapy Association (see http://www.aota.org/Practitioners/Advocacy/State/Resources/PracticeAct/36445.aspx). It is very important for therapists and therapist assistants to understand their state's statutes that regulate assistant practice.

Informed consent and patient confidentiality during health care interactions are fundamental patient rights that have emerged in the law over the last half-century. Annas (1998) has identified five core patient rights in health care: the right to information, the right to privacy and dignity, the right to refuse treatment, the right to emergency care, and the right to an advocate. Occupational therapists and physical therapists are legally required to obtain informed consent prior to treatment. This means that the patient needs to be provided with information in order to decide whether to accept or refuse treatment. Specifically, the therapist needs to inform the patient of the type of procedures to be employed, any risks or hazards involved, the anticipated outcome of the intervention, whether alternatives to the treatment exist, and the consequences of not receiving treatment. Two other forms of informed consent are an advanced directive and a durable power of attorney. An advanced directive is a legal document that details what treatment a patient does or does not wish to be given when the patient is no longer able to make a decision about such matters. Examples of an advanced directive are a living will and a "do not resuscitate" order in a hospital setting. A durable power of attorney is a legal document that designates another person to make health care decisions if the patient becomes unable to do so.

In 2003, new patient privacy standards for the protection of "individually identifiable" health information went into effect (U.S. Department of Health and Human Services 2002). These federal regulations apply provisions of the 1996 Health Insurance Portability and Accountability Act (HIPAA). Providers are required to identify and track the flow of personal health care information in their practices and systems, and take the necessary steps not to disclose information for nontreatment, nonpayment purposes. In general, patient consent (authorization) is not required when personal health information is used for treatment, payment, and routine health care operations (e.g., the education of students). Other uses, however, require patient authorization for release of information. Examples of other uses include the marketing and business relationships a practice may have with other providers (except insurance companies). In addition, providers are required to disclose the minimum necessary information to achieve the business objective. The regulations provide for specific consumer rights to their personal health information and a record of how it has been disclosed. Therapists must take specific steps to prevent the oral release of personal health information, as well as its technical release (e.g., via a computer screen in a waiting area). Civil and criminal penalties for unauthorized disclosure have been defined in the regulations.

In addition to professional licensure discipline, remediation for medical error or medical negligence is also available through civil court action. An action by a therapist that produces a wrong (called a tort) resulting in injury is termed medical negligence or malpractice. The law provides for relief from this wrong by permitting the injured party to sue the provider for damages caused by the action. To prove medical negligence, the injured party must prove that the therapist failed to perform those duties and functions that would be done by a similarly trained therapist in the same situation. In addition, the person suing the therapist must demonstrate that the actions of the therapist caused the harm and that damages or injuries were suffered by the patient. If one of these duties or harms is not demonstrated, a court will not find medical negligence. Standards of care, accreditation policies, organizational policies and procedures, clinical pathways, expert opinion, and professional publications are all key measuring sticks to determine the ability and actions of the provider accused of medical negligence. Good patient-communication skills, insurance, and legal representation are necessary for adequate protection of the therapist in a medical negligence situation (Scott 1991). The incidence of malpractice by physical therapists and occupational therapists is low. A study of the National Practitioner Data Bank public use data file found that the incidence of physical therapist malpractice was 2.5 cases per 10,000 therapists (Sandstrom 2007). A typical physical therapist malpractice settlement was treatment related and occurred in an urban state by a physical therapist age 30 to 50 for an amount between $10,000 and $15,000. A recent report by C.N.A./HPSO insurance reported 162 closed claims from 56,971 insured therapists in 2005 (2.8 closed claims/ 1000 insured therapists). The average indemnity payment for physical therapist claims was $39,857.

The Future of Health Care Quality

In *Crossing the Quality Chasm*, the Institute of Medicine (2001) identified six areas of care in need of improvement in the United States health care system: safety, effectiveness, patient-centeredness, timeliness, efficiency, and equitability. Among the recommendations to achieve progress in these areas is to increase accountability and transparency of the system, promote evidence-based practice, increase use of information technology, and align payment policies with quality initiatives. As we have discussed in this chapter, several of these recommendations have already been initiated, and significant progress has been made. Over the last decade, the integration of quality and payment has increased. The public now has Internet access to basic quality report cards on organizational providers (e.g., hospitals, nursing homes, and home health agencies). Evidence-based clinical practice guidelines are widely available for many conditions. **Pay for performance** is emerging as a strategy to reward (or penalize) providers who do not meet basic quality expectations (see Chapter 7). Public policies such as the Tax Relief and Health Care Act of 2006, which includes a quality measures reporting system, address pay for performance (AOTA 2007). Medicare will continue to look at quality measures and outcomes as mechanisms to determine the appropriateness for Medicare payments (Dan Jones, personal communication, 12/20/2006), and other insurers will pay close attention to these changes. Physical and occupational therapists can expect changes to occur impacting all areas of health care, and these changes will likely impact therapy practice (see Chapter 8).

A second major challenge for the health care system will be to make progress in health status for all Americans and to decrease and eliminate **health disparities.** A health disparity is "a significant disparity in the overall rate of disease incidence, prevalence, morbidity, mortality, or survival rate" between population groups (NIH 2001, p.3). Braveman (2006) has defined a health disparity as the "difference in which disadvantaged social groups—such as the poor, racial/ethnic minorities, women, or other groups who have persistently experienced social disadvantage or discrimination—systematically experience worse health or greater health risks than more advantaged social groups. 'Social advantage' refers to one's relative position in a social hierarchy determined by wealth, power, and/or prestige" (p.167).

Examples of health disparities include racial disparities, age disparities, and disparities experienced by persons with disabilities. African-Americans experience greater rates of morbidity and mortality in several disorders including cardiovascular disease, cancer, diabetes, and disability (Centers for Disease Control and Prevention 2005; Oliver and Muntaner 2005; Siminoff and Ross 2005). It has been demonstrated that children with juvenile arthritis (Brunner et al. 2006), children with intellectual disabilities (Havercamp et al. 2004; Krahn, Hammond, and Turner 2006), and children from socially disadvantaged backgrounds (Bauman et al. 2006) experience more health problems than other children. Finally, a study by Nosek et al. (2006) found that women with disabilities experience an average of 14.6 secondary conditions compared with 75 percent of their community-based sample reporting over 10 conditions. Strategies are needed to comprehensively address these differences in health status. Among the major causes of disability and illness worldwide, Michaud et al. (2001) identified occupational hazards and physical inactivity. Occupational and physical therapists have important contributions to make to address these issues (see Chapter 13). A goal of the PPACA of 2010 is to address lack of health insurance and its adverse affect on health status as a method to reduce health disparities.

Active Learning Exercise

Read more about disparities in health status and the quality of health care in the United States at http://www.ahrq.gov/qual/qrdr11.htm. Look at the State Snapshots. What is the quality of care for your state?

Conclusion

In this chapter we have introduced and reviewed several principles and concepts related to the definition, measurement, and utilization of quality in the development and implementation of health services. Occupational therapists and physical therapists will encounter the quality principle when utilizing patient outcome management systems, payment reporting systems, and in the legal system related to their license to practice. Increasingly, quality measurement will be used to determine the appropriateness of payment. In Chapters 6–9 we will explore in some detail the payment systems encountered by therapists. As you do so, consider these policies from the perspective of how they affect access, cost, and quality of health care. Prior to this section, we are going to introduce and discuss policies that address social disablement and the advocacy process, or the purpose and method for effecting policy change.

Chapter Review Questions

1. Compare and contrast the personal- and population-based definitions of quality health care. Review their strengths and weaknesses.

2. Define and provide examples for structure, process, and outcomes as measures of health care quality.

3. What are "report cards" in health care, and how are they used? Provide one example of a report card.

4. Define "accreditation," and review the major accrediting agencies for health care–related organizations in the United States.

5. What is the purpose of professional regulation?

6. What are expectations for privacy of health information in the U.S. health care system?

7. Review the four standards that must be demonstrated to prove medical negligence and the strategy for a successful defense of an allegation of medical negligence.

8. Define "pay for performance" and how it is used in health care policy.

9. Define health disparities and identify reasons for why they exist.

Chapter Discussion Questions

1. Review the chapter reading about evidence-based practice. Describe your impressions of the barriers and opportunities to employing evidence-based practice in your work.

2. Public reporting of health provider quality data is increasing. Outpatient therapists are reporting patient quality of care data to Medicare. While not currently public information, discuss your perceptions of the strengths and weaknesses of a public report card system on the quality of health care.

3. Access to medical records is restricted by patient privacy laws. Discuss the purpose of these laws and how you are going to ensure that you do not access patient records for unacceptable reasons.

4. Discuss how physical therapists and occupational therapists can work to reduce health disparities in your community.

References

Amato, A., E. Dobrzykowski, and T. Nance. 1997. The effect of timely onset of rehabilitation on outcomes of outpatient orthopedic practice. *J Rehabil Outcomes Meas* 1(3): 32–38.

American Occupational Therapy Association (AOTA). 2007, January 26. Medicare quality measures for occupational therapy coming soon. http://www.aota.org/nonmembers /area1/links/link22.asp (accessed April 9, 2007).

Annas, G. J. 1998. A national bill of patient rights. *N Engl J Med* 338(10): 695–99.

Bauman, L.F., E.F Silver, and R.E. Stein. 2006. Cumulative social disadvantage and child health. *Pediatrics* 117(4): 1321–28.

Bennett, S., K. McKenna, T. Hoffmann , L. Tooth , A. McCluskey, and J. Strong. 2007. The value of an evidence database for occupational therapists: An international online survey. *Int J Med Inform* 76(7): 507–13.

Braun, B.L., E.A. Kind, J.B. Fowles, and W.G. Suarez. 2002. Consumer response to a report card comparing healthcare systems. *Am J Manag Care* 8(6): 522–28.

Braveman, P. 2006. Health disparities and health equity: Concepts and measurement. *Ann Rev Public Health* 27: 167–194.

Bridges, P.H., L.L. Bierema, and T. Valentine. 2007. The propensity to adopt evidence-based practice among physical therapists. *BMC Health Serv Res* 7: 103.

Brunner, H.I., J. Taylor, M.T. Britto, M.S. Corcoran, S.L. Kramer, P.G. Melson, U.R. Kotagal, T.B. Graham, and M.H. Passo. 2006. Differences in disease outcomes between Medicaid and privately insured children: Possible health disparities in juvenile rheumatoid arthritis. *Arthritis Rheum* 55(3): 378–84.

Casarett, D., and C. Helms. 1999. Systems errors versus physicians' errors: Finding the balance in medical education. *Acad Med* 74(1): 19–22.

Centers for Disease Control and Prevention. 2005. Health disparities experienced by black or African Americans—United States. *MMWR Morb Mortal Wkly Rep* 54(1): 1–3.

C.N.A. HealthPro. 2006. Physical therapy claims study. http://www.cna.com/vcm_content/CNA/internet/Static%20File%20for%20Download/Risk%20Control/Medical%20Services/Physical_Therapy_Claims_Study.pdf (accessed on December 5, 2012).

Commission on the Accreditation of Rehabilitation Facilities. 2008. http://www.carf.org/ (accessed May 20, 2008).

Crowell, M.S., B.S. Tragord, A.L. Taylor, and G.D. Deyle. 2012. Integration of critically appraised topics into evidence-based physical therapy practice. *J Orthop Sports Phys Ther* 42(10): 870–79.

Dobrzykowski, E. 1997. The methodology of outcomes measurement. *J Rehabil Outcomes Meas* 1(1): 8–17.

_____ and T. Nance. 1997. The Focus on Therapeutic Outcomes (FOTO) outpatient orthopedic rehabilitation database: Results of 1994–1996. *J Rehabil Outcomes Meas* 1(1): 56–60.

Donabedian, A. 1966. Evaluating the quality of medical care. *Milbank Q* 44: 166–203.

_____. 1988. The quality of care: How can it be assessed? *JAMA* 260(12): 1743–48.

_____. 1990. The seven pillars of quality. *Arch Pathol Lab Med* 114(11): 1115–18.

Dysart, A.M., and G.S. Tomlin. 2002. Factors related to evidence-based practice among U.S. occupational therapy clinicians. *Am J Occup Ther* 56(3): 275–84.

Ellwood, P. 1988. Shattuck Lecture. Outcomes management: A technology of patient experience. *N Engl J Med* 318(23): 1549–56.

Epstein, A.J. 2006. Do cardiac surgery report cards reduce mortality? Assessing the evidence. *Med Care Res Rev* 63(4): 403–26.

Field, M.J., and K.N. Lohr, eds. *Guidelines for clinical practice: From development to use.* Washington DC: National Academy Press.

Focus on Therapeutic Outcomes, Inc. 2012. http://www.fotoinc.com/ (accessed December 8, 2012).

Focus on Therapeutic Outcomes, Inc. (FOTO). 2012. http://www.fotoinc.com/ (accessed December 8, 2012).

Guccione, A.A., T.J. Mielenz, R.F. DeVellis, M.S. Goldstein, J.K. Freburger, R. Pietrobon, S.C. Miller, L.F. Callahan, K. Harwood, and T.S. Carey. 2005. Development and testing of a self-report instrument to measure actions: Outpatient Physical Therapy Improvement in Movement Assessment Log (OPTIMAL). *Phys Ther* 85(6): 515–30.

Havercamp, S.M., D. Scandlin, and M. Roth. 2004. Health disparities among adults with developmental disabilities, adults with other disabilities, and adults not reporting disability in North Carolina. *Public Health Rep* 119(4): 418–26.

Institute of Medicine. 1999. *To err is human: Building a safer health system.* Washington DC: National Academy Press.

Institute of Medicine. 2001. *Crossing the quality chasm: A new health system for the 21st century.* Washington DC: National Academy Press.

Joint Commission on the Accreditation of Healthcare Organizations. 2007. About Accreditation. http://www.jointcommission.org/GeneralPublic/About_Accreditation.htm (accessed February 1, 2007).

Krahn, G.L., L. Hammond, and A. Turner. 2006. A cascade of disparities: Health and health care access for people with intellectual disabilities. *Ment Retard Dev Disabil Res Rev* 12(1): 70–82.

Leape, L.L. 1997. A systems analysis approach to medical error. *J Eval Clin Pract* 3(3): 213–22.

Lenz, G. 2008. Managed Care. In W. Kirch, ed., *Encyclopedia of Public Health* (876–79). New York: Springer. doi:10.1007/978-1-4020-5614-7.

Maher, C.G., C. Sherrington, M. Elkins, R.D. Herbert, and A.M. Moseley. 2004. Challenges for evidence-based physical therapy: Accessing and interpreting high-quality evidence on therapy. *Phys Ther* 84(7): 644–54.

McCluskey, A., and M. Lovarini. 2005. Providing education on evidence-based practice improved knowledge but did not change behaviour: A before and after study. *BMC Med Educ* 5: 40.

Meenan, R.F., P.M. Gertman, and J.H. Mason. 1980. Measuring health status in arthritis. The arthritis impact measurement scales. *Arthritis Rheum* 23(2): 146–52.

Michaud, C.M., C.J., Murray, and B.R. Bloom. 2001. Burden of disease—Implications for future research. *JAMA* 285(5): 535–39.

Mu, K., H. Lohman, and L. Scheirton. 2006. Occupational therapy practice errors in physical rehabilitation and geriatric settings: A national survey study. *Am J Occup Ther* 60(3): 288–97.

National Board for Certification in Occupational Therapy. About Us. http://www.nbcot.org/index.php?option=com_content&view=article&id=40&Itemid=14 (accessed March 27, 2013).

National Committee for Quality Assurance. About NCQA. http://www.ncqa.org/about/about.htm (accessed February 1, 2007).

Nosek, M.A., R.B. Hughes, N.J. Petersen, H.B. Taylor, S. Robinson-Whelen, M. Byrne, and R. Morgan. 2006. Secondary conditions in a community-based sample of women with physical disabilities over a 1-year period. Arch Phys Med Rehabil 87(3): 320- 327.

Oliver, M.N., and C. Muntaner. 2005. Researching health inequities among African Americans: The imperative to understand social class. *Int J Health Serv* 35(3): 485–98.

Rothschild, J.M., D.W. Bates, and L.L. Leape. 2000. Preventable medical injuries in older patients. *Arch Intern Med* 160(18): 2717–28.

Rotter, T., L. Kinsman, E.L. James, A. Machotta, H. Gothe, J. Willis, P. Snow, and J. Kugler. 2010. Clinical pathways: Effect on professional practice, patient outcomes, length of stay and hospital costs. *Cochrane Database of Systematic Reviews* Issue 3. Art No: CD006632 DOI: 10.1002/14651858.CD00632.pub2.

Sackett, D.L., S.E. Strauss, W.S. Richardson, et al. 2000. *Evidence based medicine: How to practice and teach EBM* 2nd ed. Edinburgh Scotland: Churchill Livingstone.

Salbach, N.M., S.B. Jaglal, N. Korner-Bitensky, S. Rappolt, and D. Davis. Practitioner and organizational barriers to evidence-based practice of physical therapists for people with stroke. *Phys Ther* 87(10): 1284–303.

Sandstrom, R. 2007. Malpractice by physical therapists: Descriptive analysis of reports in the National Practitioner Data Bank Public Use Data File, 1991–2004. *J Allied Health* 36(4): 201–08.

Schmitt, K., and G. Shimberg. 1996. Demystifying occupational and professional regulation: Answers to questions you may have been afraid to ask. Council on Licensure, Enforcement and Regulation.

Schultz, J., K. Thiede-Call, R. Feldman, and J. Christianson. 2001. Do employees use report cards to assess health care provider systems? *Health Serv Res* 36(3): 509–30.

Schwartz, W. B., and D. M. Mendelson. 1994. Eliminating waste and inefficiency can do little to contain costs. *Health Affairs* 13(1): 224–38.

Scott, R.W. 1991. The legal standard of care. *Clin Management* 11(2): 10–11.

Seiden, D. J. 1994. Health care ethics. In. A. R. Kovner, ed., *Health care delivery in the United States* (486–531). New York: Springer.

Siminoff, L.A., and L. Ross. 2005. Access and equity to cancer care in the USA: A review and assessment. *Postgrad Med J* 81(961): 674–79.

Thomas, E.J., and T.A. Brennan. 2000. Incidence and types of preventable adverse events in elderly patients: Population-based review of medical records. *BMJ* 320(7237): 741–44.

United States Department of Health and Human Services. Office for Civil Rights. Medical privacy: National standards to protect the privacy of personal health information. http://www.hhs.gov/ocr/hipaa/finalreg.html (accessed January 6, 2003).

Ware, J.E., and C.D. Sherbourne. 1992. The MOS 36-item short-form health survey (SF-36) I. Conceptual framework and item selection. *Med Care* 30(6): 473–83.

Werner, R.M., and D.A. Asch. 2005. The unintended consequences of publicly reporting quality information. *JAMA* 293(10): 12–44.

Wicks, E.K., and J.A. Meyer. 1999. Making report cards work. *Health Affairs* 18(2): 152–55.

4

Public Policies Addressing Social Disablement

CHAPTER OBJECTIVES

At the conclusion of this chapter, the reader will be able to:

1. Discuss different societal perspectives about disabilities.

2. Describe the focus of key public policies for people with disabilities.

3. Explain how therapists can access each of the public policies about disabilities.

4. Apply concepts in this chapter to a case study or active learning exercise.

ABBREVIATIONS FOR PUBLIC POLICIES DISCUSSED IN THIS CHAPTER

ADA: Americans with Disablities Act

ATA: Assistive Technology Act

DDA: Developmental Disabilities Act

FHA: Fair Housing Act

IDEA: Individuals with Disabilities Education Improvement Act

OAA: Older American Act

RA: Rehabilitation Act

SSA: Social Security Act

SSDI: Social Security Disability Insurance

SSI: Supplemental Security Income

WIA: Workforce Investment Act

KEY WORDS

Assistive Technology
Barriers
Empowerment
Inclusion
Independent-Living
Reasonable Accommodations
Related Services
Vocational Rehabilitation

CASE EXAMPLE

Larry, a physical therapist, and Martha, an occupational therapist, work collaboratively in a school-based setting. Both follow Amanda, a pleasant, shy 10-year-old girl with a severe developmental disability, who has some mental and more motor impairment. Because of the Individuals with Disabilities Education Improvement Act (IDEA) Amanda receives added services to allow her to integrate into and benefit from the school environment. Even before Amanda entered school, she had home-based physical therapy and occupational therapy services under Part C of the IDEA. When she entered kindergarten, Amanda was placed in a special classroom with five other children and gradually integrated into a few classes in the general classroom. Over the years, Amanda continued to receive occupational therapy and physical therapy under Part B of the IDEA. Amanda benefits immensely from the IDEA. If she had been born prior to the enactment of the law, she would likely have not attended school. Now she receives services until she is 22 years old, and there will be a plan for her to transition into employment.

Yet, Amanda has concerns beyond the classroom environment that are not addressed by the IDEA. She needs an electric wheelchair and other low-tech assistive technology to assist with doing activities of daily living (ADL) at home. She would benefit from training and computer software to help her at home. Amanda is the only child of a single mother who has limited financial resources.

Amanda's astute therapists recognize that many of her needs can be helped by other public policies and related community resources beyond the IDEA, so they do their research. In their state, Amanda can receive a new electric wheelchair funded by Medicaid. Her low-tech ADL needs can be arranged by a community-based church lending service. Her computer software training can be acquired through the State Assistive Technology Project. People from Amanda's State Assistive Technology Project are even able to assess Amanda's home and school for suggested modifications. Amanda's mother is given the opportunity to buy adaptive equipment, including the computer software, at a discounted cost. Martha and Larry network with staff from their state office funded by the Developmental Disability Act. There they find additional resources to help Amanda and her mother. Through resources available because of various public policies and with the help of her therapists, Amanda is able to have an optimal quality of life. Larry and Martha reflect that as a result of their networking for Amanda, they enhanced their knowledge of broader community resources to help their clients based on public and private policies. They share this information with their peer therapists in an in-service program and develop an informative poster for a presentation at their state therapy conferences.

Case Example Questions:

1. What effects do the Individuals with Disabilities Education Improvement Act, the Assistive Technology Act, and the Developmental Disability Act have on Amanda's experience of disablement?

2. How can you find out about additional policy resources in your state to service clients that you work with?

Introduction

In Chapter 1 we introduced the social disability model as an important paradigm with which to understand disablement. The social disability model defines disablement as a sociopolitical experience resulting from the marginalization of people with disabling conditions by policies, social structures, attitudes, and (**barriers**) of the nondisabled population. The source of the disablement experience is not in the individual, but rather in the community. In this chapter, we focus on public policies that developed to address the isolation of, and discrimination against, people with disabling conditions—people like Amanda in the case study.

U.S. citizens historically held different perspectives about people with disabilities. For example, at the beginning of the 20th century, it was considered humane to place people with disabilities in institutions to be protected from society. Our current perspective is to encourage people with disabilities to be included in societal, school, work, and living activities. In current terminology, this philosophy is called **inclusion** or integration. It is written into many policies and approaches. For example, a position paper from the American Physical Therapy Association states, "People with disabilities share the same rights as all other individuals to have access to and opportunities for full economic, social, and personal development. The American Physical Therapy Association (APTA) shall advocate for full inclusion for people with disabilities in all aspects of community life and within the profession of physical therapy" (APTA 2009). The American Occupational Therapy Association (AOTA) developed over the years several position papers related to disability and inclusion (e.g., AOTA 1993; AOTA 1995; AOTA 2000; AOTA 2009; Hansen and Hinojosa 2004).

Thoughtful readers may question the different perspectives about disabilities adopted from the beginning of the 20th century until now. However, societal perspectives are never right or wrong; rather, they reflect the beliefs and knowledge of what people thought was the best approach at the time. For example, in the United States, a paradigm shift about disabilities occurred between 1968 and 1988. Several factors contributed to this different perspective. People with disabilities were living longer. There was more community exposure, and disability organizations that advocated for the rights of people with disabilities emerged. In addition, a disability rights movement and an **independent-living** philosophy were strong contributing factors. The disability movement considered the civil rights of the "minority" group of people with disabilities (Bristo 1996). The independent-living philosophy was based on self-rule and self-help, and political and economic rights (Bristo 1996). Therefore, a paradigm shift occurred, from viewing people with disabilities solely from a medical perspective to an inclusion model. With the medical model, people with disabilities were perceived as "sick" or "impaired" and needing a cure. The newer perspectives incorporated people with disabilities into a community-based model emphasizing inclusion and **empowerment**. Thus, disability began to be seen as a larger societal problem requiring societal intervention, and this perspective is reflected in many of the recent disability laws, including the Americans with Disabilities Act (ADA) (Bristo 1997). Table 4-1 describes the paradigm switch from a medical model perspective to the current perspective.

The perspectives of a society about important issues like disability are supported by public policy, which is the codification of the shared values of a society (McClain 1996. Policies develop when society does not deal appropriately with perceived issues. Policies about disabilities can also be viewed as regulatory and allocative tools mandated by the government (McGregor 2001). Therefore, it is relevant for therapists to become aware of the different policies about disabilities, how they are regulated and allocated, and the values influencing them. Therapists commonly work with some, but not all, of society's health care and disability-related policies. For example, therapists working in school systems provide services to children through the Individuals with Disabilities Education Improvement Act (IDEA). IDEA supports the education of children and youths with disabilities. However, therapists may not be as familiar with the Developmental Disabilities Act (DDA) or the Rehabilitation Act (RA). Yet these acts offer services that help similar clients, and therapists can educate people with disabilities and their caregivers about the benefits of these acts.

Table 4-1 Contrast of Paradigms

	Old Paradigms	New Paradigms
Definition of disability	The individual is limited by impairment or condition	The individual with an impairment requires an accommodation to perform functions to carry out life activities
Strategy to address disability	Fix the individual, correct the deficit	Remove barriers, create access through accommodation and universal design, promote wellness and health
Method of addressing disability	Provision of medical, vocational, or psychological rehabilitation services	Provision of supports (e.g., assistive technology, personal assistance services, job coach)
Source of intervention	Professionals, clinicians, and other rehabilitation service providers	Peers, inclusionary service providers, consumer information services
Entitlements	Eligibility for benefits based on severity of impairment	Eligibility for accommodations seen as a civil right
Role of disabled individual	Object of intervention, patient, beneficiary, research subject	Consumer or customer, empowered peer, research participant, decision-maker
Domain of disability	A medical "problem"	A socioenvironmental issue involving accessibility, accommodations, and equity

Source: Adapted by Betty Jo Berland from materials prepared for the NIDDR's Long-Range Plan by Gerben DeJong and Bonnie O'Day and reprinted with permission from NIDRR, Washington DC (NIDDR 2000).

The public policies presented in this chapter are divided into three main sections based on the people they serve and the societal values they represent. In the first section, policies representing two specific age groups—youths and older adults in our society—are presented and discussed. The second section represents civil rights policies that focus on people who work and live in our society, and includes an examination of the Americans with Disabilities Act and federal income replacement or supplementation programs through the Social Security Administration. The third section represents a policy related to technology, which helps people of all ages with disabilities, and a policy that helps people with disabilities obtain fair housing. We consider the following public policies: the ADA, the Assistive Technology Act (ATA), Developmental Disabilities Act (DDA), Fair Housing Act (FHA), Individuals with Disabilities Education Improvement Act (IDEA), Older American Act (OAA), Rehabilitation Act (RA), and the Work Investment Act (WIA). In addition, we discuss two income replacement programs: Supplemental Security Income (SSI) and Social Security Disability Insurance (SSDI). The premise behind these policies correlates well with the therapy profession's belief in the value and dignity of people with disabilities and the recognition of a need for a quality of life. Table 4-2 overviews the prime focus of each of these laws. The chapter presents the main considerations about each law and how they are relevant to helping therapy clients.

Public Policies Supporting Youths and Older Adults

Public policies support the societal value of helping the future of our youth and children. Historically, Americans have also valued helping older adults with public policy. In this section, we will discuss the Individuals with Disabilities Education Improvement Act (IDEA), the Developmental Disabilities Act (DDA), and the Older Americans Act (OAA).

The Individuals with Disabilities Education Improvement Act (IDEA) (P.L. 108–446) is rooted in earlier legislation enacted in 1975 called the Education for All Handicapped

Table 4-2 Focus of Disability Policies

Disability Policy	Focus
Americans with Disabilities Act (ADA)	A major civil rights act that provides protection not only in employment, but in transportation and public accommodations, in telecommunications, and with state and local governments, for people with disabilities. Expanded coverage to areas not previously covered by other federal disability acts.
Assistive Technology Act (ATA)	Supports state programs for public-awareness programming to increase access to technology.
Developmental Disability Act (DDA)	Services those with intellectual impairments and other developmental disabilities. Provides protection and advocacy. Promotes "independence, productivity, integration and inclusion into the community."
Fair Housing Act (FHA)	Federal act that prohibits housing discrimination, includes discrimination against people with disabilities.
Older Americans Act (OAA)	Federal, state, tribal, and local collaboration for "organizing, coordinating and providing community-based services and opportunities for older Americans and their families" (AOA, n.d. ß2).
Rehabilitation Act (RA)	Helps people with disabilities maximize their employment abilities and independent living abilities, and supports inclusion in society.
Workforce Investment Act (WIA)	Supports federal job training for many populations. Addresses "employment services, adult education, and literacy programs, welfare-to-work, vocational education, and vocational rehabilitation" (AFL-CIO 2011).

Source: Administration on Aging (AOA) (n.d.). Fact Sheets: Older Americans Act. Retrieved from http://www.aoa.gov/AoA_programs/OAA /Introduction.aspx; AFL/CIO (2011). The Workforce Investment Act. Retreived from http://www.workingforamerica.org/documents/workforce.htm; L.F. Rothstein. *Disability and the law* (1992); K. Jacobs (1996). Work assessments and programming. (1996).

Children Act (EAHCA, P.L. 94–142) (NICHCY 2000). This legislation resulted from the strong advocacy efforts of parents and advocacy groups, such as the Association of Retarded Citizens later known "The Arc." These groups were interested in children with disabilities receiving better educational opportunities. Prior to the EAHCA, many children with disabilities, especially those with moderate to severe disabilities, did not get an education, and families had to find their own means for educational services (Bristo 1996; Mellard 2000). IDEA and its predecessor, EAHCA, are considered to be landmark legislation that helped integrate youth with disabilities into American society (Bristo 1997; Mellard 2000).

IDEA supports special education in the least restrictive environment (LRE) for children and youth, from 3 though age 21. LRE means that as much as possible, children with disabilities are educated alongside children without disabilities in the classroom and that "removal of children with disabilities from the regular educational environment occurs only if the nature or severity of the disability is such that education in regular classes with the use of supplementary aids and services cannot be achieved satisfactorily" (U.S. Department of Education n.d.). IDEA enables children with disabilities to receive a free appropriate public education (FAPE) (Special Education Advisor 2010). FAPE is defined as "special education and related services that (A) have been provided at public expense, under public supervision and direction, and without charge; (B) meet the standards of the state educational agency; (C) include an appropriate preschool, elementary school, or secondary school education in the state involved; and (D) are provided in conformity with the individualized education program required under Section 1414 (d) of this title" (U.S. Department of Education n.d.)." It is important to note that in addition to the IDEA, each state has its own laws and regulations regarding school-based services.

Every few years the IDEA is amended; the purpose of amending this or any legislation is to focus on achieving its original goals and making sure that it reflects current issues. The 2004 revisions addressed accountability and prevention of academic or social/behavioral problems. The revisions focused on students achieving better academic success, functional outcomes, and postsecondary achievement. Overall there was an emphasis on utilization of evidence with practice (Jackson 2007).

The current IDEA has four parts (Part A General Provisions, Part B Assistance for Education of all Children with Disabilities, Part C Infants and Children with Disabilities, and Part D National Activities To Improve Education of Children with Disabilities [P.L. 108–446]). Each of the four parts has specific regulations. Therapy practice is strongly influenced by Parts B and C.

Therapy is defined as a related service in Part B. Part B is "permanently authorized" by the IDEA (Jackson 2007, p.12) and provides special education and related services for children ages 3 through 21 who have disabilities (AOTA 2006a). Under Part B, a student's needs and the services provided are outlined in an individualized education program (IEP). The IEP is completed by a team of school staff and the child's parents/family members. Parents/family members should play an active role in deciding on intervention goals and activities to shape the IEP. More details about the application of the IEP are discussed in Chapter 12. Examples of other regulations addressed in Part B are FAPE, nonacademic services, hearing aid checks, methods of ensuring services, and personnel qualifications.

With the reauthorization of the IDEA in 2004, two major regulatory changes involving Part B assisted children in the general classroom and influenced therapy practice. One change called *early intervening services (EIS)* integrated academic and behavior supports for students in grades kindergarten through 12 not identified as needing special education (AOTA 2006b; U.S. Department of Education 2007). Linked to the EIS is a provision that allows for a Response to Intervention (RtI) approach. RtI, is also part of the No Child Left Behind Act (NCLB, P.L. 107–110), which is a law that establishes educational standards in the U.S. school system. RtI is defined as "tools that enable educators to target instructional interventions to children's areas of specific need as soon as those become apparent" (U.S. Department of Education 2007). Key to the RtI is the application of "research-based, scientifically validated instruction and interventions" (Clark and Polichino 2010). Although originally aimed at children with specific learning disabilities (SLD), the RtI process involves identification of children in the general classroom and utilizes a systematic curricular approach to address instructional or social/behavioral issues (Clark, Brouwer, Schmidt, and Alexander 2008; Clark and Polichino 2010).

A three-tiered approach to RtI is suggested (IDEA Partnership Project 2012) for screening and intervention in the classroom. The first tier involves a baseline of universal interventions with "strong core instruction and screening for all students" (Clark et al. 2008). An example of a universal intervention is generally addressing ergonomic concerns for all children in the classroom. From the screening process, students with concerns are pinpointed to be addressed by the second tier. The second tier includes targeted approaches, such as providing adaptive equipment to some students to increase participation in an art group (AOTA n.d.a, p.2). The third tier focusing on individual students involves intensive interventions for specific needs, such as addressing handwriting for a student struggling in the classroom (AOTA n.d. a, p.2).

The provision of the RtI is not mandated by the IDEA or NCLB but highly encouraged by the US. Department of Education. Programs vary from state to state (Clark and Polichino 2007), and as benefits are recognized by school systems, more states have implemented an RtI framework (61 percent in 2010 as compared to approximately 25 percent in 2007) (Samuels 2011).

Part C is a voluntary federal grant program (Clark 2008) which requires states to "maintain and implement a statewide, comprehensive, coordinated, multidisciplinary, interagency system to provide early intervention services for infants and toddlers with disabilities and their families" (IFSPweb n.d.). Funding for Part C is discretionary and controlled by the annual Congressional appropriations process (Jackson 2007; Streeter

2007). Thus, it is up to the discretion of the legislators whether or not to fund Part C on an annual basis. States have more flexibility with Part C than with Part B, resulting in program variability (Clark 2008). There are 16 components required to be met by states. One of these components, reflecting a growing expectation for evidence-based practice, is that services are based as much as possible on research. (This expectation for more evidenced-based practice is also true with therapy practice under Part B.) Other exemplars of components with Part C are multidisciplinary evaluations of the child and family and provision of services in the child's natural environment (Clark 2008). The intervention team is required to complete an Individualized Family Service Plan (IFSP) for each eligible child and family. The IFSP identifies services that a child will receive, and is done in conjunction with the child's parent(s). Therapists working with infants and toddlers with Part C should become familiar with all components of this multidisciplinary program.

Legislative amendments involve the political process and compromises between the political parties within the Senate and Congress. Over the years, bills have been introduced by Congress to amend the IDEA to provide full funding, but to date these bills have not passed. Achieving full funding is an issue as without full funding the costs for IDEA fall back on the local school district and taxpayers (Steve Milliken, personal communication, 4/7/2012). Bills addressing full funding have kept in the forefront a commitment when IDEA was first enacted for Congress to meet its promise of funding up to 40 percent of the *excess cost* of educating students with disabilities (the amount above and beyond what a given state spends on educating its students without disabilities). As of 2011, federal funding totaled 16.1 percent of these costs (Diament 2011).

Regulations from the Department of Education implement the policies set forth in the law. With the 2004 amended IDEA, regulations focused on aligning the bill with the NCLB (AOTA n.d.b). AOTA is calling for further alignment of these two bills with the reauthorization of NCLB (AOTA 2010). It is not unusual for related bills to have similar language or to align together on the basis of the political climate and attitudes of the time.

Finally, anytime a major bill is amended, coalitions lobby for issues that are important to their members. Examples of coalitions involved with IDEA are the National Education Association, the American Association of School Administrators, and professional organizations such as American Occupational Therapy Association and the American Physical Therapy Association.

The current IDEA has accomplished many of its original goals. Most children with disabilities are now educated in their neighborhood schools and are integrated into regular classrooms. Most children are enrolled in postsecondary education, and there has been an improvement in high school graduation rates and employment rates. Data indicates that 217,905 students with disabilities aged 14 to 21 graduated from high school with a diploma in 2007–2008, which was a 16 percent increase from 1996–1997 (U.S. Department of Education 2010, p.2). Additionally, employment rates for young adults with disabilities increased about 15 points. However, the percentage working 35 hours or more per week decreased (U.S. Department of Education 2010, p.2).

IDEA and Therapy

IDEA supports services for children with intellectual disability, hearing impairments (including deafness), speech or language impairments, visual impairments (including blindness), serious emotional disturbances, orthopedic impairments, autism, traumatic brain injury, other health impairments, or specific learning disabilities (Section 602 (3)(A)(i)).

Under IDEA Part B, therapists provide **related services**. Related services are interventions needed to help children benefit from special education. Therefore, in the school setting, therapy is not perceived as, nor should it be, a medically based intervention. Thus, therapists trained in traditional medical settings adapt to a different therapy focus. Physical and occupational therapy services can follow children as long as the Individualized Education Program (IEP) process determines a need for intervention. All children eligible for services under IDEA receive an IEP, and there are guidelines to which therapists must adhere to address the required areas of an IEP. Some of these guidelines changed with the 2004 reauthorization (AFB n.d.; FAPE 2004). Therapists can work within the general classroom as part of the RtI process to address academic and behavioral issues (U.S. Department of Education 2007). In addition, although not specifically stated in the law, nothing precludes therapists from providing evaluation and intervention as an early intervening service (Jackson 2007).

Occupational and physical therapists also work under Part C of the IDEA or the early intervention program for infants and their families from birth to 36 months. The regulations for early intervention services mention therapy and clearly indicate that individual therapy services can stand alone (Leslie Jackson, personal communication, 3/15/2012). Therapists provide input to the plan of care, or Individualized Family Service Plan (IFSP). Specific guidelines exist for what is included in the IFSP (Clark 2008). The IFSP is a "family-centered practice approach" (Clark 2008, p.CE-3) with parents guiding the priorities of services. State regulations determine whether the family needs to co-pay for services or whether there can be a health insurance subsidy (Opp 2007).

Under Part C, therapists provide intervention for young children in their natural context or their typical environment, which can be the home, day care, or even a playground (Opp 2007). Thus, the setting for therapy need not be the school system, as in Part B.

Therapists should keep abreast of legislative changes related to the IDEA and how they affect therapy. They need to learn how the IDEA is regulated in their state and in their school system. A proactive stance is beneficial before and when the law is reauthorized, especially since so much of school-based practice is defined and largely funded by the IDEA. Advocacy efforts can be made with school systems, organizations, Congress, and the Department of Education. Therapists also need to be aware of related legislation such as NCLB because it too influences school-based therapy practice. In Chapter 12 we will further describe the system created by this law: special education.

The Developmental Disabilities Act (DDA)

In the United States, there has been a long history of people with developmental disabilities and intellectual impairments not getting adequate services. However, it was in the 1960s, during President Kennedy's administration, that treatment of people with developmental disabilities and intellectual disabilities became a high-priority societal concern. This concern corresponded with an overall societal interest in civil rights and a change in the societal view of developmental and intellectual disabilities from being congenitally caused to resulting from a societal problem related to poverty, prenatal care, and other social influences (Hightower-Vandamm 1979). The legislative roots of the modern-day Developmental Disabilities Act began in 1963 with two federal laws: P.L. 88–156 aimed at helping higher-risk mothers, and P.L. 88–164 aimed at providing federal funds for building facilities for people with intellectual impairments (Hightower-Vandamm 1979). Since the 1960s, the DDA has been reauthorized several times with the most current reauthorization in 2000. These reauthorizations reflect the societal evolution of viewing developmental and intellectual disabilities within a social model. Although many gains have been made as a result of the DDA, barriers still remain for societal inclusion of people with developmental disabilities (National Council on Disability 2011).

The current Developmental Disabilities Act (P.L. 106–402), is divided into several titles. Title I has four parts, which include (1) state councils on developmental disabilities, (2) protection and advocacy systems, (3) university-affiliated programs, and (4) projects of national significance. States have some discretion under the law to design their own systems for the councils, protection and advocacy agencies, and university-affiliated programs. As a result, these programs take different forms in the various states (Gordon 2000), and the perceived "quality" and "effectiveness" of these programs vary (National Council on Disability 2011, p.7). The state councils help advocate for people with developmental disabilities (Graney 2000). State councils assist with consumer empowerment, advocacy, systems change, obtaining recourses for people with developmental disabilities and their family members, and promoting community inclusion

(National Association of Councils on Developmental Disabilities [NADDC] 2013). The protection and advocacy agencies mediate and handle legal situations for people with developmental disabilities. The university-affiliated programs provide interdisciplinary education and training for professionals, conduct applied research, and provide training and technological assistance for people with disabilities, their families, and others. The projects of national significance involve research, evaluation, and demonstration projects (Graney 2000).

Title II provides support to families with children who have disabilities. Examples of family support are respite care and subsidies (Title II, Section 202). Title III is a limited scholarship program for staff assisting individuals with developmental disabilities. At the time of writing this chapter, the DDA remains the same, as it has not been reauthorized; however, organizations such as "The Arc" are calling for the act to be reauthorized by Congress (The Arc 2011).

The DDA and Therapy

There are approximately 7–8 million individuals with intellectual and developmental disabilities in the United States (The Arc 2011). Many of these people can benefit from the DDA. The intent of the DDA is to manage the arrangement of services and advocacy efforts on behalf of those with developmental disabilities and not to provide direct services (Graney 2000). Therefore, most therapists are not directly involved with the act, and it does not reimburse therapy services. The DDA has much the same philosophical intent as therapy services, namely, helping people achieve maximal independence and potential (Gordon 2000).

Nevertheless, over the years, the American Occupational Therapy Association has taken an active role in lobbying for different amendments (Boyd et al. 1996). Therapists should become familiar with the parts of the act that help the clients they serve. On behalf of clients they may utilize protection and advocacy (P & As) services to "protect the legal and human rights of individuals with developmental disabilities" (National Council on Disability, n.d.). For example, P & A services might be assessed for a client with developmental disabilities whose IEP is not being implemented. Therapists may utilize resources from their state Councils on Developmental Disabilities. Therapists can become involved in interdisciplinary training programs through the University Centers on Excellence in Developmental Disabilities (Maureen Fitzgerald, personal communication, 11/7/2011). University centers offer excellent programming related to therapy practice. For example, many university centers offer programming about autism such as the Center on Human Development and Disability at the University of Washington. Through this center, "research, training, outreach, and advocacy" about autism is offered (Cooper 2011, p.18). Other examples of programming from university centers focus on assistive technology, employment, transportation, and housing (Cooper 2011). Therapists can find out more information by contacting their local University Centers on Excellence. Centers can be located through the Association of University Centers on Disabilities on the Internet.

Finally, therapists need to understand that the majority of funding support for people with developmental disabilities (National Council on Disability 2011) and other disabilities is from Medicaid. Medicaid provides medical and other supports for people with disabilities. Qualified individuals receive a baseline of medical benefits such as laboratory and X-ray services, and inpatient hospital services. Optional medical benefits, including therapy, vary among states. Medicaid helps finance long-term care services for people with disabilities in institutions or in community-based group homes (Elizabeth M. Boggs Center on Developmental Disabilities 2011). Medicaid may finance direct support workers for people with disabilities. There is a strong push with state programs to provide community-based options. Although people with disabilities along with older adults make up approximately 25 percent of Medicaid enrollees, they account for two-thirds of Medicaid spending (The Arc n.d.). Therefore, in times of economic cutbacks it is important to advocate for state Medicaid funds to help people with disabilities. (More details about Medicaid can be found in Chapter 9.)

Table 4-3 Summary of the Objectives of the Older Americans Act

- Adequate income for older adults in retirement
- Best mental and physical health for all older adults
- Suitable housing considering special needs and costs
- Full restorative services for long-term care and a variety of community-based services to support older adults
- Nondiscriminatory employment
- "Retirement in health, honor, and dignity" (Section 101)
- Participation in meaningful activities
- Adequate community services and resources
- Benefits from research
- "Freedom, independence, and the free exercise of individual initiative in planning and managing their own lives" (Section 101)

Adapted from: Title I: Declaration of Objectives for Older Americans. Retrieved from http://www.aoa.gov/AoA_programs/OAA
/oaa_full.asp#_Toc153957625.

Before moving on to the next sections, review again the initial case example about Amanda. Consider the details provided in this chapter about the IDEA and the DDA in terms of the case example, and reflect on how these acts can benefit Amanda and similar clients.

The Older Americans Act (OAA)

The Older Americans Act (OAA) (P.L. 89–73) was enacted originally in 1965, along with other programs that support older Americans, such as Medicare and Medicaid. (Medicare and Medicaid are discussed in Chapters 8 and 9.) The purpose of the OAA, a federal, state, tribal, and local collaboration (AOA 2006), is to enhance the quality of life for older Americans. This is reflected by its 10 broad objectives, outlined in Title I (Texas Department of Aging and Disability Services 2012) and summarized in Table 4-3. The OAA created many benefits for older Americans, including the Administration on Aging, state grants for programs and services, and research and training (AOA n.d.). The current OAA includes a national aging services network of "56 state agencies on aging, 629 area agencies on aging, nearly 20,000 service providers, 244 tribal organizations, and 2 native Hawaiian organizations representing 400 tribes" (AOA 2010). These different divisions oversee programs for older adults. State programs funded by the OAA provide a variety of services for older adults, including housing, nutrition, health, employment, retirement, health promotion, protection and advocacy services, as well as other social and community services (AOA n.d.).

Therapists should consider referring patients/residents that they work with to their local office on aging, state units, or one of the tribal organizations for many beneficial services. Therapists often observe the positive impact of the act on the patients they serve. For example, in home health environments, some of the patients followed may be receiving Meals on Wheels. Therapists may provide programming at senior centers funded by the OAA to help with activities of daily living, health promotion, life transitions, and with education about function with specific conditions (AOTA 2011). Some therapists received grants from their OAA for such programming (T. Nanof, personal communication, 11/6/2007). As of the writing of this chapter, the OAA was last reauthorized in 2006 and may soon be reauthorized.

Active Learning Exercises

Martha is a 68 year-old client with the diagnosis of left cerebrovascular accident whom you follow in home health care practice. She lives alone in a one-story home. She has many needs to remain in her home. Among these needs are difficulties making meals, help with putting in place home modifications, and finding transportation to get to physician appointments. On the web, locate your local Office on Aging and identify what services can help Martha and other clients.

Work-Related Policy Acts

Case Example

Maria is a therapist who works in a program financed by her state vocational rehabilitation program.

Maria was trained as an occupational therapist in traditional practice. Her first position was at an acute care hospital, where she specialized with orthopedic patients. Maria enjoyed the position, but felt that she wanted to do more with her skills, talents, and interests. Her dream was to reach out to Hispanic people who had work injuries. Therefore, she started researching opportunities and found that therapists can become case managers and work towards certification through the Commission for Case Management Certification. Being proactive, she researched the requirements for the certification on the web (refer to ccmcertification.org). She learned that some therapists are involved in work programs. Maria found a therapist to be a mentor and then assumed a position as a case manager helping Hispanic people at a work-training program financed by the state's vocational rehabilitation program. Eventually Maria fulfilled the certification requirements to become a certified case manager.

Maintaining or promoting the ability of people to work is a strong value associated with self-worth, status (Baker and Jacobs 2003), and a sense of productivity that has consistently been part of American society. People with disabilities want to be productive working members of our society (National Council on Disabilities 2004) (see Chapter 1). Therefore, it is not surprising that a large number of public policies are related to encouraging or maintaining the abilities to work. Examples of these public policies are the Rehabilitation Act, Workforce Investment Act, the Americans with Disabilities Act, and the Work Incentive Improvement Act of 1999. This section overviews these public policies. We will also discuss the Social Security programs that provide vital income support for persons with disabilities who cannot work.

The Rehabilitation Act (RA) and the Workforce Investment Act (WIA)

The Rehabilitation Act (RA) (P.L. 93–112, 1987) and the Workforce Investment Act (WIA) (P.L. 105–22) are based on the strong American value of promoting productive work among members of our society. These laws are rooted in earlier policies related to work at the beginning of the 20th century (Vocational Rehabilitation Act and Worker's Compensation Laws) when work conditions were a major concern in industrial settings.

Modern policy for the Rehabilitation Act is traced to the 1970s when the Vocational Rehabilitation Act was amended to become the Rehabilitation Act of 1973. Historically, it is important to know that Sections 501, 503, and 504 of the Rehabiliation Act were foundational for the subsequent Americans with Disabilities Act (ADA). Section 501 established "a federal interagency committee on employees who are individuals with disabilities" (Tucker 1994, p.48). A key part of section 501 is the requirement that federal agencies have an affirmative action plan for the employment of people with disabilities. Section 503 requires nondiscrimination on the basis of disability and puts an affirmative action plan in place for federal agencies that contract for $10,000 or more. Section 504 prohibits discrimination in federal agencies, employment, education, architectural accessibility, and health, welfare, and social services for recipients of federal funding (Tucker 1994). Section 504 was landmark legislation, as it was the first civil rights declaration for people with disabilities. Section 504 states that "no qualified individual with a disability in the United States shall be excluded from, denied the benefits of, or subjected to discrimination under" any program receiving federal assistance or conducted by any executive agency or the United States Postal Service" (U.S. Department of Justice 2005, p.17). For the "first time in federal legislation, discrimination was defined as the failure to provide a reasonable accommodation to a qualified person with a disability" (Conyers 2002, as cited by Conyers and Ahrens 2003, p.59). With the elevation of the RA to a civil rights act, people with disabilities were allowed a legal means of advocating for their rights. Because of the controversies about this regulation, people in the disabilities movement attained increased public visibility (Bristo 1997).

The RA was amended in 1986 to include Section 508. This section established non-binding regulations for people with disabilities regarding usage of technology in federal workplaces (United States Access Board n.d.) With the 1998 amendments, Section 508 was strengthened to require that people with disabilities in federal workplaces, including employees and members of the public, have "access to electronic and informational technology" (The Rehabiliation Act Amendments 1998; U.S. Department of Justice 2005).

A related but different law is the WIA (P.L. 105–220, 1998). The purpose of the WIA is "to provide workforce investment activities, through statewide and local workforce investment systems, that increase the employment, retention, and earnings of participants, and increase occupational skill attainment by participants, and as a result, improve the quality of the workforce, reduce welfare dependency, and enhance the productivity and competitiveness of the nation." The WIA is considered to be the "largest single source of federal funding for workforce development activities," and because of this act, there are sites for "training and employment services" for many workers, including those who lose their jobs or are impoverished according to federal standards (Williamson 2009). In 2009, Congress made additional investments in this act, and it will soon be up for reauthorization (National Skills Coalition n.d.).

The Rehabilitation Act, the Workforce Investment Act, and Therapy

The RA is instituted in a community-based and not a medically based model. **Vocational rehabilitation** specialists, funded by the Rehabilitation Act, work primarily with people who have disabilities and need services. These specialists help people with disabilities obtain employment through assessment, consultation, mentoring, training, job placement, and assistive device provision. The 1998 amendments more clearly defined the RA as an employment program, which results in even less involvement from therapists. The amendments specify that therapy can be involved only if therapy services cannot be funded by another source (Dunn 2000). Thus, if Medicaid (see Chapter 9) covers rehabilitation services, the RA does not reimburse for rehabilitation. However, some therapists work in partnership with employment specialists to assist with "assessment and skill development" (Stein and Cutler 2002, as cited by Winstead 2009, p.16). Finally, since the RA is a state–federal program and state programs vary (Dunn 2000), therapists should have a good understanding of the focus of their state agencies.

The WIA of 1998 helps clients with work-related concerns, and it includes many beneficial services. It is difficult to gauge how involved physical therapy and occupational therapy are with this act. However, familiarity with WIA helps clients access services. Section 103 of the WIA (Workforce Investment Act of 1998, 105–220, § 404) lists many services, including, but not limited to, training programs and centers, vocational rehabilitation services, prosthetic and orthotic services, diagnosis and treatment for mental and emotional disorders, and transportation services. Section 103 mentions visual services and reading services for people who are blind and interpreter services for people who are deaf. In addition, Section 103 lists technical and consultation assistance for individuals seeking self-employment, establishing a small business, or needing job assistance. This act provides consultative and technical assistance to educational programs to help students with disabilities make the transition to post-school activities and employment (see Section 103 of the act for a full listing of the available services covered).

Work Incentives Improvement Act of 1999 (P.L. 106–170) and Ticket to Work (TWWIIA) and Self-Sufficiency Program

The Work Incentives Improvement Act of 1999 (P.L. 106–170) provides an opportunity for therapists to intervene with disabled persons to facilitate return to work. This act helps eliminate some *disincentives* to finding employment, such as losing the federal subsidized health insurance of Medicaid and Medicare, with the *incentive* of continual insurance coverage at work. It also provides exceptions for further review of disability (National Council on Disabilities 2004).

The Work Incentives Improvement Act includes a voluntary nationwide program (TTW and Self-Sufficiency Program) to "increase opportunities for SSA disability beneficiaries aged 18 to 65 to obtain employment, vocational rehabilitation, and support services, ultimately to replace their SSA benefits with benefits from work" (National Council on Disabilities 2004, p.86). With the Ticket to Work program "tickets are provided to entitled [Social Security] beneficiaries who may assign them to an Employment Network (EN) of their choice to obtain employment services, vocational rehabilitation services, or other support services necessary to achieve a vocational (work) goal" (SSA n.d.). Examples of services that people access through this law are therapy, job training and placement, counseling, and obtaining adaptive equipment (Brown 2008). The Ticket to Work program encourages "state and private parties to work together with Social Security Disability clients toward getting them into full- or part-time paying jobs" (Brown 2011).

The Future of Work-Related Public Policies

It is obvious that much progress has been made through public policies to meet the need for people with disabilities to work and be engaged in society. However, people with disabilities still remain behind the nondisabled population with employment and other areas such as medical insurance (National Council on Disabilities 2009). According to a report from the Bureau of Labor Statistics (2011) people with disabilities have lower employment rates than the nondisabled American population. (18.6 percent of people with disabilities are employed versus 63.5 percent of people without a disability).

Some suggestions by the National Council on Disabilities (2004) to encourage more people with disabilities to obtain employment are for increased usage of technology, improved employer awareness about disabilities, and hiring people with disabilities within governmental agencies. Other suggestions are for providing more funding and removing barriers to finding work, such as loss of health insurance.

The Americans with Disabilities Act (ADA)

The broadest reforming civil rights act, helping disabled people of all ages, is the Americans with Disabilities Act (ADA) (P.L. 101–336) of 1990. The ADA is a federal antidiscrimination law guaranteeing equal opportunity, and not just equal treatment, for those with disabilities (Wells 2000). Previous acts, such as the Civil Rights Act of 1964, the RA, and the EAHCA, established the climate for the development of the ADA (Bristo 1997; Wells 2000). The Civil Rights Act of 1964 was the first federal act to consider discrimination in public places and tie nondiscrimination to the receipt of federal funds (Wells 2000). The perspective of inclusion under the EAHCA helped influence public opinion about the ADA (Bristo 1997). The ADA expanded some of the premises of the RA, especially Section 504 (Rothstein 1992).

The Americans with Disabilities Act was revolutionary in many ways. One was its use of language. The act changed the verbiage of public policy from "handicapped" people to people "who have disabilities" (Rothstein 1992). To qualify as having a disability with the ADA, the person must "[have a] physical or mental impairment that substantially limits one or more major life activities, [have] a history or record of such an impairment, or is regarded as having such an impairment" (U.S. Equal Employment Opportunity Commission 2008). The ADA does not list specific disabilities (U.S. Department of Justice 2005).

The "people first" language of the ADA reflected a change in societal values toward empowerment and respect for people with disabilities. Another unique aspect was the focus on the abilities and aptitudes of people with disabilities, with an emphasis on societal inclusion (Bowman 1992). Thus, the ADA considered work, along with other related societal areas, as a way to keep people with disabilities working and included in the larger fabric of society. For example, the act dealt with the dilemma of people who might be able to work at a job but not successfully access the transportation system to get there or be able to get to the actual jobsite in a facility. The act made public areas accessible, even for disabled persons who were not working. Therefore, the inclusion of public transportation and architectural accessibility in the ADA reflects the law's broad perspective. As stated, a primary purpose of the ADA is to help people with disabilities be employed and have the same advantages as others who are not disabled (Goren 1999).

The ADA has four titles. Title I deals with employment and requires employers who have 15 or more employees to provide equal employment opportunities to qualified individuals with disabilities. This title mentions protection against discrimination in hiring, promotion, pay, and other rights of employment. It provides restrictions on questions about disabilities before the job is offered. In addition, Title I requires that employers make "**reasonable accommodations**" to allow the person to work, unless there is "undue hardship." *Reasonable accommodations* is defined as "any modification or adjustment to a job or work environment that permits a qualified applicant or employee with a disability to participate in the job application process, to perform the essential functions of a job, or to enjoy benefits and privileges of employment equal to those enjoyed by employees without disabilities" (U.S. Department of Justice 2012). Undue hardship is defined as "action requiring significant difficulty or expense." Factors include the nature and cost of the accommodation in relation to the size, resources, nature, and structure of the employer's operation (U.S. Equal Employment Opportunity Commission 2008).

Title II covers state and local governments. It requires that people with disabilities be provided with equal opportunity to benefit from services such as public education, employment, transportation, health care, social services, courts, voting, and town meetings. Title II requires that governments follow architectural standards in new construction and renovation of buildings. In addition, Title II requires reasonable modification of policies and procedures to avoid discrimination against those who have disabilities. Another part of Title II is the provision of coverage for public transportation so that there is no discrimination against people with disabilities in using services. Title III covers public accommodations in businesses such as retail stores, hotels, and restaurants. Public accommodations must comply with standards and requirements with architecture and access. Title IV covers telephone and television accessibility for people with hearing and speech disabilities. It requires telephone companies to enable people with hearing and speech disabilities to use special adaptive phones, such as telecommunications devices for the deaf (TDDs). Closed captions on television of federally subsidized public service announcements are required by this title (AOTA 1993; U.S. Department of Justice 2005).

Massive public policy like the ADA does not solve all of society's problems, but provides a framework for improvement. Still, in spite of improvement in many areas of life for people with disabilities, issues remain that are related to the ADA. Examples of workplace issues are the exclusion of people with disabilities from the social life on the job, the existence of interpersonal problems in the workplace, and stereotyping people with disabilities (Gupta 2006). People who have severe mental health conditions experience discrimination in the workplace because of having the two labels of a mental illness and a disability (Conyers and Ahrens 2003). However, people with disabilities who experience discrimination can voice their concerns through the Equal Employment Opportunity Commission (EEOC), which implements the employment descrimination parts of the ADA. (Gupta 2006; U.S. Equal Employment Opportunity Commission n.d.). In many communities, cost issues exist related to the adjustment of the physical environments for accessibility. Finding reliable, reasonable, and accessible transportation is still a problem in some communities (National Council on Disabilities 2004).

Therapy and the ADA

Therapists can help people qualified for the ADA with maximizing functioning in ADL and performance skills, assisting with activity demands and client factors, and a consideration of all aspects of a person's contextual environment (AOTA 2000). In different ways, the ADA impacts therapists and therapy practice (AOTA 2000). From a manager's perspective, the ADA influences hiring decisions. Direct questions concerning a disability cannot be asked during an interview. The manager should be interested in whether the qualified person can perform the "essential functions" of a job in the therapy department. As discussed, the ADA requires employers to make "reasonable accommodations" to allow the qualified person to work, as long as these accommodations do not entail "undue hardship." Therefore, managers of therapy departments may be involved in the process of implementing reasonable accommodations.

Consulting is a unique way for therapists to get involved with the ADA (Fontana 1999; Hanebrink and Brown-Parent 2000). Therapists have skills to be ADA consultants. However, it is important that therapists have a strong knowledge base about the law to implement it in practice. It is helpful to review the law, attend training seminars, network with ADA advocacy organizations, and read relevant newsletters (Fontana 1999). Hanebrink and Brown-Parent (2000) suggest that therapists increase their knowledge by participating on local private and government committees for people with disabilities and by attending continuing education courses. Simply networking with people involved in implementing the act is beneficial.

With a knowledge base about the ADA, therapists can consult about legislation and architectural codes, assist local government agencies, and provide suggestions for reasonable accommodations (AOTA 2000). Consulting with human resource departments may involve doing jobsite analysis and writing job descriptions (Wells 2000). Jobsite analyses and job descriptions describe the important job functions and help to identify reasonable accommodations (Gupta, Gelpi, and Sain 2005). Through performing work assessments, therapists address ergonomic adaptations (Stockdell and Crawford 1992) and adaptive equipment needs so that the person works in a safe environment (Gupta 2006; Schreuer, Myhill, Aratan-Bergman, Samant, and Blanck 2009). Providing expert-witness testimony involves consultation skills (Hanebrink and Brown-Parent 2000). With consultation, therapists may choose to conduct research for intervention strategies and programs that address the ADA objectives (Bowman 1992). Other avenues for consultation include government agencies, public transportation and communication bodies, businesses, and individuals who have disabilities (Hanebrink and Brown-Parent 2000). Therapists may consider working as a team with architects, engineers, and others to help meet the requirements of the ADA (Wells 2000). Another form of consultation is "mediating the interactive process between employer and employee" with workplace accommodations (Schreuer, Myhill, Aratan-Bergman, Samant, and Blanck 2009, p.149).

The ADA is so broad that it helps people of all ages and types of disabilities. Adaptations help older adults and children (Asher and Rosenthal-Pollak 2009) remain part of society. Especially as society ages, worksite adaptations may help older adults who choose to continue working (Bachelder and List-Hilton 1994). Adaptations can be made to help children and adolescents with disabilities stay in appropriate environments (Kalscheur 1992). Some suggested areas for interventions to meet ADA requirements with youth are play, sports, education, gathering places, and entertainment environments (Kalscheur 1992). Therapists can assist with emergency preparedness for children in school systems (Asher and Rosenthal-Pollak 2009). Therapists may also help qualified disabled students in higher education (Bowman and Marzouk 1992). Furthermore, occupational therapists with a background in mental health may become involved with making reasonable accommodations for those with mental health diagnoses. Mental health accommodations may focus on the psychosocial aspects of employment, such as communication skills, time management, multitasking, concentration, and self-efficacy (Crist and Stoffel 1992). Other areas for mental health accommodations include addressing memory, endurance, stress management, and managing medical needs (Winstead 2009).

The National Institute on Disability and Rehabilitation Research (NIDRR) established regional centers "to provide information, training, and technical assistance to employers, people with disabilities, and other entities with responsibilities under the ADA" (My Company 2007, p. 1). These centers offer resources that therapists can use to help their clients access employment, public services, public living situations, and communications (My Company 2007). The ADA was reauthorized in 2010 with changes to Title II. Some of these changes include standards for accessible design (NICHCY 2010), ticketing, service animals, and wheelchairs and other power-driven mobility devices (Department of Justice 2011).

Social Security Income Programs

Readers may be familiar with the traditional Social Security program. This program based on Social Security taxes paid by workers benefits "retirees, disabled persons, and families of retired, disabled, or deceased workers" (National Academy of Social Insurance, n.d.). The Social Security program offers two disability benefit packages: Social Security Disability

Income (SSDI) and Supplemental Security Income (SSI). Each of these programs provides important income protection and supplementation for persons with disabilities. These programs make available a benefit "floor" for the workforce to prevent a person with a disability from becoming financially destitute and are vitally important for persons experiencing severe and persistent disablement where work is not possible.

SSDI provides a monthly income for a person who is considered to be permanently disabled (i.e., "has a qualifying medical condition that is expected to last at least one year or to result in death or has lasted or is expected to last for a continuous period of not less than 12 months") (Social Security Administration 2011). The way monthly payments for SSDI are figured is based on average lifetime work earnings. In short, this amount of income is dependent upon the income received when one was working. In some cases, spouses and unmarried children are eligible for benefits. To qualify, a person has to meet a "recent-work test" and a "duration-of-work test." The recent-work test requires the person to have worked at least half of the time in the recent past (which varies by the person's age). The duration-of-work test requires a person to have worked a minimum number of years. If the person meets these tests, then medical information is ascertained and a state disability determination office decides whether or not the person qualifies for SSDI.

SSI provides income protection for persons who are elderly (age 65 or older), blind, disabled, and meet the income requirements (Social Security Administration 2011). Income limits vary from state to state and include all forms of income (e.g., Social Security payments, pensions, insurance benefits). Financial assets must be less than $2,000 ($3,000 for a married couple), excluding a house, car, burial account, and small life insurance policies. Persons who meet the criteria for SSI receive an additional monthly income and, in many states, may qualify for Medicaid (Social Security Administration 2011). To encourage people on SSI as well as SSDI to return to the workforce, the government instituted the Ticket to Work program (previously discussed in this chapter) that provides vouchers for persons on SSDI for vocational training and counseling.

Although the SSDI and SSI programs share a lot of similarities, such as the same definition of disability, there are differences. One major difference is that health insurance for the SSDI is covered by Medicare whereas health insurance for the SSI program is covered by Medicaid (Social Security Administration 2011). It is important to note that to qualify for Medicare a person must have received the SSDI benefit for a minimum of two years.

Active Learning Exercise

Changes in the Social Security disability programs encourage persons to return to work without having their important benefits revoked. Visit http://www.ssa.gov/pubs/10095.html and read about these initiatives. What are the incentives offered, and how do they reflect societal values?

Housing Programs for Persons with Disabilities

Therapists work in the community with people who have disabilities. Being an advocate may involve educating people with disabilities about public policies related to housing. A key law is the Federal Fair Housing Act of 1968 (FFHA) (P.L. 100–430), amended in 1988 to include discrimination in housing based on many factors, including disability. The FFHA covers public-assisted and some private housing. The act requires that property owners "make reasonable exceptions to accommodate people with disabilities" such as allowing a guide dog for a person who is blind living in a rented house in which the landlord has established a rule for no pets (Family Center on Technology and Disability n.d. p.3; U.S. Department of Justice 2005). The FFHA requires property owners to "make reasonable access-related modifications to the property if necessary" (Family Center on Technology and Disability n.d. p.3), such as widening doorways for wheelchairs (U.S. Department of Justice 2005). Along with this law, therapists should consider the ADA, as it too includes accessibility guidelines for buildings and other facilities.

Active Learning Exercise

Roger is a client you are following in home health care. Along with being post total hip fracture he has a history of diabetes. Because of the visual condition of diabetic retinopathy, Roger would like to obtain a guide dog. He inquires about finding appropriate housing in a public assisted facility to address his mobility needs and to support having a guide dog. Go to the U.S. Department of Housing and Urban Development website, http://www.hud.gov/groups/disabilities.cfm, and review the material on helping people like Roger with their housing needs.

Technology and Persons with Disabling Conditions

Therapists recognize the importance of technology to enhance client independence. They use a variety of low-tech devices, such as long-handled reachers, and high-tech devices, such as electric wheelchairs and computer technology, as part of practice. Society, too, recognized the need for promoting the usage of technology for people with disabilities to maximize their independence. This recognition came with the **Assistive Technology** Act of 1998, one of the most recent bills aimed at helping people with disabilities.

The Assistive Technology Act of 1998

The Assistive Technology Act (ATA) (P.L. 105–394) promotes an evaluative process along with the usage of technology to improve function, independence, and quality of life of persons with disabilities. The ATA reflects the rapidly changing and increasingly sophisticated development of technology for people with disabilities. Many of these changes came about after World War II, when advancing technology for health care became a societal value (Lenker 2000). As Bristo states, "for people with disabilities…technology changes the most ordinary of life activities from impossible to possible" (National Council on Disabilities 2000, p.1).

The intent of the original act was "systems change," to be initiated by state technology-assistance programs. The focus was on advocacy for and modeling of changes in systems, such as school systems, that increase access to and funding of assistive technology. Amendments in 1994 improved the focus on advocacy as a strategy for systems change. The 1998 act shifted the focus to systems-capacity building. This shift, while not removing the responsibility to conduct systems-change activities, appears to allow for activities that enhance or expand the delivery of assistive technology services (as well as the development of new assistive technology and alternative financing systems) (Schultz 2000).

The Assistive Technology Act includes three types of programs. The first is the creation of assistive technology centers (demonstration, informational, equipment loan, referral services). The second is protection and advocacy services. The third is federal/state loan and financing options for assisted technology (Family Center on Technology and Disability n.d.)

The Assistive Technology Act of 2004

The 2004 amendments made state programs more consistent, ensuring the likelihood that persons with disabilities make informed decisions about assistive technology through equipment demonstrations and loans. These amendments allow people with disabilities to acquire assistive technology through reutilization and alternative financing programs (Mark Schultz, personal communication, 2/5/2007). The ATA may soon be reauthorized (The Arc 2011).

Therapists and the ATA

The original purpose of the ATA was for education and awareness rather than for the provision and funding of technology. However, changes in the ATA allow for clients to access and acquire assistive technology. As defined by the 2004 act, assistive technology is "Any item, piece of equipment, or product system, whether acquired commercially, modified, or customized, that is used to increase, maintain, or improve functional capabilities of individuals with disabilities" (PL 108–364, Section 3). The utilization of resources provided by this act helps therapists understand current assistive technology, especially because technology is such a rapidly developing area. Therapists may refer their clients to state centers established by this law, to familiarize them with the most current technology available. People in state centers encourage client access to technology, provide technological assistance and education, and possibly provide loaner equipment programs (Brachtesende 2003). In addition, the act may help therapy clients through funded research for the development of new technology. At the state level, therapists may become involved with educational programs about assistive technology.

Yet, in spite of federal legislation, such as the ATA, access to assistive technology for therapy clients remains a challenge as few insurance companies in the traditional medical system cover many devices (Brachtesende 2003). For example, Medicare does not pay for bathroom adaptive equipment such as grab-bars, elevated toilet seats, and shower seats (Medx Publishing 2008). Therefore, therapists should examine all community options to obtain essential equipment. Suggested community options include state agencies for assistive technology; local drug stores; local community lending closets, often through churches; local health-related organizations, such as the Arthritis Foundation; local chapters for disability organizations, such as Easter Seals; and community-service organizations, such as Lions Clubs (Brachtesende 2003). Therapists interested in assistive technology should also become aware of and network with the Rehabilitation Engineering and Assistive Technology Society of America (RESNA). The purpose of this interdisciplinary organization is "to contribute to the public welfare through scientific, literary, professional, and educational activities by supporting the development, dissemination, and utilization of knowledge and practice of rehabilitation and assistive technology in order to achieve the highest quality of life for all citizens" (RESNA n.d.).

Active Learning Exercise

Find the assistive technology project for your state on the Internet.

a) Identify its location(s) and what services the project provides. Remember that there is some leeway on how services are provided from state to state.

b) Next, find an assistive technology site for another state website, and compare and contrast services offered by your state with those offered by the other state.

c) (For practicing therapists) Think about the clients from your current case load to determine whether any can be helped by the assistive technology project in your state.

d) (For students) You are following a 42-year-old man Thomas with the diagnosis of multiple sclerosis who is blind in his left eye due to glaucoma. Thomas ambulates with a walker and displays some difficulty with fine motor tasks. Thomas would like to work from home on his computer doing freelance accounting. Yet he finds that working on his computer is difficult due to problems with vision, coordination, and endurance. Research your State Assistive Technology Project and find out what supports Thomas can receive to help him do work and life tasks.

e) Tour an assistive technology project site and find out about technology options for clients.

Working with Policies Addressing Social Disablement

As care becomes more integrated across settings, it is beneficial to become aware of policies that address social disablement. Even if therapists do not receive direct reimbursement from some of the relevant acts, they can advise their patients by being familiar with various programs available in their communities.

Therapists can learn how to access and work with policies through networking and advocacy skills. An understanding of the legislative process is essential. Therapists must recognize that disability policies are laws that can be changed by legislative systems on both the federal and state level. As with any law, the revision of a policy involves the identification of the pertinent issues, the design of the policy, public support, and legislative decision making (McGregor 2001). Historically, disability policies have gone through many changes over time. Prior to each amendment, therapists should advocate for their concerns on the state and national level (see Chapter 5 for a discussion of advocacy and the legislative process).

Therapists should understand the philosophy and priorities of the state agencies that institute these policies. Each state program institutes policies a little differently. It takes networking to find out a given state's priorities regarding disability policies. Networking helps locate special-interest groups that influence these policies. State agencies often have grant funding for research, and therapists might choose to access that funding. Furthermore, therapists must understand that the federal laws are superseded by any state statutes that provide greater protection for people with disabilities (Wells 2000).

It is important to be aware that for any federal law with state mandates there is a constant tension between federal and state control, especially related to funding issues, as funding controversies are an economic certainty (Reed 1992). With programming on a state level, therapists should work closely with their state agencies.

Therapists must be aware of trends in public policy related to disability. For example, all these acts profess to hold the philosophy of inclusion or integration of a person with a disability into the "least restrictive environment" and to enhance function. This paradigm switch increases the quality of life and participation of people with disabilities in our society, which has been well illustrated with the exemplars of IDEA and ADA. Most of these laws have similar definitions of disability and specific requirements that a person must meet to qualify (Rothstein 1992). With amendments, some policies may adapt parts of other policies. For example, several policies have adapted protection and advocacy boards. Societal trends will change, and, as discussed at the beginning of the chapter, views about disability will change.

Finally, even though federal laws are available to help people with disabilities, there remain many barriers, controversies, and room for improvement. Several plausible explanations exist for problems with policies. First, the history of legislation for people with disabilities has not been a planned effort, but rather a piecemeal attempt to deal with concerns (Bowman 1992). Thus, many of the discussed policies overlap in some areas and became similar over the years. Also, services can be piecemeal. For example, someone with a developmental disability might benefit from services from the DDA, the IDEA, the ATA, Medicaid, and Medicare. Yet unfamiliarity with state resources may result in the individual missing beneficial services. Second, public policies may involve multiple levels of federal and state bureaucracies (McGregor 2001). Bureaucracies are "a body of nonelective government officials" (Merriam-Webster n.d.) working in state and federal agencies that make rules to implement the state and federal laws/acts. It is the bureaucrats who actually institute the policies, and interpretations can vary. As Bristo (1997, p.25) states, "The customer with disabilities seeking services faces a maze of programs, requirements, and bureaucratic obstacles." Furthermore, decisions regarding the provision of services continue to be made by bureaucrats rather than by people with disabilities, thus promoting dependence (Bristo 1997). Third, because public policies are federal laws, compromises are made during the debates in the House and Senate (Reed 1992). These compromises often deal with the funding aspects of the policies. As discussed, the IDEA has never been fully funded. Fourth, the written language and regulations of the acts may include limitations (Nosek 1992). For example, the terminology "essential functions of the job and reasonable accommodation" is not clearly defined in the ADA and can be interpreted in many ways (Gupta, Gelpi, and Sain 2005). Fifth, even though these policies are in effect, people in society may not understand the issues related to the provision of services for disabilities (Wells 2000). For example, people who are minorities and have a disability may encounter dual discrimination and have trouble obtaining services (Wells 2000). Even members of Congress may present a barrier because of a lack of understanding of, and a failure to support, disability policies (Bristo 1996). Last, the real power of all these laws depends on how they are actually implemented and not on how they are described on paper (Nosek 1992). For even with such policies, people with disabilities are older, more impoverished, and less employed and less educated than those without disabilities (American Psychological Association 2011; Bristo 1996). Thus, the end analysis of all these policies is how they really benefit the disabled members of our society.

Active Learning Exercise

Interview a contact person (either in person, on the phone, or through technology) from a state agency funded by public policy that helps people with disabilities. Determine how the selected agency can help clients. Prepare a minimum of two to three questions to ask. Examples of state agencies are vocational rehabilitation projects and assistive technology projects.

Sample Questions:

What types of clients does your organization work with?

What does your organization do?

What type of referrals to your organization would be appropriate from therapy?

Are there services that therapy can access to help clients?

Are there any educational opportunities offered by your organization that may help the clients I serve?

Conclusion

Numerous public policies enacted in the last 50 years address social disability by reducing social barriers and empowering persons with disabling conditions. We discussed the history, purpose, effectiveness, and relationship to therapy practice of many of these policies. Together, such policies create a more inclusive society. To provide comprehensive care, therapists need to consider these discussed policies to help the clients they serve.

Chapter Review Questions

1. Define "inclusion," "barriers," and "empowerment."
2. Review the purpose of the following disablement-related laws:
   a. Individuals with Disabilities Education Act
   b. Developmental Disabilities Act
   c. Older Americans Act
   d. Rehabilitation Act
   e. Workforce Investment Act
   f. Americans with Disabilities Act
   g. Social Security income programs
   h. Assistive Technology Act

Who is eligible for services? What types of services are provided? How are physical and occupational therapists involved in delivering services to eligible populations?

Chapter Discussion Questions

1. Reflect on the paradigm switch in the 20th century regarding views about disability. What were the different values influencing disability prior to the 1960s and after the 1960s? How do you feel that people with disabilities currently are viewed in today's society?

2. Briefly describe the focus of policies discussed in this chapter. What are some of the similarities and differences between the different disability policies?

3. Discuss why it is beneficial for therapists to know about policies (such as the DDA and the ATA), even though they do not provide direct services through these laws.

References

Administration on Aging (AOA). 2010. Older American's Act. Retrieved from http://www.aoa.gov/aoaroot/aoa_programs/oaa/index.aspx.

AFB. n.d. Summary of key sections of the Individuals with Disabilities Education Improvement Act (IDEA) of 2004, Public Law 108–446: 2005. Josephine L. Taylor Leadership Institute National Education Program. Retrieved from http://www.afb.org/Section.asp?SectionID=58&TopicID=264&DocumentID=2768.

AFL-CIO Working for America Institute. 2011. The Workforce Investment Act. Retrieved from http://www.workingforamerica.org/documents/workforce.htm.

American Occupational Therapy Association (AOTA). 1993. The role of occupational therapy in the independent living movement. *Am J Occup Ther* 47: 1079–80.

_____. 1995. Occupational therapy: A profession in support of full inclusion. *Am J Occup Ther* 50: 855.

_____. 2000. Occupational therapy and the Americans with Disabilities Act (ADA). *Am J Occup Ther* 54: 622–25.

_____. 2006a. Section-by-section analysis of IDEA 2004 Part B regulations. Retrieved from http://www.aota.org/Archive/Advocacy/FedReimbA/Issues/IDEA/Id04/Regs/36304.aspx.

_____. 2006b. The new IDEA: Summary of the Individuals with Disabilities Education Improvement Act of 2004 (P.L. 108–446). Retrieved from http://www.aota.org/nonmembers/area21/index.asp.

_____. 2009. Occupational therapy's commitment to nondiscrimination and inclusion. Retrieved from http://ajot.aotapress.net/content/63/6/819.full.pdf.

_____. 2010. AOTA principles for the reauthorization of Elementary and Secondary Education Act: Submitted to the Committee on Education and Labor. Retrieved from http://www.aota.org/Practitioners/Advocacy/Federal/Testimony/2010/ESEA.aspx?FT=.pdf.

_____. 2011. Occupational therapy's role in senior centers. Retrieved from http://www.aota.org/Consumers/Professionals/WhatIsOT/PA/Facts/39477.aspx?FT=.pdf.

_____. n.d.a. Occupational therapy: Response to intervention. Retrieved from http://www.aota.org/Practitioners-Section/Children-and-Youth/New/RtI-Brochure.aspx?FT=.pdf.

_____. n.d.b. The New IDEA 2004: Section-by-section analysis of Part B regulations as they relate to occupational therapy. Retrieved from http://www.aota.org/Archive/Advocacy/FedReimbA/Issues/IDEA/Id04/Regs/36304.aspx

American Office on Aging. 2006. Choices for independence: Modernizing the Older Americans Act. Retrieved from http://www.aoa.gov/AOARoot/AoA_Programs/OAA/Aging_Network/pi/docs/AoA-PI-06-01_Attachment_D.pdf.

American Office on Aging. n.d. Older American Act. Retrieved from http://www.aoa.gov/AoA_programs/OAA/.

American Physical Therapy Association (APTA). 2009. Americans with disabilities: role of the American Physical Therapy Association in advocacy, promotion, and accommodation: HOD P06-04-12-12. Retrieved from http://www.apta.org/uploadedFiles/APTAorg/About_Us/Policies/HOD/Health/AmericansDisabilities.pdf.

American Psychological Association. 2011. Disability & socioeconomic status. Retrieved from http://www.apa.org/pi/ses/resources/publications/factsheet-disability.aspx.

The Arc. 2011a. Developmental Disabilities Act Legislative Agenda for the 112th Congress (2011-2012). Retrieved from http://www.thearc.org/page.aspx?pid=2998.

_____. 2011b. Still in the shadows with their future uncertain: A Report on Family and Individual Needs for Disability Supports (FINDS). Retrieved from http://www.thearc.org/document.doc?id=3140.

_____. n.d. Medicaid block grant information. Retrieved from http://www.thearc.org/page.aspx?pid=3085.

Asher, A., and J. Rosenthal-Pollak. 2009. Planning emergency evacuations for students with unique needs: Role of occupational therapy. *OT Practice* 14(21): CE-1–CE-8.

Bachelder, J. M., and C. List-Hilton. 1994. Implications of the Americans with Disabilities Act of 1990 for elderly people. *Am J Occup Ther* 48: 73–81.

Baker, N.A., and K. Jacobs. 2003. The nature of working in the United States: An occupational therapy perspective. *Work* 20: 53–51.

Berland, B.J., and K.D. Seelman. 2000. "Introduction and background." In *Overview of NIDRR's long range plan*. Retrieved from http://web.archive.org/web/20000815200959/http//www.ncddr.org/rpp/lrp_ov.html.

Bowman, O.J. 1992. Americans have a shared vision: Occupational therapists can create the future reality. *Am J Occup Ther* 46(5): 391–96.

_____. and D.K. Marzouk. 1992a. Implementing the Americans with Disabilities Act of 1990 in higher education. *Am J Occup Ther* 46(6): 521–33.

_____ and _____. 1992b. Using the Americans with Disabilities Act of 1990 to empower university students with disabilities. *Am J Occup Ther* 46(5): 450–56.

Boyd, K., C. DeMarco, K. Figetakis, S. Robinson, S. Sullivan, J. Young, C. Custard, M. DiCarlo, M. Laners, K. Serfas, and K. Vigil. 1996. Developmental Disabilities Act. Unpublished ms., Creighton University, Omaha, Nebraska.

Brachtesende, A. 2003. Helping clients obtain funding for assistive technology. *OT Practice* 5(8): 18–21.

Bristo, M. 1996. *Achieving independence: The challenge for the 21st century.* Washington DC: National Council on Disabilities.

_____. 1997. *Equality of opportunity: The making of the Americans with Disabilities Act.* Washington DC: National Council on Disability.

_____. 1999. *lift every voice: modernizing disability policies and programs to serve a diverse nation.* Washington DC: National Council on Disabilities.

Brown, E.J. 2008. Will new changes save Ticket to Work? Retrieved from http://occupational-therapy.advanceweb .com/Article/Will-New-Changes-Save-Ticket-to-Work-2 .aspx.

_____. 2011. SSA wants you to get on the TTW express. Retrieved from http://occupational-therapy.advanceweb .com/Article/SSA-Wants-You-to-Get-on-the-TTW -Express-2.aspx.

Bureau of Labor Statistics. 2011. Labor force characteristics of persons with a disability in 2010. Retrieved from http://www.bls.gov/opub/ted/2011/ted_20110628.htm.

Clark, G.F. 2008. The infants and toddlers with disabilities program (Part C of IDEA). *OT Practice* 13(1): CE-1–CE-8.

Clark, G.F., A. Brouwer, C. Schmidt, and M. Alexander. 2008. Response to Intervention model: Using the print tool to develop a collaborative plan. *OT Practice* 13(14): 9–13.

Clark, G.F., and J.E. Polichino. 2008. FAQ on Response to Intervention. Retrieved from http://www.rsoi.org /Documents/9-TIES%202010%20KEYNOTE--AOTA%20 FAQ%20on%20Response%20to%20Intervention%20 Final%20Revise%2012-21-08.pdf.

_____. 2010. Response to intervention & early intervening services: Occupational therapy roles in general education. *OT Practice* 15(1): CE-1–CE8.

Conyers, L.M., and C. Ahrens. 2003. Using the Americans with Disabilities Act to the advantage of people with severe and persistent mental illness: What rehabilitation counselors need to know. *Work* 21: 57–68.

Cooper, R.E. 2011. Realizing the intent of the DD Act: How the DD network advances the independence, productivity, and integration of people with intellectual and developmental disabilities. Retrieved from http://www.acf.hhs.gov/sites /default/files/add/DDNetworkPaperFINAL.pdf.

Cornell University Law School: Legal Information Institute. n.d. Definitions. Retrieved from http://www.law.cornell.edu /uscode/text/20/1401.

Crist, P.A., and V.C. Stoffel. 1992. The Americans with Disabilities Act of 1990 and employees with mental impairments: Personal efficacy and the environment. *Am J Occup Ther* 46(5): 434–43.

DeJong, G., and B. O'Day. 2000. Contrast of paradigms: "Old" paradigms vs "new" paradigms. Retrieved from www.ncddr.org.

Department of Justice. 2011. Fact Sheet: Highlights of the final rule to amend the Department of Justice's regulation implementing Title II of the ADA. Retrieved from http:// www.ada.gov/regs2010/factsheets/title2_factsheet.html.

Diament, M. 2011. Lawmakers push for full funding of IDEA. Retrieved from http://www.disabilityscoop.com/2011/07/22 /lawmakers-full-funding-idea/13577/.

Dunn, D. 2000, November. Personal communication.

Elizabeth M. Boggs Center on Developmental Disabilities. 2011. Why does Medicaid matter to people with disabilities and their families? Retrieved from http://www.drnj.org/pdf /Medicaid%20fact%20sheet%20_3rd%20edition_.pdf.

Family Center on Technology and Disability. n.d. Retrieved from http://www.fctd.info/resources/ATlaws_print.pdf.

Fontana, P. 1999. Pushing the envelope: Entering the industrial arena. *OT Practice* 4(12): 20–22.

Gordon, M. 2000, November. Personal communication.

Goren, W.D. 1999. *Understanding the Americans with Disabilities Act: An overview for lawyers.* Chicago: ABA Publishing Co., General Practice, Solo, and Small Firm Section, American Bar Association.

Graney, P.J. 2000. RS20194: Developmental Disabilities Act: 106th Congress legislation. Washington DC: Domestic Policy Division. Congressional Research Service, Library of Congress.

Gupta, J. 2006. Workplace accommodations: Challenges and opportunities. *OT Practice* 11(11): 14.

_____, T. Gelpi, and S. Sain. 2005. Reasonable accommodations and essential job functions in academic and practice settings. *OT Practice* 10(15): CE-1–CE-8.

Hanebrink, S., and B. Brown-Parent. 2000. ADA consulting opportunities. *OT Practice* 5(17): 12–16.

Hansen, R.H., and J. Hinojosa. 2004. Nondiscrimination and inclusion position paper American Occupational Therapy Association, Inc.: Occupational Therapy's commitment to nondiscrimination and inclusion. Retrieved from http://ajot.aotapress.net/content/63/6/819.full.pdf.

Hightower-Vandamm, M.D. 1979. Nationally speaking: Developmental Disabilities Act: An historical perspective, Part 1. *Am J Occup Ther* 33(6): 355–59.

IDEA Partnership. 2012. Response to intervention: Fundamentals for educators. Retrieved from http:// ideapartnership.org/media/documents/RTI-Collection /rti-intermediate-ppt.pdf.

IFSPweb. n.d. Individuals with Disabilities Education Act. Retrieved from http://www.ifspweb.org/idea.html.

Individuals with Disabilities Education Improvement Act of 2004, Pub. L. No. 108-446. Retrieved from http://frwebgate .access.gpo.gov/cgi-bin/getdoc.cgi?dbname=108_cong_public _laws&docid=f:publ446.108.pdf (accessed May 25, 2008).

Jackson, L.L., and American Occupational Therapy Association. 2007. Occupational therapy services for children and youth under IDEA. Bethesda MD: American Occupational Therapy Association.

Jacobs, K. 1996. "Work assessments and programming." In H. L. Hopkins and H. D. Smith, eds., *Willard and Spackman's occupational therapy* (226–48), 8th ed. Philadelphia: J.B. Lippincott.

Kalscheur, J.A. 1992. Benefits of the Americans with Disabilities Act of 1990 for children and adolescents with disabilities. *Am J Occup Ther* 46(5): 419–27.

Kelley, M. 2000, November. Personal communication.

Lenker, J.A. 2000. Certification in assistive technology. *OT Practice* 5(16): 12–16.

McClain, J. 1996, January. Personal communication.

McGregor, D. 2001. "Health policy." In L. Shi and D.A. Singh, eds., *Delivering health care in America: A systems approach.* Gaithersburg MD: Aspen.

Medx Publishing. 2008. Medical equipment and supplies covered by Medicare. Retrieved from http://www.medicare.com /equipment-and-supplies/medical-equipment-and-supplies -covered-by-medicare.html.

Mellard, E. 2000. Impact of federal policy on services for children and families in early intervention programs and public schools. In W. Dunn, ed., *Best practice occupational therapy : In community service with children and families.* Thorofare NJ: Slack Inc.

Merriam-Webster. n.d. bureaucracy. Retrieved from http://www. merriam-webster.com/dictionary/bureaucracy.

My Company, Administrator. 2007, February 7. ADA & IT centers. Retrieved from http://www.otinfo.org/index .php?option=com_content&task=view&id=15&Itemid=1.

National Academy of Social Insurance. n.d. What is Social Security? Retrieved from http://www.nasi.org/learn /socialsecurity/overview.

National Association of Councils on Developmental Disabilities (NADDC). 2013. What are Councils on Developmental Disabilities? Retrieved from http:// www.nacdd.org/about-nacdd/councils-on -developmental-disabilities.aspx/.

National Council on Disability (U.S.). 2000. *Federal policy barriers to assistive technology.* Washington DC: National Council on Disability.

National Council on Disability. 2004. Livable communities for adults with disabilities. Retrieved from http://www .ncd.gov/NCD/publications/2004/12022004#a7fd685f _3ec8_4388_a86a_e4ccbcdeed77.

National Council on Disabilities. 2009. The current state of health care for people with disabilities. Retrieved from http://www.ncd.gov/publications/2009/Sept302009.

National Council on Disabilities. n.d. Rising expectations: The Developmental Disabilities Act revisited. Retrieved from http://www.ncd.gov/publications/2011/Feb142011.

National Skills Coalition. n.d. Workforce Investment Act. Retrieved from http://www.workforcealliance.org/ federal-policies/workforce-investment-act.

Nosek, M.A. 1992. The Americans with Disabilities Act of 1990: Will it work? *Am J Occup Ther* 46(5): 466–67.

Opp, A. 2007. Occupational therapy in early intervention: Helping children succeed. AOTA. Retrieved from http:// www.aota.org/Consumers/Professionals/WhatIsOT/CY /Articles/40021.aspx.

P.L. 108–364. Retrieved from http://www.gpo.gov/fdsys /pkg/STATUTE-118/pdf/STATUTE-118-Pg1707.pdf.

Reed, K.L. 1992. History of federal legislation for peoples with disabilities. *Am J Occup Ther* 46(5): 397–409.

———. 1993. "The beginnings of occupational therapy." In H.L. Hopkins and H.D. Smith, eds., *Willard and Spackman's occupational therapy*, 8th ed. (26–39). Philadelphia: J. B. Lippincott.

Rehabilitation Act Amendments (Section 508) (1998). Retrieved from http://www.access-board.gov/sec508/guide/act.htm.

RESNA. n.d. About RESNA. Retrieved from http://web.resna .org/aboutUs/aboutResna/index.dot.

Rothstein, L.F. 1992. *Disability and the law.* Colorado Springs, CO: McGraw-Hill.

Samuels, C.A. 2011. RTI: An instructional approach expands its reach. *Education Week* 30(22): 52–58.

Schreuer, N., W.N. Myhill, T. Aratan-Bergman, D. Samant, and P. Blanck. 2009. Workplace accommodations: Occupational therapists as mediators in the interactive process. *Work* 34(2): 149–160.

Schultz, M. 2007, December. Personal communication.

Social Security Administration (SSA). n.d. About Ticket to Work. Retrieved from http://ssa.gov/work/aboutticket.html.

Social Security Online. 2011. 2011 Redbook: Overview of our disability programs. Retrieved from http://www .socialsecurity.gov/redbook/eng/overview-disability.htm.

Special Education Advisor. 2010. FAPE vs. FAPE: IDEA and Section 504. Retrieved from https://www .specialeducationadvisor.com/fape-vs-fape-idea-section-504/.

Stockdell, M., and M.S. Crawford. An industrial model for assisting employers to comply with the Americans with Disabilities Act of 1990. *Am J Occup Ther* 46(5): 427–33.

Streeter, S. 2007. The Congressional appropriations process: An introduction. Retrieved from http://www.senate.gov /reference/resources/pdf/97-684.pdf**.**

Texas Department of Aging and Disability Services. 2012. Older Americans Act summary: Declaration of objectives for older Americans. Retrieved from http://www.dads.state .tx.us/rules/oaa_summary.html.

Tucker, B.P. 1994. *Federal disability law.* St. Paul MN: West Publishing Co.

U.S. Department of Education. Sec. 300.114 LRE requirements. Retrieved from http://idea.ed.gov/explore/view/p/,root,regs ,300,B,300%252E114.

United States Access Board. n.d. Questions & Answers about Section 508 of the Rehabilitation Act Amendments of 1998. Retrieved from http://www.access-board.gov/sec508/faq.htm.

U.S. Department of Education. 2004. Building the Legacy: IDEA 2004 Section 602 definitions. Retrieved from http://idea.ed.gov/explore/view/p/,root,statute,I,A,602.

U.S. Department of Education. 2007. Questions and answers on Response to Intervention (RtI) and Early Intervening

Services (EIS). Retrieved from http://idea.ed.gov/explore /view/p/,root,dynamic,QaCorner,8.

U.S. Department of Education, Office of Special Education and Rehabilitative Services. 2010. *Thirty-five years of progress in educating children with disabilities through IDEA.* Washington DC. http://www.acf.hhs.gov/programs/add /ddact/DDC.html.

U.S. Department of Justice. 2005. A guide to disability rights laws. Retrieved from http://www.ada.gov/cguide.htm.

_____. 2008. Americans with Disabilities Act: Questions and Answers. Retrieved from http://www.ada.gov/q&aeng02.htm.

_____. 2012. Questions and answers: The Americans with Disabilities Act and persons with HIV/AIDS. Retrieved from http://www.ada.gov/aids/ada_q&a_aids.htm.

U.S. Equal Employment Opportunity Commission. 2008. Americans with Disabilities Act: Questions and answers. Retrieved from http://www.ada.gov/q%26aeng02.htm.

U.S. Equal Employment Opportunity Commission. n.d. Overview. Retrieved from http://www.eeoc.gov/eeoc/.

Wells, S.A. 2000. The Americans with Disabilities Act of 1990: Equalizing opportunities. *OT Practice* 5(6): CE-1–CE-8.

Winstead, S. 2009. Workplace accommodations for people with mental illness. *OT Practice* 13(4): 15–17.

Williamson, J. 2009. The Workforce Investment Act: What's covered, and how can it help you? Retrieved from http:// www.distance-education.org/Articles/The-Workforce -Investment-Act--What-s-Covered--and-How-Can-it-Help -You--176.html.

Workforce Investment Act of 1998, P.L. 105–220, § 404, 112 Stat. 936, 1148–49 (codified as amended at 29 U.S.C. § 723 Supp. IV 1998).

Workforce Investment Act of 1998: P.L. 105–222 (1998). Retrieved from http://www.doleta.gov/usworkforce/wia /wialaw.pdf.

5

Effecting Policy Change: Therapist as Advocate

CHAPTER OBJECTIVES

At the conclusion of this chapter, the reader will be able to:

1. Recognize the role of the physical therapist and occupational therapist as an advocate.

2. Discuss the ethical responsibilities of the therapist as a patient/client advocate.

3. Relate the basic skills of effective advocacy.
   a. Self-reflection/attitude
   b. Knowledge
   c. Assertive communication

4. State the responsibilities of the therapist in patient/client advocacy.

5. State the responsibilities of the therapist in advocating in professional organizations.

6. Discuss methods of effective advocacy in the health care environment.
   a. Policy analysis
   b. Lobbying
   c. Legislative process
   d. Use of evidence
   e. Use of social media

KEY WORDS

Advocacy
Coalitions
Empowerment
Lobbying
Reflection
Social Media
Testimony

CASE EXAMPLE ···

Marc is a physical therapist who works full time in a skilled nursing facility. Mary is an occupational therapist who recently obtained employment working part time in a home health agency and part time in the same skilled nursing facility. The following scenario illustrates how passion about policy issues motivated and benefited both of them to work together.

Mary became aware of some of the issues related to public policy and advocacy from practice experience and after attending the American Occupational Therapy Association (AOTA) annual conference. In her home health practice there was a patient Sally, a 78-year-old female who required solely occupational therapy services. Yet it was frustrating for Mary to find out that occupational therapy could not initially qualify Sally for therapy because by Medicare regulations the case needed to be opened by another health care professional. Mary also learned that she could not complete the initial comprehensive rehabilitation assessment on Sally. At conference, Mary learned more about the specific regulations related to occupational therapy practice in home health and about the current advocacy efforts by AOTA in home health and other areas. Mary learned that AOTA had been working for over 30 years to get occupational therapy to be a qualifying service for Medicare eligibility with home health care and about a change in strategy to advocate for occupational therapists to be allowed to "conduct the initial assessment visit and comprehensive assessment for Medicare [rehabilitation] patients" (Vance, Zahoransky, and Kohl 2011). Mary learned about advocacy efforts related to the therapy cap, an arbitrary amount established by the Centers for Medicare & Medicaid Services (CMS), for outpatient therapy services under Medicare Part B. Mary was impressed by the advocacy efforts put forward by the AOTA to lobby for a better solution to the limited amount of money allocated for therapy. She learned about conditions for allowing therapy extension and other suggestions to fix the therapy cap.

Mary came back from the conference energized and ready to advocate for occupational therapy services. She learned that occupational therapy was not alone with advocacy efforts about the therapy cap, so she partnered with Marc, a physical therapist, working at the same skilled nursing facility. From Marc she learned that the therapy cap is a matter of great concern for physical therapists due to the fact that the law requires physical therapists and speech therapists to share the same pool of money, whereas occupational therapy receives the full cap amount. Thus patients/clients are not getting the complete benefit of physical therapy or speech therapy services. Additionally, Marc explained that much of PT practice is with outpatient Medicare Part B, so the limited therapy cap amount hugely influences practice. Further discussion was about a history of proposed cuts with the fee schedule for outpatient therapy. Mary and Marc decided to partner together to advocate for therapy benefits with Medicare, for after all, they remarked, "We are in this together." They networked with their state associations and organized legislative visits with their senator or congressional representatives when they were in town. Along with representatives from their state organizations, Mary and Marc presented at an AARP meeting about

Medicare issues; organized a letter/e-mailwriting campaign; and developed a statewide Facebook page, which had a very positive response. Additionally, Mary worked with other occupational therapists in her state association to advocate for therapy in home health. She educated peers that were practicing in other areas about the advocacy issues in home health, and many agreed to help in a letter-writing campaign. Mary even inspired some of her patients/clients to write letters. Mary and Marc reflected that these efforts between the two state associations strengthened their professional relationship and ultimately helped their advocacy efforts. Mary was pleased that members of the state physical therapy association were willing to write letters of support for the home health issue.

Case Example Questions

1. What motivated Mary and Marc to get involved in advocating for policy change?

2. What methods did they utilize to advocate for policy change?

3. What are the benefits of the state physical therapy and occupational therapy associations working together on advocacy issues?

Introduction

Thus far, the material in this book focused on policy and systems. This chapter takes these discussions one step further by emphasizing **advocacy** skills. Therapy practitioners often encounter situations in which they can make a difference through advocacy skills. To be effective in today's health care system, therapists must develop and use advocacy skills. The importance of having advocacy skills is emphasized by several significant documents from the American Physical Therapy Association (APTA) and the American Occupational Therapy Association (AOTA). For example, advocacy is mentioned in the APTA's *Guide to Physical Therapy Practice* (2003) and the *Physical Therapy Code of Ethics* (APTA 2010). Advocacy is mentioned in the *Occupational Therapy Practice Framework II* (AOTA 2008a) and the *Occupational Therapy Code of Ethics* (AOTA 2010a). Advocacy is part of the educational standards for both professions (AOTA 2012; APTA 2011).

This chapter is divided into several sections. The first part looks at research/literature related to advocacy and the integration between advocacy and the professional codes of ethics in physical and occupational therapy. The ethical discussion grounds the reader in how fundamental advocacy is to our professional values. The next sections provide therapists with pragmatic skills for advocacy. A key consideration throughout is how advocacy can take place on many levels including at a patient/client level, at a professional level, and in the health care environment. Specific skills and knowledge are required for these levels. Assertiveness, self-awareness, and critical thinking are helpful, along with application of evidence. Essential to advocacy on a professional level or in the health care environment is understanding the political process. Throughout this chapter, the terminology "patient/client" is used as both terms are applied in practice. As you read this chapter, consider how you can become an advocate for your patients/clients and profession.

Research and Literature Related to Advocacy

Little research has been completed on the impact of client advocacy in the rehabilitation fields. Sachs and Linn (1997) studied client advocacy to determine when occupational therapists advocated and what affected their advocacy behavior. From their qualitative research, they identified three advocacy themes. The first advocacy theme was that therapists viewed themselves as "guardians of morals" for individual, professional, and social misbehavior aimed at their clients. The second advocacy theme involved representing the client's functional abilities to health and community agencies. This kind of representation allowed the therapists to increase public awareness about helping people with disabilities. The third theme was working with the interdisciplinary team, which resulted in either support or restriction of advocacy efforts. Thus, as this research study illustrates, advocacy is multileveled.

A more recent qualitative research study (Dhillon, Wilkins, Law, Stewart, and Tremblay 2010) considers the meaning of advocacy for occupational therapists. This study, completed in Canada, recognized the influence that therapists have on clients with advocacy. Several themes were identified as to why therapists advocate, including "personal fulfillment, having the power and influence to help people with disabilities, and advocating to engage clients in occupation." Additional themes were "advocacy and client-centered practice, advocacy for client rights and needs, and advocating to help clients with quality of life" (Dhillon, Wilkins, Law, Stewart, and Tremblay 2010). The therapist subjects felt that they learned advocacy skills on the job, and although many encountered challenges, they valued advocacy enough to be willing to deal with related adversity. Finally, based on the results of the study, the authors defined advocacy as "a client-centered strategy involving a variety of actions taken by the client and therapists, directed to the client's environment to enact change for the client such that engagement in occupation is enhanced through meeting basic human rights or improving quality of life" (p. 246).

Pollard, Kronenberg, and Sakellariou (2009) coined the term "padl" an acronym for "political activities of daily living" (p. 3). The concept of "padl" involves the "development and integration of political literacy and political engagement" (p. 3) within all areas of practice, including research and education. The interpretation of "padl" is different from considering advocacy with legislators as it involves citizenship to help the clients' that therapists serve and considers the complexity of political engagement with others. Thus, critical reasoning and reflection are essential skills to utilize with "padl."

Advocacy and Ethics

The advocacy process is closely tied to professional ethics. Therefore, it is important to understand ethical principles and ethical reasoning and their application to public policy (Lohman, Gabriel, and Furlong 2004). Both the Physical Therapy Code of Ethics (APTA 2010) and the Occupational Therapy Code of Ethics (AOTA 2010a) address advocacy. The Physical Therapy Code of Ethics (APTA 2010) highlights advocacy in several principles. Refer to Table 5-1 to review the ethical principles of the Physical Therapy Code of Ethics and its relationship to policy and practice.

The Occupational Therapy Code of Ethics (AOTA 2010a) addresses advocacy. Refer to Table 5-2 to review the ethical principles of the Occupational Therapy Code of Ethics and its relationship to policy and practice.

Therapist Skills for Advocacy

To advocate successfully, therapists need to have a correct attitude and self-understanding. A proper attitude involves embracing the idea of being capable of making changes and being proactive. Proactivity, rather than reactivity, is an important skill in today's ever-changing health care environment. In addition, therapists need to understand their personal perspectives and motivations for approaching client advocacy. Are they concerned about the client's well-being? Are they concerned about quality of care? Are they advocating because of concerns for the profession? Understanding one's self-motivation requires **reflection**. Perhaps, from self-reflection, the therapist discovers that the motivation for advocacy comes from a personal reason, such as meeting an unfulfilled need, rather than from a client-centered or professional reason. In that case, the therapist needs to further reflect about one's motivation for advocacy. Consider the questions in Table 5-3 to better understand personal motivation and advocacy.

In addition to possessing self-understanding, therapists need to be knowledgeable about different systems and processes. For example, to advocate successfully with the legislature, therapists should understand the legislative process. (Advocacy with the legislature will be discussed later in the chapter.) Furthermore, assertive communication skills are imperative for successful advocacy with all levels of advocacy. Therefore, it is beneficial to review these skills.

Table 5-1 The Relationship of the Physical Therapy Code of Ethics to Policy and Practice

Principle	Examples of Relationship to Policy and Practice
Principle 1: Physical therapists "shall respect the inherent dignity and rights of individuals (core values: compassion, integrity)" (APTA 2010, p. 1).	Respect personal differences when approaching advocacy in practice. Recognize own biases when approaching advocacy.
Principle 2: "Physical therapists shall be trustworthy and compassionate in addressing the rights and needs of patients/clients (core values: altruism, compassion, professional duty)" (APTA 2010, p. 1).	Advocate for clients in ways that benefit clients by acting in their "best interests." Providing "information necessary to allow (clients) to make informed decisions about physical therapy" (APTA 2010, p. 1). "Collaborating with clients to empower them in decisions about health care" (APTA 2010, p. 1). "Protection of confidential patient information" (APTA 2010, p. 1)
Principle 3: "Physical therapists shall be accountable for making sound professional judgments (core values: excellence, integrity)" (APTA 2010, p. 1).	Applying "professional judgment in the patient/client's best interest" (APTA 2010, p. 1) with advocacy efforts. "Communicating with, collaborating with, or referring to peers or other health professionals when necessary" (APTA 2010, p. 1).
Principle 4: "Physical therapists shall demonstrate integrity in their relationships with patients/clients, families, colleagues, students, research participants, other health providers, employers, payers, and the public (core value: integrity)" (APTA 2010, p. 2).	"Providing truthful, accurate, and relevant information" (APTA 2010, p. 2) with advocacy efforts. Reporting "misconduct" or "illegal and unethical acts" (APTA 2010, p. 2) of peers or suspected abuse involving children or vulnerable adults.
Principle 5: "Physical therapists shall fulfill their legal and professional obligations (core values: professional duty, accountability)" (APTA 2010, p. 2).	Reporting peer professionals who are not skilled or who are unsafe. Encouraging colleagues to seek counseling when helpful. Providing alternatives for care when a person is discharged.
Principle 6: "Physical therapists shall participate in efforts to meet the health needs of people, locally, nationally, or globally (core value: social responsibility)" (APTA 2010, p. 2).	Providing pro bono services. Advocating "to reduce health disparities and health care inequities, improve access to health care services, and address the health, wellness, and preventive health care needs of people" (APTA 2010, p. 2).

Table 5-2 The Relationship of the Occupational Therapy Code of Ethics to Policy and Practice

Principle	Examples of Relationship to Policy and Practice
Principle 1: "Occupational therapy personnel shall demonstrate a concern for the well-being and safety of the recipients of their services (beneficence)" (AOTA 2010a, p. 3).	Referring clients to other health care practitioners. Reporting unethical or illegal acts.
Principle 2: "Occupational therapy personnel shall intentionally refrain from actions that cause harm (nonmaleficence)" (AOTA 2010a, p. 4).	Applying professional judgment with all advocacy efforts. Applying the Code of Ethics in volunteer roles, such as with advocacy efforts.
Principle 3: "Occupational therapy personnel shall respect the right of the individual to self-determination (autonomy and confidentiality)" (AOTA 2010a, p. 5).	Working collaboratively with the client and others with advocacy efforts.

(continued)

Table 5-2 *continued*

Principle	Examples of Relationship to Policy and Practice
Principle 4: "Occupational therapy personnel shall provide services in a fair and equitable manner (social justice)" (AOTA 2010a, p. 6).	Education of the public about occupational therapy services. "Providing activities that benefit the health status of the community" (AOTA 2010a, p. 6). Providing pro bono or reduced-cost interventions. Advocating for "just and fair treatment" (AOTA 2010a, p. 6). Providing therapy services when necessary.
Principle 5: "Occupational therapy personnel shall comply with institutional rules, local, state, federal, and internal laws and AOTA documents applicable to the profession of occupational therapy (procedural justice)" (AOTA 2010a, p. 7).	Familiarity and application of the Code of Ethics by self and others. Familiarity of laws and policies from AOTA. Familiarity and adherence to policies and procedures for handling ethical complaints. Participating in policy and procedural formation with employers "to ensure legal, regulatory, and ethical compliance" (AOTA 2010a, p. 8).
Principle 6: "Occupational therapy personnel shall provide comprehensive, accurate, and objective information when representing the profession (veracity)" (AOTA 2010a, p. 8).	Being truthful with advocacy efforts is essential to oneself and to the profession. "Refraining from using or participating in the use of any form of communication that contains false, fraudulism [*sic*], deceptive, misleading, or unfair statements or claims" (AOTA 2010a, p. 8).
Principle 7: "Occupational therapy personnel shall treat colleagues and other professionals with fairness, discretion, and integrity (fidelity)" (AOTA 2010a, p. 9).	Respecting own and other professionals. Exposing any nonadherence of the Code of Ethics to the proper boards. Applying "conflict resolution and/or alternative dissolute resolution resources" (AOTA 2010a, p. 10).

Assertive Communication

Assertive communication is empowering. It allows people to speak up for their rights without stepping on others. To understand what assertive communication is, one must understand what it is not. Assertive communication is not aggressive communication. Aggressive communication is acting out or being angry to get one's way. Aggressive communication does not respect the rights of others. Assertive communication is not being

Table 5-3 Critical Reflective Questions for Advocacy

I advocate because of
Concern for client's well-being
Concern for quality of care
Concern for the profession
Concern for the health care environment
Personal reasons
Other reasons (please list)

quiet or passive. Being quiet about issues of importance allows others to achieve what they want to achieve at the expense of one's position. Assertive communication is not passive-aggressive communication or undermining others, such as talking about a person without the person being present.

Assertive communication involves clearly expressing feelings, beliefs, and attitudes. Different methods for assertive communication are presented in the literature (Alberti and Emmons 1978). Davis (1998) provides one option: the DESC communication model. DESC is an acronym for *describing* the circumstance, *expressing* feelings, *specifying* the change, and identifying the *consequences*. The example of communication between a therapist and a physician in the accompanying box illustrates how a therapist uses the DESC method to advocate for a client who is an aspiration risk (inhalation of a foreign substance into the respiratory tract placing the person at risk for choking [Farlex 2013]).

DESC Methodology with Professional-Level Advocacy

Description: I observed Mr. C. in room 210 eat lunch. He was noted to pocket food in his right cheek and not fully chew his food. In addition, I noted that he coughed with each bite.

Expression: I feel that Mr. C. might have an aspiration risk.

Specification of change: Mr. C. would benefit from a swallowing study.

Consequences: Such a study may provide the necessary information to help prevent him from being an aspiration risk.

Assertive communication skills accompany advocacy skills and can be used with various levels of advocacy for clients. Clients in the medical system are often in dependent and vulnerable roles, having minimal control over their situation. Therapists can advocate, using assertive communication skills, for them. Therapists can encourage family members and caregivers to advocate assertively for the client. In addition, assertive skills can be used on the professional level. Therapists can advocate for appropriate referrals to help patients/clients when therapy is not being utilized. Assertive communication skills are used with the legislature to articulate professional concerns. Let us now examine advocacy skills on these different levels.

Patient/Client Advocacy Skills

A traditional view of advocacy with patients/clients involves helping vulnerable people who cannot effectively help themselves (Carpenter 1992; Namerow 1982). Advocacy in this sense helps people who lack the ability to self-advocate, such as children, people with disabilities, the sick, or people who are unaware of available resources (Carpenter 1992; DiGiacomo 2006). Sometimes, for a person who is sick and vulnerable in the hospital or in some other institution, it is beneficial to suggest having a caregiver present to advocate for that person's needs. Through developing a rapport with clients, therapists learn about situations that may require advocacy. Reporting someone for elder abuse is an example of advocating for a vulnerable client (Foose 1999).

As discussed, advocacy should be a reflective process. Reflection involves in-depth problem-solving or clinical-reasoning. Therapists may ask themselves the following questions:

- Is it necessary that I intervene?
- Does the client want me to intervene?
- Can the client self-advocate without my help?
  - What would empower the client to self-advocate?
  - What resources are available to help the client?
- Can the client's caregiver advocate for the client?

These reflective questions bring up an important topic: When should a therapist intervene, and how can therapists empower clients to be their own self-advocates? A theme from the Dhillon, Wilkens, Law, Stewart, and Tremblay (2010) study was partnering with clients for advocacy efforts. Going one step further allowing clients to self-advocate is empowering, and providing resource information may be all that the therapist will have to do. For example, one pediatric therapist recalls a situation when an adolescent 12-year-old boy with cerebral palsy wanted to participate in the regular gym class rather than with his special education classmates. He consulted his therapist who gave him suggestions for how to advocate within the system. Ultimately his efforts helped other students be mainstreamed into the regular gym class and helped make therapy more visible.

Another basic form of advocacy is knowledge about what gets reimbursed, and how therapy gets reimbursed, so that clients do not end up with unnecessary out-of-pocket expenses. Simply documenting clients' visits according to insurance standards often enables appropriate reimbursement. Advocacy with payers may include appealing a denial of therapy coverage, which involves understanding an insurance company's appeal policies. Providing excellent intervention so that clients choose to pay for therapy out of pocket or pay from the deductible of a consumer-based health care plan is a form of advocating for the profession. Table 5-4 addresses some areas in which therapists help with client advocacy. The list is not all-inclusive, and the reader may identify other areas.

The American Physical Therapy Association (APTA) and the American Occupational Therapy Association (AOTA) have government affairs departments that assist practitioners with client advocacy. Through the Trialliance of Health Rehabilitation Professions, consisting of the presidents of AOTA, APTA, and the American Speech-Language-Hearing Association (ASHA), advocacy efforts influence health care policy. Ultimately, these health policies benefit client care. In addition, both associations pledged their support for outcome or efficacy studies that improve client care. Informal collaboration between these associations is often done at the staff level.

Professional Level of Advocacy

On the professional level, therapists advocate with peer professionals and others. An example of professional-level advocacy is with employers to improve therapy benefits. In employment settings, therapists identify concerns about peer professionals that could involve advocacy. Sometimes, a therapist identifies unethical conduct in a peer professional's interaction with clients. Perhaps a peer professional acted rudely toward a client or made the wrong intervention decision. Working in an environment that allows open communication and the disclosure of issues encourages a reduction in errors, better client care (Joint Commission on Accreditation of Healthcare Organizations 2007), and better advocacy on behalf of clients. When appropriate, unethical conduct is reported internally

Table 5-4 Ways Therapists Help Clients through Advocacy

1. Suggesting legal advice and where to get it.
2. Providing an explanation of insurance plans.
3. Suggesting counseling and where to get it.
4. Providing information to help make an informed decision (Sachs and Linn 1997).
5. Providing helpful information about services offered from public policies.
6. Suggesting referrals to specialists for better medical care.
7. Referring to social services for assistance (e.g., with housing).
8. Suggesting resources that enable the ability to remain at home.
9. Educating how to write Congress about key issues.
10. Educating about how to appeal a denial of coverage.
11. Educating and communicating with managed care organizations (MCOs) or other payers on behalf of clients.
12. Educating a potential client about the value of paying for and receiving therapy.
13. Acting as an expert witness in court.

or to an outside agency (e.g., the state licensure board) for review. In some cases, states require reporting of harmful behaviors through "mandatory reporting" laws. In other cases, a therapist may learn that therapy is not provided to a client who could benefit from services. In that scenario, the therapist advocates for a referral with the client's physician. Handling situations with peer professionals involves diplomacy and assertive communication skills. Complete Exercise 5-1 to reflect about how you would handle advocacy situations involving peer professionals.

Active Learning Exercise 5-1

Answer the following questions as a self-reflecting individual or in a group:

1. Describe how you would handle a situation in which a physician ordered an intervention that is contraindicated. You are aware that this physician does not like to ever be seen as wrong.

2. Describe how you would handle a situation in which you feel that a patient/client being reviewed on a treatment team would benefit from therapy services.

3. Describe how you would handle a situation in which you observe a peer therapist not providing the best intervention or providing an inappropriate intervention.

4. Describe how you would demonstrate patient/client advocacy after making a practice error.

5. Describe how you would handle a situation in which you observe a peer engaging in unethical behavior.

In employment settings, sometimes employers who self-insure do not understand the benefits and cost savings of therapy and may decide not to include therapy in their employee insurance plan. In such cases, meeting with appropriate personnel can make a difference for insurance coverage. In addition, professional advocacy may involve educating other professionals, such as the staff of an MCO, about the benefits of therapy services. Communication and education can make a difference with case managers, or other insurance representatives.

Advocacy with Professional Organizations

The following discussion illustrates several reasons why therapists need to be members of their professional organizations. Therapists' membership fees support lobbyists and advocacy efforts by the associations. Membership fees also support staff that assist with consultation and resources. Without professional membership, these vital supports would not be possible.

Both the APTA and AOTA have legislative bodies that allow professional members to voice their opinions and influence the position of the organization. The APTA House of Delegates is the organization's deliberative policy-making body. It meets annually to discuss and debate professional issues and to communicate policy positions of physical therapists to the outside community (APTA 2013). AOTA has a legislative body called the Representative Assembly (RA). It is the governing and policy-making part of the association. Just as in Congress, state representatives debate and vote on important issues. It is important for therapists to communicate their stance on resolutions that are up for discussion to their state representatives.

Both the APTA and the AOTA have government affairs departments to help lobby for issues. The APTA Department of Government Affairs maintains web-based legislative action centers for both federal and state legislative affairs (APTA, n.d.). At the federal level, the APTA maintains a Federal Government Affairs and Payment Policy & Advocacy division that advocates for the profession in the Congress and in the Executive Branch of the federal government. The Payment Policy & Advocacy division of the APTA's Department of Government Affairs "is responsible for Medicare policy and advocacy issues affecting physical therapists" (APTA n.d.). At the state level, the State Government Affairs division monitors and advocates for issues affecting physical therapists (e.g., legislation, licensure, scope of practice). The Government & Payment Advocacy Department sponsors an annual State Government Affairs Forum, and an Advocacy Forum to allow members to meet, discuss, and mobilize for legislative action. A federal government affairs committee advises the department on critical legislative and regulatory issues facing the profession. The Physical Therapy Political Action Committee (PT-PAC) is the political fundraising arm of the profession and makes contributions to the political campaigns of candidates running for public office. Finally, the APTA supports a strong grassroots advocacy network. The PTeam is a program that develops and implements local advocacy efforts at state and federal levels. At the head of the grassroots network, the Federal Affairs Liaisons (FAL) includes representatives from each state chapter who serve as liaisons between the APTA and the state chapter regarding federal issues. The Key Contact grassroots effort involves physical therapy practitioners who are the primary contact about physical therapy issues with legislators (APTA 2011b).

AOTA has a Public Affairs Division that includes a State Affairs Group, a Federal Affairs Group, and a Reimbursement and Regulatory Affairs Group. Overall, the Public Affairs Division "supplies research, policy analysis, and supports state affiliates and individual members on public policy issues" (AOTA n.d., p. 1). Staff members from the State Affairs Group provide "research, technical assistance, and consultation on a wide range of state legislative and regulatory issues and function as a clearinghouse for information useful to state regulatory boards" (AOTA 2010b). Staff members from the Federal Affairs Department "monitor and lobby the U.S. Congress and selected federal agencies" (AOTA 2010c). The staff members from the Reimbursement and Regulatory Policy Group analyze federal regulations and policies affecting occupational therapy practice, such as Medicare. They act as advocates with federal agencies, payers, and external organizations, and they educate AOTA members about reimbursement and regulatory issues (AOTA n.d.).

AOTA sponsors an annual Capitol Hill Day, which involves occupational therapy practitioners going to the AOTA headquarters for a legislative briefing and meetings with members of Congress and/or staff. Therapists learn the logistics of how to meet with members of Congress and/or staff about issues relevant to occupational therapy. AOTA also serves as a year-round resource for occupational therapy practitioners interested in going to Washington, DC, to meet with their congressional representatives and senators. AOTA offers educational activities on issues when needed.

AOTA has a political action committee, called AOTPAC, or the American Occupational Therapy Political Action Committee. This legally sanctioned "voluntary, nonprofit unincorporated committee" (AOTA 2008b, p. 1) has the "purpose of furthering the legislative aims of the [AOTA] by influencing or attempting to influence the selection, nomination, election, or appointment of any individual to Federal public office, and of any occupational therapist, occupational therapy assistant, or occupational therapy student member of AOTA seeking election to public office at any level" (AOTA 2008b, p. 1). The AOTPAC is the only PAC representing the interests of occupational therapists (AOTA 2009) and is primarily financed by volunteer contributions from AOTA members (AOTA 2008b). Overall, AOTPAC helps ensure the visibility of occupational therapy in Washington, DC, and in politics generally.

Finally, all the major rehabilitation associations in the Trialliance (APTA, AOTA, and ASHA) maintain websites with up-to-date information about legislative and advocacy issues relevant to their members. These websites are great resources for updates and calls for action about important political issues. APTA, for example, has a Legislative Action Center. It includes information on federal and state advocacy as well as a "take action" link and information about the PT-PAC. AOTA also has a Legislative Action Center. This action center provides legislative contacts, information about federal issues, advocacy resources, and a media center to spur political action. Both APTA and AOTA's websites contain information about how to network with members of Congress by e-mailing or writing them about important issues or simply by identifying whether a member of Congress supports a legislative issue. In the associations' professional magazines (e.g., *PT Magazine*,

OT Practice) one can find articles about legislative issues. At professional conferences, the associations provide workshops related to legislative and reimbursement issues.

Beyond working with or utilizing advocacy resources from national professional associations, therapists should consider involvement with their state therapy associations and with other health care or disability state organizations. Many state therapy associations include a legislative committee that works on state and national issues. Therapists benefit by becoming involved in the advocacy efforts of related state organizations, as it expands therapy influence and provides another perspective. Therapists should consider their area of work and passion to find the appropriate state organizations. For example, therapists working with an older adult clientele might consider involvement in their state AARP organization or in the state chapter of an organization for a specific condition, such as the American Stroke Association or the Alzheimer's Association. Therapists working with pediatric populations might become involved with advocacy efforts of their state chapter of the Autism Society. In these organizations, therapists can advocate for the role of therapy and show how they can help the clients that the organization serves.

Advocacy with the Health Care Environment

In the United States, the state and federal legislatures allow citizens to advocate for their concerns. As Scott-Lee (1999, p. 5) states, "The framers of the Constitution believed so strongly in the people's right to participate in government, that they preserved that right, among others, for themselves, their fellow colonials, and the future generations of Americans." Today, therapists advocate by **lobbying** for concerns that have an impact on therapy practice. Sometimes, physical and occupational therapists take on direct roles as hired lobbyists. As Amy Lamb (2004), an occupational therapist who worked as a state lobbyist, reflected, "On the surface, being a lobbyist may seem unusual for an occupational therapist; however, I see it as a natural fit.... In the discussion of our field, occupational therapists and occupational therapy assistants are the experts" (p. 1).

Advocacy occurs in the legislative process (legislative advocacy) and the regulatory process (regulatory advocacy). Legislative advocacy encompasses being informed about legislative issues, lobbying through personal visits or letters, and involvement in political campaigns. Regulatory advocacy means providing input when rules that implement legislation are written.

A good example of the legislative advocacy process and the impact that advocacy can have are the efforts that the APTA, AOTA, and ASHA put forth for their members and for other consumer groups with the Medicare Part B outpatient therapy cap. The therapy cap passed with the Balanced Budget Act of 1997 (P.L. 105–33). Since 1997, the monetary limit established for therapy Part B ($1,900 for 2013) has been widely recognized as inadequate for providing necessary therapy services. Massive lobbying efforts by the professional organizations, along with individual efforts by therapists and clients, managed to successfully place a moratorium or temporary stoppage of the therapy cap several times. Always at issue are finances and limited funding from Medicare. APTA, AOTA, ASHA and other provider and consumer groups have consistently worked with Congress and the Centers for Medicare and Medicaid Services (CMS) to find an appropriate long-term solution. However, a short-term solution that has been enacted by Congress over the past several years is an exceptions process to the cap. This process enables therapy services for those eligible beneficiaries who need services costing more than the cap. The exceptions process resulted from the large amount of feedback from therapists and clients, as well as from lobbying efforts by the therapy associations. This example illustrates several points. First, therapists must stay aware of what happens in the larger health care environment that affects practice, and they need to advocate for client concerns. Second, sometimes advocacy efforts only partially work, but if none are made, then compromises like the exceptions process for certain diagnoses would not happen. Lastly, therapists need to pay close attention to regulations related to public policy, such as the exceptions process, as changes will be made in the future for an appropriate permanent fix.

Now let us consider a regulatory advocacy example. One of the authors of this book (H.L.) made a difference on the state level by successfully advocating for legislative changes in the state workers' compensation law to increase therapy coverage.

After reviewing the state law, she went to the billing officer of the hospital to express her concerns about limitations in therapy payment for key workers' compensation codes. The billing officer immediately connected her with the lawyer for the State Workers' Compensation Court so that she could voice her concerns. From this communication, she learned about an upcoming hearing. Along with a representative from the state occupational therapy organization, she prepared and presented testimony that resulted in increased payment for therapy services. Thus, successful changes because of advocacy can and do occur on the state and national levels, and behind every successful advocacy effort are the power of motivation, passion about issues, and the desire to make changes.

Therapists advocate with representatives of state and federal governments to promote issues that help therapy practice. Advocacy is most effective when done in **coalitions**, or groups of people with similar concerns. Although first attempts at advocacy may seem overwhelming, sometimes making the effort results in successful changes. Even if the effort is unsuccessful, getting involved is a learning experience. Therapists should know the positions of the stakeholders and the majority and minority parties on important health care issues (Callahan 2000). Timing is essential. Obviously, a legislator will be most interested in learning the various viewpoints before a vote is taken. The next section highlights one method for promoting advocacy with state and federal legislatures. As noted in this discussion, there are many points in the sequence of events where therapists will need to critically analyze the political process.

Sequence for Advocacy

Step I: Knowledge

Therapists become aware of key issues that concern state or national therapy practice. Knowledge comes from state and national professional associations, professional Internet sites, state agencies, and the media.

Step II: Research

Through research therapists develop a clearer understanding of many aspects about the bill. Table 5-5 lists some questions to consider when doing this research. It helps to understand the full history of the bill, including any previous legislative history (Callahan 2000). Research involves critical analysis of the state of society at the time that the bill was introduced, and with the current bill. Some considerations are the status of the economy, the majority party in the legislature, and the overall priorities of society. For example, one consideration might be the priorities for spending of the national budget: Is more money being spent on war efforts or international affairs over domestic issues, such as health care? Or is the country in an economic downturn that is impacting the progression of domestic bills related to health care?

It helps to understand whether the bill addresses a feature of a problem or the actual problem (Callahan 2000) and what may be missing from the current legislation. It is interesting to consider how the issue is presented by the media (Callahan 2000). Are the real facts or biases presented? Reading the legislative language of bills (refer to http://thomas .loc.gov/home/thomas.php) and comparing similar bills help to clarify different opinions. It is important to understand and articulate reasons for opposing viewpoints. Therapists determine who (e.g., professional organization, coalition, or political party) is behind the proposed legislation and who is against the proposed legislation, and their viewpoints. This awareness involves identifying and networking with the key people involved with the proposed legislation. Securing their cooperation as allies encourages successful changes. Attending coalition meetings with allies can be highly beneficial in clarifying the political picture about the legislation. Members of a coalition may share research about the legislation that benefits all members. Network with other rehabilitation professionals. For example, an occupational therapist in charge of legislative issues for a state occupational therapy organization networks with the legislative representative in the state physical therapy association about an issue of common concern. Completing additional journal or Internet research helps therapists better understand a bill. Internet sites often provide analyses of legislation. However, critical readers need to consider the source of

Table 5-5 Questions to Consider when Researching a Bill

What is the history of the bill?
What is the current state of society at the time when the bill is introduced?
What societal values and trends does the bill address?
Does the bill address a feature of a problem or the entire problem?
What content is in the current bill, and what is missing?
What facts, fallacies, or biases about the bill are presented by the media?
What is the opposing viewpoint about the bill?
Who (e.g., a professional organization, a coalition, or a political party) is behind the bill, and who is against the proposed legislation?
What is the future impact of the bill on society, if passed?

Source: Callahan 2000; Lohman 2003.

the information: Is the source supportive of one's viewpoints, and even if it is supportive, does it provide accurate information? Finally, one must contemplate the impact of a bill, if passed, on future generations. (Lohman 2003). Step I is completed when therapists are ready to take positive action because they clearly understand and have critically thought through all issues related to a bill, for a "key means for understanding public policy is by using a critical analysis approach" (Lohman 2003).

Step III: Implementing Political Action

To implement political action, therapists must identify their state and national legislative representatives and their stances. If therapists do not have this information, they can get it from many sources, including various coalitions, the library, newspaper articles, and Internet sites. The APTA, AOTA, and ASHA Internet sites, as well as other sites, have links that enable finding one's legislative representatives. Newspaper articles quote the key players and their stances on the legislation, as well as public opinions. Internet sites for the *Washington Post* or the *New York Times* are helpful resources. The Internet site of one's senator and representative can help determine positions on an issue.

A key to successful advocacy and implementing political action involves communicating with the appropriate legislative personnel, such as the legislative staff. Legislative staff are the gatekeepers for the legislative representative and should be treated with respect. Furthermore, therapists should network with representatives from their own constituency as legislators value the opinions of their constituents.

Writing or e-mailing letters are popular and effective communication methods with legislators, especially if they are original, well-timed, relevant, and well-written. Writing an original letter or e-mail is viewed as preferable. Most websites from professional associations include sample form letters, which therapists can send or adapt. Members of Congress are very interested in knowing the opinions of their constituents. An understanding of where a bill is at in the legislative process is helpful. To influence the legislative process, write a detailed letter to a member of a committee, as much of the actual work on developing legislation takes place in committees. If an issue is being discussed for a vote, a brief message sent to one's representative with a suggested stance may be all that is necessary (Weingarten 1996). Since 2001, it is considered quicker to fax or e-mail letters to Washington, DC, offices rather than mailing them, as mailed letters are held for inspection. Table 5-6 lists hints for writing about a specific act or bill.

A Legislative Visit

Another highly successful advocacy technique is scheduling a visit with one's federal or state legislator. Ideally, it is helpful to visit someone who supports a bill or is undecided. Sometimes, however, meeting with a person who opposes a bill can provide a clearer picture of another perspective, which is important for critical analysis. This meeting may result in changing the legislator's opinion or, at the very minimum, making the persons aware of

Table 5-6 Writing a Letter or E-mail to a Legislator about a Specific Act or Bill

1. For letters, use a personal letterhead if your home is in the legislator's district and the address is in a district different from that of your work. Use a professional letterhead only if you obtain permission from your employer or the association you are representing.

2. Addressing correspondence:

To a Representative

The Honorable (full name)
_____ (Rm.#)_____(name of) House Office Building
United States House of Representatives
Washington, DC 20515
Dear Representative:

To a Senator

The Honorable (full name)
_____ (Rm.#)_____(name of) Senate Office Building
United States Senate
Washington, DC 20510
Dear Senator:

To a Committee Chair or Speaker

Dear Mr. Chairman or Madam Chairwoman (Or Dear Mr. Speaker):

3. Clearly state in the first paragraph the number and name of the bill and your position with respect to it. It is helpful to begin the letter on a positive note by thanking the person. This sets the tone and helps to garner the person's support. The thank you can be as simple as thanking the person for commitment to public service, even if you disagree with his or her position on an issue.

4. Clearly state who you are (a constituent, a stakeholder, someone directly affected by an issue, an expert about an issue, or an organizational representative) and what perspective you are representing. It is especially helpful to identify yourself as a constituent.

5. Make the letter clear and concise, usually no longer than one page. Limit issues presented and state facts, as your credibility is important. Include any research evidence that supports your stance as evidence is viewed positively in today's society. If the purpose of the letter is to influence a vote, clearly describe what you want the person to do.

6. Use specific examples to support your views. If applicable, provide examples or a story from your practice area as that can communicate a very persuasive message. Discuss any new information that may help the congressperson form a viewpoint or provide information that is relevant to his or her interests.

7. Try to use your own words and not copy a form letter. Accessing a form letter can be a good beginning resource, but develop from there.

8. In representing an organization, it is important that everyone have the same stated stand.

9. Be constructive and provide solutions, not just complaints.

10. Thank the person for time and attention

11. Include contact information (name, address, phone number, and e-mail address).

12. Double-check grammar and spelling before sending. Spell out any abbreviations.

13. The same guidelines apply for writing e-mails to congressional representatives as with writing letters. Remember to keep the e-mails original.

14. Faxes or e-mails are the most expedient and preferred methods for communication with Washington, DC, offices. Fax numbers and e-mail addresses can be obtained from the website of a legislator.

Sources: AOTA 2000c; Autism Society 2004–2011; www.learn2.com; http://www.propeople.org/advocate.htm; http://www.apha.org/NR/rdonlyres/58CDD03C-DCAC-4CE0-8821-40360BD202B7/0/TipsForWritingToYourPolicy.pdf; Dodge 2005; Weingarten 1996.

your concerns. Offering solutions not just criticism is a helpful approach. Visiting legislative offices is important, as legislators are quite sensitive to public opinion, especially from their constituents. Often, therapists meet with staff members rather than the legislators. However, as stated earlier, never underestimate the power of a staff member. Table 5-7 provides hints for talking with legislative personnel. Legislators on the federal level always have staff personnel. On the state level, legislators may or may not have a staff representative.

Table 5-7 Communicating with Legislators or Staff Members

1. Make an appointment and clearly state the reason for the visit. Stating that you are a constituent makes the legislator or staff member more willing to meet with you. If telephoning, after identifying yourself, briefly state your position on the specific bill.

2. For an appointment with a staff member, ask to meet with the staff person who handles the issue that you are addressing, such as about health care public policy.

3. Research the legislator's position and background about the issue before the meeting. Consider ideology, past votes, committee service, and length of service and whether the legislator is up for reelection. If up for reelection, the legislator may be more willing to examine positions. Also consider the stance of the legislator's political party about a bill. Only ask for the legislator's position if you do not know it.

4. Be aware of the timing of congressional recesses, as members often return to their home states during that period, and it may be easier to make an appointment.

5. Work as part of the state and/or national therapy association (APTA or AOTA). As discussed, lobbying as part of coalitions is powerful. If going on your own, advise the state and/or national organization. Staff at the organization can provide resources and advice on how to present your stance if it differs from that of the legislator with whom you are meeting.

6. Sometimes it helps to attend a meeting along with representatives from a coalition of professionals from other disciplines to coordinate efforts.

7. Practice your presentation with someone not familiar with the issues. Monitor for clarity, professionalism, and timeliness.

8. Be prompt and dress professionally.

9. Be patient and flexible. It is not unusual for a meeting to be interrupted with other business.

10. Have the facts clearly outlined on a handout to provide to the legislator or staff member. It is best to research the literature and have clear evidenced-based facts rather than an emotionally based handout.

11. Be prepared to explain physical or occupational therapy. Tailor the explanation to the area that you are advocating for. Consider bringing an additional general fact sheet about the profession.

12. To present clearly, stay with the key points on the handout. Presenting different stories can undermine the power of the communication. If the conversation gets off issue, go back to the points on the handout.

13. Think of the session as an educational opportunity, and bring educational materials to the meeting. Often, legislator or staff members are not familiar with the nuances of a situation, as they usually specialize in a few areas. Therapy practitioners are experts on the impact of legislation on patient/client care.

14. View the meeting as an equal discussion, not as a lecture. Offer ideas for solutions to the issue.

15. Remember the bigger picture by articulating the linkage between your position and the interests of people in the legislator's constituency. Be aware that you are only one of many individuals/groups visiting on a daily basis to advocate.

16. Describe how you or your professional group can help the legislator.

17. If appropriate, ask for a commitment to your stance.

18. If relevant, share a patient/client story that relates to the issues of the bill.

19. Be polite and respectful. Consider the visit as the beginning of an ongoing relationship, so keep communication channels open.

20. Do not monopolize the legislator's or staff member's time. Plan on taking 15 minutes, as legislators and their staff members are busy people.

21. Provide a prompt thank-you letter clearly restating the key points covered in the meeting. Include any requested materials or information with the letter.

Sources: Amputee Coalition 2009; AOTA 2000b; AOTA 2000d; AOTA 2000e ; Vermithrax 2000.

Appearing at Hearings and Preparing Testimony

Table 5-8 summarizes the legislative process. Although it seems straightforward, there can be many nuances in how a bill progresses or is held up in the political process. Therefore, it is important to know where a bill is at in the legislative process to appropriately advocate. When a bill goes to a committee, there are often hearings in which appropriate citizens, including therapists, provide testimony. Therapists should be aware that legislation can change quickly and that bills can be reintroduced with changes. Therefore, it is important with testimony to find out any last-minute changes that have occurred. Table 5-9 provides hints for preparing and presenting testimony.

Table 5-8 Legislative Process: How a Federal Bill Becomes a Law

House	Senate
1. Bill is introduced in the House Bill is titled HR _____.	**1. Bill is introduced in the Senate** Bill is titled S _____. (Senate follows the same steps as House, with exception of the "rules" step.)
2. Bill is referred to committee Bill is carefully analyzed. If the committee takes no action, the bill is killed.	**2. Bill is referred to committee**
3. Bill is referred to a subcommittee At this point, therapists and others can provide testimony at a scheduled hearing. The specialized subcommittee may "mark up" the bill, or make changes to it, prior to recommending it back to the full committee. If the subcommittee votes not to report legislation to the full committee, the bill is killed.	**3. Bill is referred to a subcommittee**
4. Bill is reported by full House committee After obtaining the subcommittee's report, the full committee may do further study and hearings, which is again a time for testimony. The full committee votes, or "orders a bill to be reported," on its recommendations.	**4. Bill is reported by full Senate committee**
5. Publication of written report After the full committee votes favorably to have a bill reported, the chairperson allocates staff to prepare a written report that includes the intent and scope of the legislation, its influence on existing laws, the position of the executive branch, and dissenting views.	**5. Publication of written report**
6. Rules Committee action Many bills go to this committee for a "rule" to accelerate floor action and set conditions for discussion and amendments on the floor. Some "privileged" bills go directly to the floor for debate.	**6. Rules Committee action** In the Senate, the "rules" step is skipped. In addition, some bills may skip committee discussions and go to the Senate floor for debate.
7. Debate/Floor vote The bill is debated, is often amended, or can be killed. If passed, it goes on to the Senate to follow the same route.	**7. Debate/Floor vote** The bill now goes on to the next step: conference action.

Conference Action

After the Senate and House have passed related bills, a conference occurs with representatives from both divisions to reconcile any differences between the bills.

If the conference does not reach a compromise, the bill is killed. If differences are reconciled, a written conference report is prepared, which both divisions must approve. The bill is then sent to the president.

Presidential Action

The president has four options:

Option 1: Sign the bill, and it becomes law.

Option 2: Take no action for 10 days while Congress is in session, and the bill automatically becomes law.

Option 3: Veto the bill. If the bill is vetoed, Congress can override the veto by a two-thirds vote in both houses.

Option 4: Take no action after the Congress has adjourned for its second session, and the bill is killed.

Sources: AOTA 2000a; AOTA 2000e; APTA 2000c; OT Advocate Packet; PT Advocacy.

Table 5-9 **Preparation of Testimony**

- Testimony involves research and clear, credible facts. As with finding evidence to support intervention, the same concepts apply. Consider the level, validity, reliability, and statistical significance of the presented evidence.
- Read a draft of the testimony aloud and have others review it.
- Role-play presenting and timing of the testimony. Be aware that usually there is a time limit to provide testimony, so stick to the key points. Practice presenting in a calm and friendly tone. To test for clarity, practice with people who are unfamiliar with the issue.
- Prepare to answer questions or provide supplementary knowledge. Have someone role-play an adversarial stance to practice answering difficult questions. Know the opposition's position to be prepared with counterarguments.
- Know the names of all the legislators on the committee and something about their positions on the topic. Do your research!
- Address committee chairpersons as Mr. Chairman, Madam Chairwoman, Mr. Speaker, etc., depending on the person.
- Be clear and to the point. Do not use vague terminology such as "it seems" or "it appears."
- If possible, include relevant patient/client stories to make the testimony meaningful.
- Present what the committee wants to hear, such as fiscal issues and evidence. Clearly define any medical jargon.
- Complete a prehearing briefing to determine that everything is organized.
- Make sufficient copies of the testimony to bring, and provide copies to members of the committee before the hearing.

Presentation of Testimony

- Dress professionally.
- Address comments to the members of the committee.
- In your introduction, identify yourself, your professional background, and the organization you represent. Relate the importance of the issue, and thank the members of the committee for allowing you time to present your case. Always be polite.
- Ask that your testimony be included in the hearing record.
- Articulate loudly and clearly. Do not read your testimony word for word; rather, provide a presentation.
- Do not repeat information that has already been stated in prior testimony.

Answering Questions and Conclusion of the Testimony

- Close the testimony with a brief summary of your position, and offer to answer any questions.
- Be clear and consistent, and not evasive, in your answers to questions.
- If you do not know the answer to a question, admit it, but offer to provide the answer in writing at a later date.
- Do not appear intimidated.
- Promptly follow up with members of the committee. Be sure to write thank-you letters. In the letters, include key points covered in the testimony and any requested materials.

Sources: Dodge 2005; Vermithrax 2000.

Implementing Political Action on the State Level

Most of what has been discussed applies to advocacy on federal and state levels. However, what is unique about advocacy on the state level is that it is easier to contact state personnel about issues and to maintain ongoing relationships. Also unique on the state level is that some public policies, such as Medicaid, are combined federal-state laws that are regulated at the state level. Therefore, state departments will have the responsibility for determining the regulation of the state law. Therapists can have a strong influence when they advocate with these state-level agencies. Table 5-10 presents some questions to ponder.

Step IV: Critical Thinking/Reflection

This step involves applying critical thinking to evaluate what was and was not successful with the advocacy effort. Alternative strategies may be tried if the initial effort was unsuccessful (Callahan 2000). Although reflection is written into the advocacy sequence as a

Table 5-10 Critical Reflection Questions after an Advocacy Effort

1. Were we proactive rather than reactive with our advocacy efforts?
2. Did we follow the steps for successful advocacy?
3. Which of our efforts worked and why?
4. Which of our efforts didn't work and why?
5. What would we do differently next time?
6. Who are the key people to stay in contact with? Did we promptly provide requested information? Did we properly and promptly thank them for their help?

final step, therapists should be critically analyzing the advocacy process throughout, as advocacy is not a linear process.

Policy Making, Advocacy, and Evidence

Considering evidence with all areas related to health care including advocacy and policy making is important (Anderson et al. 2005). For busy therapists, it may seem easier to hear another person's report of relevant policy information rather than researching the information to find the facts. Yet learning information in a secondhand manner can result in misconceptions. With the availability of laws and regulations and other reliable sources on the Internet, such as on professional websites, therapists can ascertain the correct information. The key is finding the reliable sources.

Furthermore, in a time of scarce resources, payers, regulators, legislators, and our clients not only value evidence but may demand it (AOTA 2010d; Lieberman and Scheer 2002). Additional factors that encourage use of evidence with policy making is the increase of information with the World Wide Web and the need for considering evidence with ethical issues and decision making (Anderson et al. 2005). Both the APTA (2011a) and the AOTA (2011a) include evidence as part of their organizational visions. The AOTA vision describes the profession as "science-driven, and evidence-based (AOTA 2011a)." The APTA Vision 2020 mentions evidence, and under the descriptors of the elements of the vision, it includes the integration of evidence-based practice with "health care policy decision making" (APTA 2011a).

Applying evidence impacts all three discussed levels of advocacy: patient/client, professional, and the health care environment. On a client level, therapists can provide clients with evidence about interventions to help with self-advocacy efforts for payment or referrals. On a professional level, therapists can apply evidence with advocacy efforts that support and justify the need for therapy with payers and other health care professionals. Therapists can use evidence of effective intervention to help advocate for referrals. In the larger health care environment, therapists can effectively use evidence with lobbying efforts. Simply having relevant statistics about constituents from a legislative district is effective use of evidence. Including evidence is also very effective with professional presentations and or publications about advocacy issues, as therapists can reach a larger audience with these approaches (Field-Fote as cited by DiGiacomo 2006).

Beyond using evidence to support therapy practice, representatives from our professional associations model use of evidence with their lobbying efforts and other initiatives. For example, the AOTA, under a contract with the U.S. Center for Disease Control and Prevention's National Center for Injury Prevention and Control, used the results of an evidence review for a policy analysis about Medicare coverage with fall-prevention services. This evidence review was the basis for the American Geriatric Society/British Geriatric Society's *Clinical Practice Guideline: Prevention of Falls in Older Persons* (2010). A subsequent report, (AOTA 2010d) contained recommendations to change Medicare policy and reimbursement to be consistent with evidence-based practices regarding fall prevention (personal communication, Christina Metzler, 10/2011).

Public Policy, Advocacy, and the Social Media

Social media, or electronic communication through Internet sites such as Facebook, Twitter, YouTube, LinkedIn, and blogs, transform the way people communicate about relevant issues, including public policy. Social media have quickly taken off because they assist with interactive communication (discussion and debate) (Dobyns 2008; Eytan et al. 2011) and help build relationships (Goldner 2010). Additionally, social media facilitates easy and fast access to important information (Dobyns 2008) and encourages participation in advocacy issues (Tarloff as cited by Strzelecki 2011). Americans are actively engaged in postings and discussions about news events on social media sites (Purcell, Rainie, Mitchell, Rosenstiel, and Olmstead 2010). Social media may be a powerful place to spur social change. One author, Chappell (2010/2011), predicts that social media will be the place where movements to fix issues begin and that with a compelling message changes can occur. Usages of social media with advocacy are in their infant stage, and in time, research will determine their overall impact.

Our professional therapy associations recognize the power of social media and utilize it. The APTA has a page on their website titled "Social Media and Networking." There they list several social media venues that APTA is actively engaged in, including a "fan" page on Facebook focused on "issues, thoughts, and experiences" (APTA 2011b). AOTA has a social networking site called OT Connections. There AOTA members can find blogs, groups, and discussion forums about many subjects, including advocacy and leadership. The intent of the advocacy group on OT Connections is to "increase communication and education about advocacy and public policy for OTs in all settings" (AOTA 2011b). Other therapy initiatives such as the Facebook page "Stop the Medicare Therapy Cap" (Facebook 2011) illustrate the use of social media for advocacy efforts. On this site, therapists access discussion boards, helpful links, and pictures, and use a "wall" to "blog" their thoughts. Blog sites, such as one developed for the occupational therapy association in Washington State (Kaplan 2009) are used to "inform, empower, and inspire" (p. 19) about advocacy issues.

When considering social media usage with advocacy efforts, therapists should critically reflect about the best platform on which to present their message. A blogging site can be used for discussion and sharing of ideas (Dobyns 2008), and a YouTube video post might be used as a creative means to educate therapists and consumers about important advocacy issues. Twitter could be used to follow an advocacy event, or as a quick means to make an important announcement (Dobyns 2008). Social media are changing rapidly, and new platforms will develop.

Finally, although there are many benefits for applying social media with advocacy efforts, therapists need to be careful with postings, as inappropriately posted information becomes public knowledge and "can have unintended and far-reaching consequences" (AOTA 2011c, p. 1). Therapists need to keep aware of privacy regulations (e.g., Health Insurance Portability and Accountability Act [HIPAA]), ethical principles, and employers' policies regarding social media (Strzelecki 2011). Ultimately, therapists need to recognize that they represent themselves and their profession (Strzelecki 2011) with postings on social media sites, so professionalism and accurate information are imperative.

Conclusion

In conclusion, advocacy is an essential skill that therapists should develop and be prepared to use on many levels, whether with clients, various professional and other organizations, the state legislature, or with the U.S. Congress. Even if one does not get involved on a state or national level, advocacy can be done in one's own workplace by helping clients and promoting therapy. Essential to the advocacy process is an understanding of one's own motivation and having assertive communication and critical thinking skills. Finally, advocacy involves personal strength, for, as Lohman, Gabriel, and Furlong (2004) state, "Being an advocate for change…may be difficult. It may put the practitioner in conflict with the prevailing political climate that seems focused on the bottom line and costs, rather than quality of life for people with disabilities. Such advocacy requires moral courage."

Active Learning Exercises

Advocacy Scenarios: Identify what you would do to advocate in each situation.

Scenario 1: Mark works in an outpatient therapy clinic for a private company. He treats a large population of older adults, particularly with orthopedic concerns. Mark's main focus is patient/client care, and he does an adequate job with rehabilitation. He is, however, ignorant of the changes in the outer health care environment. If asked, he states, "I assume that the company I work for will keep me aware." Therefore, Mark is caught totally unaware with changes in the fee schedule for Medicare Part B. Subsequently, his hours are cut back due to decreases in payment. What could Mark have done differently?

Scenario 2: Melissa works in acute care practice with people who have a variety of diagnoses. On the oncology floor, she provides intervention with a middle-aged woman who seems very depressed. This woman indirectly hints of suicide. What should Melissa do?

Scenario 3: Maya works in an interdisciplinary rehabilitation department. She is the only certified hand therapist and has over 10 years experience working with hand conditions, more than anyone else in the department. Lately, a new secretary has been assigning clients as orders are processed. The secretary is now assigning clients with hand concerns to all therapists, not primarily to Maya. Maya would like to follow more of the hand patients/clients. What should she do?

Scenario 4: Melvin is the director of a small outpatient clinic. Lately he notices a decrease in client load. He ignores the situation, thinking that it is temporary. Finally, he attempts to figure out what is wrong, but by then it is too late. Melvin didn't realize that his primary admitting physician was unhappy with the care provided by one of the therapists in the department and is now admitting elsewhere. How should Melvin have handled the situation differently?

Scenario 5: You are the administrator of a therapy department. You find out that Medicaid is decreasing reimbursement for therapy services in your state. Describe the steps that you will take to obtain better reimbursement.

Scenario 6: You become aware that one of your state senators is supporting some Medicare concerns of older adults, but not concerns related to therapy. Describe the steps that you would take to educate this senator.

Scenario 7: Rick, a sixteen-year-old student at Stevenson High School, is being followed by therapy. He expresses the desire to be part of the school track team and mentions that no one in his special needs classroom has ever been involved before. Rather than you advocating for Rick's desire, discuss how you can encourage Rick to be a self-advocate.

Active Learning Exercise

Self-Reflection

Identify a situation in which you were an advocate. Reflect about the following questions:

What level of advocacy were you involved in (patient/client, professional, or in the health care environment)?

Were you successful? Why or why not?

Did you take a proactive stance in the advocacy effort? Why or why not?

What did you learn from the experience? What would you do differently?

Source for some of the above resources: http://www.apha.org/legislative/advocacylinks.htm.

Active Learning Exercises: Advocacy Activities

- Critically reflect about the reality of becoming involved in advocacy, keeping in mind that advocacy begins in small increments (DiGiacomo 2006), such as assisting a client with payment or writing a letter about a relevant policy issue.

- Access your profesional website (APTA, AOTA) and review all the advocacy resources available for members. Identify information that is new or relevant to your practice area. Then review information that is relevant to a peer therapist in another practice area.

- Utilizing the letter-writing/e-mail guidelines provided in this chapter, write a letter/ e-mail to a senator or representative based on a bill relevant to therapy.

- Utilizing the information provided on how to present testimony, simulate giving testimony about a bill relevant to therapy. Research and develop a "fact sheet" to include with the testimony. Then, in front of a mock committee, present a three-minute testimony. Be prepared to address opposing arguments. Or have someone prepare and present opposing testimony or supporting testimony from another perspective. Critique the testimony and fact sheet on the basis of the guidelines presented in the chapter.

- As a group, identify a bill relevant to therapy. Have each member of the group develop a persuasive argument based on different perspectives about the bill. Examples of these perspectives could be a constiuent's viewpoint, a health care provider's viewpoint, a senator's viewpoint, and a payer's perspective.

- Referring to the advocacy resources provided at the end of the chapter, identify an advocacy group in the community that services clients who are also followed by physical and occupational therapy. Interview the lobbyist or a representative from the association. Prepare a list of five to six questions to find out how he or she advocates for the members of the organization. Develop a fact sheet describing how physical therapy or occupational therapy relate to the focus of the association.

- Attend a meeting of an advocacy group from a different organization related to a practice interest area, such as the AARP. Critically reflect about their advocacy interests and how they relate to the patients/clients that therapists follow. Consider joining the group, becoming involved, and maybe eventually taking on a leadership role.

- Interview a representative from your state therapy association legislative committee. Find out what motivated him or her to become involved with the state committee. Identify the public policy issues relevant to therapy in your state. Find out about the background of your state lobbyist.

- Develop a "mock" Facebook or blogging site about a public policy issue. Consider the appropriate evidence to include on the site. Apply creative means to engage the audience of the site.

Chapter Review Questions

1. Describe the ethical responsibilities of therapists to be involved in advocacy.

2. Relate the basic skills of advocacy and how they affect each other:
   a. Self-reflection
   b. Knowledge
   c. Assertive communication

3. Provide an example of therapist advocacy on each of the following levels:
   a. Patient/Client
   b. Professional
   c. Organizational

4. Review the features of an effective legislative lobbying campaign:
   a. Legislative visit
   b. Letter writing
   c. Testimony provision

Chapter Discussion Questions

1. Discuss any recent changes in health care that made therapists consider the importance of advocacy skills in professional practice.

2. Reflection has been emphasized as an important component of effective advocacy. Why are self-motivation and passion about an issue important to advocacy over the long term?

3. Discuss an experience you had in trying to effect reform or bring about institutional change. What did you learn from the experience?

4. Discuss the use of evidence with advocacy.

5. Explain creative ways to apply social media with advocacy.

References

Accreditation Council for Occupational Therapy Education (ACOTE®). 2008a. Accreditation standards for a master's-degree-level educational program for the occupational therapist. Retrieved from http://www.aota.org/Educate/Accredit/StandardsReview.aspx

_____. 2008b. Accreditation standards for a doctoral-degree-level educational program for the occupational therapist. Retrieved from http://www.aota.org/Educate/Accredit/StandardsReview.aspx.

_____. 2012. 2011 Standards and Interpretive Guide (effective July 31, 2013) December 2012 Interpretive Guide Version. Retrieved from http://www.aota.org/Educate/Accredit/Draft-Standards/50146.aspx?FT=.pdf.

Alberti, R.E., and M.L. Emmons. 1978. *Your perfect right: A guide to assertive behavior,* 3rd ed. San Luis Obispo CA: Impact Publishers.

American Geriatrics Society. 2010. AGS/BGS Clinical practice guideline: Prevention of falls in older persons (2010). Retrieved from http://www.americangeriatrics.org/health_care_professionals/clinical_practice/clinical_guidelines_recommendations/2010/.

American Occupational Therapy Association. 2000a. How a bill becomes a law. In C. Metzler and C. Willmarth, eds., *Public Policy 101.* Bethesda MD: American Occupational Therapy Association.

_____. 2000b. Guidelines for a site visit for members of the U.S. Congress. In *OT Advocate Packet.* Bethesda MD: American Occupational Therapy Association.

_____. 2000c. Tips for writing a letter to your member of Congress. In *OT Advocate Packet.* Bethesda MD: American Occupational Therapy Association.

_____. 2000d. Tips for meeting with your members of Congress. In *OT Advocate Packet.* Bethesda MD: American Occupational Therapy Association.

_____. 2000e. AOTA expands your influence. Retrieved from http://www.aota/org/.

_____. 2008a. *Occupational therapy practice framework: Domain & process,* 2nd ed. Bethesda, MD: American Occupational Therapy Association.

_____. 2008b. AOTPAC fact sheet. Retrieved from http://www.aota.org/Practitioners/Advocacy/AOTPAC/About/36338.aspx?FT=.pdf.

_____. 2009. Why should I donate to AOTPAC? Retrieved from http://www.aota.org/Practitioners/Advocacy/AOTPAC.aspx.

_____. 2010a. Occupational therapy code of ethics and ethics standards. Retrieved from http://www.aota.org/Consumers/Ethics/39880.aspx.

_____. 2010b. AOTA's State Affairs Group. Retrieved from http://www.aota.org/Practitioners/Licensure/ContactUs_1.aspx.

_____. 2010c. About AOTA's Federal Affairs Department. Retrieved from http://www.aota.org/Practitioners/Advocacy/Federal/38625.aspx

_____. 2010d. AOTA's Evidenced-based practice resources: Using evidenced to inform occupational therapy practice. Retrieved from http://www.aota.org/Educate/Research/2011-EBP-Resources.aspx?FT=.pdf .

_____. 2010e. Final report on activities: Improve public policy response and Medicare coverage for fall prevention and intervention. Retrieved from http://www.aota.org/Practitioners-Section/Productive-Aging/Falls/Other/Final-Report.aspx.

_____. 2011a. The road to the centennial vision. Retrieved from http://www.aota.org/news/centennial.aspx.

_____. 2011b. OT connections. Retrieved from http://otconnections.aota.org/.

_____. 2011c. Advisory opinion for the ethics commission: Social networking. Retrieved from http://www.aota.org/Practitioners/Ethics/Advisory/51807.aspx?FT=.pdf.

_____. n.d. Public affairs division. Bethesda MD: AOTA.

AOTAction Network. 2000. *Helping to ensure the future of OT through congressional action.* Bethesda MD: American Occupational Therapy Association.

American Physical Therapy Association. 2013. Advocacy. Retrieved from http://www.apta.org/Advocacy/.

_____. 2013. House of Delegates. Retrieved from http://www.apta.org/hod/ House of Delegates Policies. http://www.apta.org/Home/Members/governance/governance.

American Physical Therapy Association. 2003. *Guide to physical therapist practice,* 2nd rev. ed. Alexandria VA: American Physical Therapy Association.

_____. 2010. Code of ethics for the physical therapist. Retrieved from http://www.apta.org/uploadedFiles/APTAorg/About_Us/Policies/HOD/Ethics/CodeofEthics.pdf.

_____. 2011a. Vision 2020. Retrieved from http://www.apta.org/vision2020/.

_____. 2011b. Social media & networking. Retrieved from http://www.apta.org/socialmedia/.

_____. 2013a. Advocacy. Retrieved from http://www.apta.org/Advocacy/.

_____. 2013b. House of Delegates. Retrieved from http://www.apta.org/hod/ House of Delegates Policies. http://www.apta.org/Home/Members/governance/governance.

_____. n.d. Federal Regulatory Affairs. Retrieved from http://www.apta.org/FederalAdvocacy/ (accessed December 5, 2012).

_____. n.d. Grassroots. Retrieved from http://www.apta.org/Grassroots/ (accessed December 5, 2012).

American Public Health Association. 2000. Face to face meetings with policymakers. Retrieved from http://www.apha.org/legislative.

Amputee Coalition. 2009. Fact sheet: Do's and don'ts of a legislative visit. Retrieved from http://www.amputee-coalition.org/fact_sheets/leg_vist.html.

Anderson, L.M., R.C. Brownson, M. Fullilove, S.M. Teutsch, L.F. Novick, J. Fielding, and G. Land. 2005. Evidence-based public health policy and practice: Promises and limitations. *Am J Prev Med* 28(58): 226–230.

Autism Society. 2004–2011. Tips for contacting your legislator. Retrieved from http://autismsociety-nc.org/index.php?option=com_content&view=article&id=109&Itemid=624.

Callahan, S. 2000. Educational innovations: Incorporating a political action framework into a BSN program. *J Nurs Ed* 39(1): 34–36.

Carpenter, D. 1992. Professional development module. P9: Advocacy. The "what" and "when" of advocacy. *Nursing Times* 88(26): i-viii.

Chappell, K. December 2010/January 2011. On our radar: The Advocate. *Ebony* 66(2/3): 23.

_____ 2011. Evaluative criteria for PT programs. Retrieved from http://www.capteonline.org/uploadedFiles/CAPTEorg/About_CAPTE/Resources/Accreditation_Handbook/EvaluativeCriteria_PT.pdf.

Commission on Accreditation in Physical Therapy Education (CAPTE). 2012. Evaluative criteria for PT Programs. Retrieved from http://www.capteonline.org/uploadedFiles/CAPTEorg/About_CAPTE/Resources/Accreditation_Handbook/EvaluativeCriteria_PT.pdf.

Davis, C.M. 1998. *Patient practitioner interaction: An experiential manual for developing the art of health care,* 3rd ed. Thorofare NJ: Slack.

Dhillon, S.K., S. Wilkins, M.C. Law, D.A. Stewart, and M. Tremblay. 2010. Advocacy in occupational therapy: Exploring clinicians' reasons and experiences of advocacy. *Can J Occup Ther* 77(4): 241–247.

DiGiacomo M. 2006. Advocating for people with disabilities. *PT Magazine* 14(11): 50.

Dobyns, K. 2008. In the clinic: Enhancing practice through online social networking. *OT Practice* 13(20): 7–9.

Dodge, J. 2005, April, 26. Effective advocacy in Nebraska. Presented at Persuading Others to Rally around the Cause. Nebraska Appleseed and Voices for Children.

Eytan, T., J. Benabio, V. Golla, R. Parikh, and S. Stein. 2011. Social media and the health system. *Permanente Journal* 15(1). Retrieved from http://www.thepermanentejournal.org/issues/2011/winter/445-social-media-and-the-health-system.html.

Facebook. 2011. Stop the therapy cap. Retrieved from http://www.facebook.com/pages/Stop-the-Medicare-Therapy-Cap/290661517047/.

Farlex. 2013. The free dictionary by Farlex. Retrieved from http://medical-dictionary.thefreedictionary.com/aspiration.

Foose, D. 1999. Elder abuse: Stepping in and stopping it. *PT Magazine* 7(1): 56–62.

Goldner, S. 2010. Take the a-path to social media success. Retrieved from http://www.econtentmag.com/Articles/Column/Guest-Columns/Take-the-A-Path-to-Social-Media-Success-71926.htm.

Joint Commission on Accreditation of Healthcare Organizations. 2007. *Disclosing medical errors: A guide to an effective explanation and apology.* Oakbrook Terrace IL: Joint Commission Resources, Inc.

Kaplan, A. 2009. Perspectives : Blogging for advocacy. *OT Practice* 14(13): 19–20.

Lamb, A. 2004. Lobbying 101. *OT Practice* 9(17): 16–19.

Lieberman, D., and J. Scheer. 2002. AOTA's evidence-based literature review project: An overview. *Am J Occup Ther* 56(3): 344–349.

Lohman, H. 2003. Critical analysis of a public policy: An occupational therapist's experience with the Patient Bill of Rights. *Am J Occup Ther* 57(4): 468–72.

Lohman, H., L. Gabriel, and B. Furlong. 2004. The bridge from ethics to public policy: Implications for occupational therapy practitioners. *Am J Occup Ther* 58(1): 109–12.

Namerow, M.J. 1982. Implementing advocacy into the gerontological nursing major. *J Geront Nurs* 8(3): 149–51.

Pollard, N., D. Sakellariou, and F. Kronenberg. 2009. *A political practice of occupational therapy.* Edinburgh: Churchill Livingstone/Elsevier.

Purcell, K., L. Rainie, A. Mitchell, T. Rosenstiel, and K. Olmstead. 2010. Understanding the participatory news consumer: How Internet and cell phone users have turned news into a social experience. Washington DC: Pew Internet and American Life Project. Retrieved from http://pewinternet.com/Reports/2010/Online-News.aspx.

Sachs, D., and R. Linn. 1997. Client advocacy in action: Professional and environmental factors affecting Israeli occupational therapists' behavior. *Can J Occup Ther* 64(4): 207–15.

Scott-Lee, S.J. 1999. Lobbying for occupational therapy. *OT Practice* 4(8): 5, 12.

Strzelecki, M. 2011. Social media sites: How practitioners can better follow, fan, and friend. *OT Practice* 16(5): 8–11.

Vance, K., M. Zahoransky, and R. Kohl. 2011. Short course: Medicare home health policy and practice. {Powerpoint Slides}. Retrieved from http://www.aota.org/member-docs/2011-conference-pa/hh-presentation.aspx.

Weingarten, F.W. 1996. Writing a member of Congress. Computing Research Association. Retrieved from http://www.cra.org/govaffairs/advocacy/writecong.html (accessed March 7, 2007).

Wynn-Gilliam, K. 2000. APTA mobilizes on manipulation: Association at work series. *PT Magazine* 8(2): 34–38.

6

Fundamentals of Insurance

CHAPTER OBJECTIVES

At the conclusion of this chapter, the reader will be able to:

1. Discuss the social purpose of health care insurance.

2. Define and relate the basic features of an insurance contract:

   a. Eligibility
   b. Covered events
   c. Covered services
   d. Beneficiary cost limits
   e. Provider cost limits
      1. Fee for service
      2. Case rate
      3. Capitation

3. Explain the organization and administration of insurance markets.

   a. Actuarial analysis
   b. Moral hazard
   c. Insurance market reform and the Patient Protection and Affordable Care Act of 2010
   d. Explain regulation of health care insurance markets

KEY WORDS

Actuarial Analysis
Actuarial Value
Adverse Selection
American Health Benefit Exchanges
Assignment of Benefits
Beneficiary
Capitation
Case Rate
Co-Insurance
Co-Payment
Community Rating
Cost Limits
Deductible
Essential Health Benefits
Favorable Selection
Fee Schedule
Guaranteed Issue
Health Insurance Portability and Accountability Act
Individual Mandate
Moral Hazard
Patient Protection and Affordable Care Act of 2010
Premium
Rescission
Risk
Underwriting

CASE EXAMPLE ···

Melissa is a certified hand therapist and has decided to develop a business plan for a private hand therapy practice. She has developed a good working relationship with local physicians who are interested in helping her by referring patients in need of therapy. As part of her business plan, Melissa needs to identify her sources of funding for her practice. She knows through experience that most of her current patients have either employment-based health care insurance or workers' compensation insurance that pays for therapy. She networks with other providers in the community and identifies the major insurance companies in the area. She contacts them and learns of their interest in her as a provider. She learns that policyholders of their plans have different out-of-pocket costs they are responsible for depending on the insurer and type of insurance. She also learns that, depending on the insurance company and the type of insurance plan, she will be paid using different methods of payment. Some insurance plans will pay her for each procedure she completes. Other insurance plans will pay her for a visit of therapy irrespective of the procedures she performs. She also realizes that each company has different paperwork to be completed. The complexity of the insurance system surprises her, but she recognizes that she will need to understand it in order to be successful in her private practice.

Case Example Question:

1. How does Melissa's situation reflect the development of policy dualism discussed in Chapter 1?

Introduction

Insurance is a financial mechanism that shares and disperses the risk of financial loss due to the occurrence of an adverse event within a population. Insurance performs an important social function by improving the financial stability of individuals and organizations. Individuals and organizations pay a fee (premium) to create a pool of resources that will provide income or service benefits to holders (beneficiaries) of an insurance contract (policy). A beneficiary who experiences an adverse event covered by the contract is eligible to receive benefits. Since insurance funds the majority of therapy services, physical therapists and occupational therapists need to understand the form and structure of insurance in order to meet contractual obligations for the reimbursement of their care.

In this chapter, we will introduce the social function of insurance, the basics of an insurance contract, a classification system of insurance contracts, and how insurance is regulated. Chapter 7 is devoted to the most common form of health care insurance today: managed care. Chapters 8 and 9 will discuss the largest social insurance programs in the world: Medicare and Medicaid. We begin the chapter with an explanation of the social purpose and organization of health care insurance.

Why Have Health Care Insurance?

Purpose of Insurance

Insurance performs an important social purpose in protecting individuals and organizations against unforeseen and severe financial loss. For many employees, health care insurance is an important part of a work-related benefit package. Without insurance, many ill or injured persons would be forced into liquidation of assets and bankruptcy to pay for the costs of medical illness and disability.

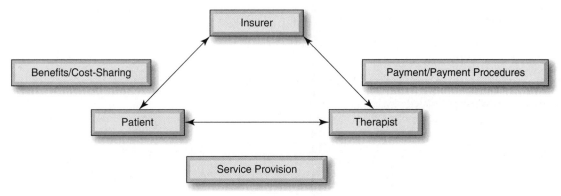

FIGURE 6-1 Relationship of Patient-Provider-Insurer

Insurance is a set of two contracts (see Figure 6-1). One contract is between the insurance company and the contract holder (the patient). This agreement defines a set of benefits that the contract holder is entitled to in the event that an event occurs covered by the contract, and it defines how the costs for these benefits will be shared. The second contract is between the insurance company and the provider of the health care service. This agreement defines the payment procedure and amount that will be reimbursed when contract holders use their insurance. In both cases, an important function of insurance is to manage the risk of an adverse event.

Risk and Insurance

The basic purpose of insurance is to share and disperse the negative consequences of an adverse event. Health care insurance prevents any one individual or group of individuals from suffering serious financial hardship or poor health due to an illness or injury. To prevent this from occurring, individuals come together to form a **risk pool** that collects a fee (**premium**) from each member (**beneficiary**) that can be disbursed to individuals who actually incur an event covered by the contract. The purchase of insurance does not guarantee that one will receive benefits equal to the amount of money contributed to the pool. In fact, if all the beneficiaries received benefits equal to or greater than the amount they contributed, the risk pool would be financially bankrupt. Implicit to the concept of insurance is the sharing of risk. Insurance exists to provide "peace of mind" in that the individual will receive benefits in case of the occurrence of the adverse event. Those without insurance are placed at risk of significant loss of financial resources and/or health.

Insurance also provides a stable source of funds for health care providers, including therapists. The money in the risk pool is available to pay for services when persons do not have the personal resources to pay. In this case, the risk of the provider not being paid is kept relatively low in contrast to the situation of care provision to the person without insurance. Insurance companies are required to maintain adequate reserves to pay for claims that are made against the risk pool. This helps to maintain a stable health care system.

Basics of an Insurance Contract

A medical care insurance contract with a beneficiary defines eligibility for benefits, what events and services are covered by the plan, what the cost limits of the insurance plan are, and how coordination of benefits will occur (see Table 6-1). Insurance contracts with providers define the mechanisms and circumstances of payment for services (see Table 6-2). It is important to understand that an insurance contract does not pay for all of the services that can be requested by a beneficiary or delivered by a provider. For example, most insurance contracts exclude payment for luxury or experimental services. Insurance contracts inform the beneficiary and the provider about what services are covered and how much of the cost of care will be paid for by the insurance company. Insurance contracts only provide benefits to eligible beneficiaries for covered events and covered services. Insurers do develop standards of care and implement review processes that determine the appropriateness of services and their eligibility for reimbursement. We will have more to say about this function of insurance in Chapter 7.

Table 6-1 Basic Features of an Insurance Contract

A. Eligibility
    1. Established by the sponsor of the plan.
B. Covered Events
    1. Medical problem diagnosed by a credentialed physician.
    2. Contract is responsible for event precipitating the illness or injury (e.g., workers' compensation insurance is responsible for work-related illness or injury).
    3. Excludes illness or injury caused by war, riot, or self-inflicted.
C. Covered Services
    1. Stated in contract.
        a. Reasonable and necessary
        b. Acceptable medical practice
    2. Excludes experimental and certain elective procedures (e.g., cosmetic surgery).
D. Beneficiary Cost Limits
    1. Plan limits: lifetime, overall limit, annual, out-of-pocket limit.
    2. First-dollar coverage: deductible or co-payment.
    3. Co-insurance: shared percentage-based reimbursement between insurer and beneficiary up to out-of-pocket limit.
    4. Limits on utilization: pre-authorization, day-dollar-visit limits, provider selection, documentation or expectation for improvement.
E. Coordination of Benefits
    1. Primary and secondary insurance: "Birthday" rule for children.

Eligibility

Eligibility is established based upon criteria set by the sponsor of the insurance plan. The United States lacks a comprehensive single source for health care insurance that is open for enrollment by all Americans. Instead, the United States has a mix of programs that determine eligibility based on the motivation of the sponsor and the willingness of the beneficiary to participate. For example, employment-based coverage is offered only to employees of a given business or members of a given labor union. The process of **underwriting** determines whether an individual's personal characteristics (e.g., age, medical history) qualify the person to purchase the insurance. Strict application of underwriting rules resulted in problems with insurance availability that were addressed by the **Patient Protection and Affordable Care Act of 2010** (PPACA). An insurance contract defines who is eligible to join the risk pool and contribute premiums.

Covered Events

Covered events are usually medical illnesses or injuries that have been diagnosed by a credentialed physician. The credentialing process is an insurance procedure that verifies that the provider has met minimum qualifications for the relevant area of practice. Typically, an insurance contract will not list events that are covered but rather events that are excluded from coverage under the contract. Events due to war, civil disturbance, or self-inflicted injuries are usually not covered. Some insurance contracts exclude preventive health services. It is important to note that the type of insurance must match the covered event. For example, if a person is injured on the job, insurance will be provided by workers' compensation insurance, not an employer-sponsored group health insurance plan.

Covered Services

Once insurance eligibility is established and a covered event has occurred, a beneficiary or provider is eligible to receive benefits for covered services from the plan. Benefits may be financial remuneration for expenses incurred due to a covered event or, more commonly, the services themselves. Services typically include physician care, hospital stays, outpatient care, rehabilitation therapy, behavioral health care, short-term nursing facility stays, and prescription drug benefits. At a minimum, services need to be "reasonable and necessary" to treat the covered event. In general, services should contribute to the recovery of the patient and meet locally acceptable standards of patient care. The precise meanings of "reasonable and necessary" and "acceptable" are determined by an internal review process (utilization review) performed by the insurer.

Cost Limits

Finally, an insurance contract will establish rules that limit the cost of services to the insurance plan. For the beneficiary, this occurs through plan limits, "first dollar coverage" limits, co-insurance, and limits on utilization of care. Insurance contracts between the insurance plan and providers will limit costs to the plan by means of fee schedules, case rates, and capitation. These limits define how the insurance plan will pay for professional services. The PPACA of 2010 requires private insurers to spend 85 percent of the premiums collected (**actuarial value**) either on clinical services or on rebates to consumers.

Beneficiary Cost Limits

Insurance contracts will establish two types of plan limits: an overall plan limit and an out-of-pocket limit. The overall plan limit is the maximum dollar amount the plan will pay over the lifetime of a covered member. An out-of-pocket limit is the maximum amount a beneficiary is responsible to pay during a plan year. The PPACA of 2010 eliminated all overall plan limits and the ability of insurers to cancel policies in force (termed **rescission**; except in the case of application fraud). In 2014, all annual plan limits are eliminated.

Second, an insurance contract will define when plan coverage begins. It is typically calculated on an annual basis by plan year. This first-dollar-coverage limit will vary by type of health care insurance plan. For example, a **deductible** is the amount of money to be paid out of pocket by the beneficiary before any reimbursement by the insurance company. In this form of insurance cost limit, the beneficiary is responsible for all covered costs during the plan year up to a set amount of money (e.g., $250). Another example of a first-dollar-coverage limit is a **co-payment**. A co-payment is a flat fee (e.g., $20) paid by the beneficiary each time a health care service is utilized. This form of first-dollar-coverage limit is common to the health maintenance organization (HMO) form of managed care. Co-payment is commonly seen in therapy practices since care usually consists of several visits over a relatively short period of time. In this example, a patient commonly would owe a co-payment for each visit.

A third form of cost limit in insurance contracts is **co-insurance**. It is used in indemnity plans and some forms of managed care to share a percentage of costs between the beneficiary and the insurance plan until the out-of-pocket limit is reached. For example, a "70–30" co-insurance means that the insurance plan is responsible for 70 percent of the costs and the beneficiary for 30 percent after the deductible is paid and before the out-of-pocket limit is reached. Once the out-of-pocket limit is reached, the insurance contract will typically pay all remaining costs for the plan year up to the overall plan limit.

A fourth form of cost limit in insurance contracts is limits on the utilization of covered services. Physical therapy and occupational therapy services typically require preauthorization by physician referral and, in some cases, by the insurer. Therapy services commonly have a day, dollar, or visit limit for the plan year. In this case, the insurer will pay for therapy services up to a defined amount of money (e.g., $3,000 per year) or number of visits (e.g., 60 visits per year). After this limit is exceeded, the patient is responsible for all therapy costs. An insurance contract may limit beneficiary selection of providers to a contracted panel. A typical standard for reimbursement of occupational therapy and physical therapy services in all insurance contracts is the expectation and documentation of improvement in function or health status in order to justify the continuation of services.

Provider Cost Limits

The various types of provider cost limits are summarized in Table 6-2. These types of limits are not seen by consumers. They are important for therapists to understand, since they have an effect on reimbursement. Consider the following formula:

$$\text{COST (REVENUE)} = \text{PRICE} \times \text{VOLUME OF SERVICES}$$

The cost (or revenue generated to a therapist) of an episode of care is dependent upon the price charged for the service and the number of services charged at various prices. In order to control growth in costs, payers (insurance companies or the government) can either limit price, volume of services, or both. Services in a clinical practice are typically defined as a list of procedures (e.g., evaluation or therapeutic exercise) that are used to communicate the charges of the patient's care to the insurer. This list is called a fee schedule.

A **fee schedule** is a predetermined list of procedure payments that are negotiated between the provider and the insurance plan. A fee schedule is used in many types of insurance contracts, including managed care and social insurance. In an insurance contract, providers and insurers negotiate an acceptable price for each service. Except for meeting other requirements for eligibility, covered events, and covered services, the volume of services provided is primarily at the discretion of the therapist. A fee schedule can limit the price for procedures but does not control the volume of services.

Another form of cost limit in an insurance contract is a **case rate**. Case rates are all-procedure-inclusive payments that take three forms: per diem (daily), per visit, and per episode. A per diem rate is a flat payment for a day of services. A per visit rate sets reimbursement for each therapy visit. A per episode rate is a negotiated fee for an entire episode of care (multiple visits and days). Each of these forms of payment "bundles" individual procedure fees into a combined rate that is often a discounted amount of money from the total of each individual fee on a fee schedule. Case rate payment is not based on the number of procedures but rather on the days, visits, or episode of therapy.

A final form of cost limit separates the episode of care from the patient. **Capitation** is a form of reimbursement that pays the provider a flat fee for a set period (typically each month) for each member of a health care insurance plan. A therapist would be paid for care of a patient regardless if that patient actually used the therapist's services. Instead of encouraging more efficient care, a capitated model incentivizes less care and more activities to improve health and wellness.

The various forms of provider cost limits share varying amounts of financial risk between the insurance company and the provider. For example, a fee schedule has low financial risk to the provider. A therapist is paid for each procedure provided to a beneficiary. As long as the cost to provide that procedure is less than the payment amount, the provider is making a profit with each procedure. Case rates "bundle" procedures together into one all-inclusive payment. The cost of providing these procedures may or may not be greater than the case rate payment. Finally, capitated contracts share the most financial risk with the provider. Acceptance of a flat rate payment for a set period of time means the provider is guaranteed a payment. This flat rate, however, is not based on actual patient visits or procedures, so the therapist is at risk of the costs of care exceeding reimbursement in a capitated contract.

Coordination of Benefits

Some individuals will be covered by more than one insurance contract. This is a common situation in marriages where both spouses have employment-based insurance for themselves and their dependents. In such cases, a coordination of benefits occurs. The policy held by the insured person seeking services is considered to be the primary insurance, and the other coverage is considered to be secondary insurance. For children with dual parental coverage, the birthday rule is commonly used. The insured parent whose birthday is the earliest in the calendar year is considered to be the primary insurer.

Organization and Administration of Health Care Insurance

The organization and administration of an insurance program is performed by private companies and by the government. Private insurance companies are regulated by state governments that, at a minimum, require insurance plans to maintain adequate financial reserves to cover the needs of the risk pool. The United States, unlike most industrialized countries, does not provide universal medical care coverage for its citizens. As a consequence, health care insurance in the United States is a dualistic mix of public and

Table 6-2 Provider Cost Limits in Health Care Insurance Contracts

A. Fee Schedules
    1. Negotiated list of payment rates by health care procedure.
B. Case Rates
    1. Per diem
        a. All-procedure-inclusive daily payment rate.
    2. Per visit
        a. All-procedure-inclusive payment rate for each visit.
    3. Per episode
        a. All-procedure-inclusive rate for a treatment episode.
C. Capitation
    1. Payment to provider based on members in health plan.

private insurers (see Chapter 1). Health insurance market reform was a major focus of the Patient Protection and Affordable Care Act of 2010 (PPACA).

Actuarial Adjustment and Insurance

In order for insurance to be a stable source of funding for therapy and medical care, the collected premiums must cover the benefits to pool members, the administrative expenses of the insurance plan, and, in the case of private insurers, generate a profit. The premium fee is determined by a process called **actuarial analysis**. Actuarial analysis commonly considers demographic factors (e.g., age, gender, medical history), past medical care utilization rates, and known cost data to make statistical decisions about future utilization and costs. An actuarial adjustment determines the premium fee based on the information included in the actuarial analysis. For example, people over the age of 65 would pay a greater amount for medical care insurance than individuals in their early 20s. Actuarial adjustment provides for equity in cost sharing based on likely need for benefits. If performed improperly, actuarial methods can result in excessive profits or losses for the insurer and can affect the availability and affordability of health care insurance to the public.

Moral Hazard and Insurance

Moral hazard is an insurance problem that can be caused by both the beneficiary and the insurer. Moral hazard is financially irresponsible behavior regarding insurance. Persons who believe that they will utilize health care want to purchase insurance. This tends to make insurance expensive since more health care results in higher plan costs. However, for the risk pool to work, persons who may not need health care need to pay a premium to cover their potential risk for needing health care. Individuals create moral hazard by choosing not to purchase health care insurance when they have the capability to do so or by utilizing unnecessary medical care services covered by the insurance. People who choose not to purchase health care insurance shift the costs of their unpaid medical care to people who pay into the risk pool. People who overutilize services raise the costs of health care for all insured individuals.

Insurance companies commit moral hazard through a biased process of actuarial adjustment. **Favorable selection** results from an actuarial process that preferentially identifies people with anticipated low health care costs. This will result in lower beneficiary premiums and higher insurer profits. Favorable selection also creates a pool of individuals with higher health care costs who may not be able to obtain affordable insurance. Individuals in this pool are affected by **adverse selection**.

By the mid-1990s, the problems of rising insurance costs and moral hazard made it increasingly difficult for some people to obtain or maintain health care insurance. To address the problem caused by insurance moral hazard, some states attempted to mandate a form of actuarial adjustment called **community rating**. Community rating requires insurance companies to set a premium fee not based on individual experience but on the experience of all persons in a given city, county, or other geographic area. Premium rate increases to cover all persons, both the healthy and the sick, resulted in many people choosing to disenroll from their insurance plans. In effect, community rating caused adverse selection. At the federal level, the 1996 **Health Insurance Portability and Accountability Act** (known as HIPAA) prevented employers from denying coverage for pre-existing conditions unless they had existed for less than six months. If the person was denied insurance coverage for a pre-existing condition, the exclusion period was limited by HIPAA to 12 months (DOL 2012).

The PPACA enacted landmark reforms aimed at reducing or eliminating moral hazard and increasing the numbers of persons covered by insurance contracts (Kaiser Family Foundation 2011b). First, PPACA reforms limit the ability of persons to not participate in the risk pool. The PPACA permits persons under age 26 to continue insurance coverage as a dependent under a parent's insurance plan. This generally healthy population has had higher rates of uninsurance. More significantly, all persons will be required to purchase "qualifying health coverage" by 2014 or pay a penalty (i.e., **individual mandate**; see Table 6-3). Both of these provisions increase the number of persons participating in the risk pool. Second, PPACA limits the ability of insurers to commit favorable selection. Insurance contracts may not deny coverage to children with pre-existing conditions, and this provision will be extended to adults in 2014 (i.e., **guaranteed issue**). It also puts limits on waiting periods for benefits.

Insurance Markets

Access to health care is heavily influenced by the availability and affordability of insurance. The large number of persons without health insurance in the late 20th and early 21st century is testimony to the problems with insurance markets in the United States. For certain populations, government organizes and sponsors health insurance (e.g., Medicare and Medicaid). We will cover those programs in later chapters. The majority of the working-age population, however, is dependent upon privately-sponsored insurance in either the employment-based or individual insurance markets. Private insurance is most commonly provided as a benefit of employment. Health care insurance sponsored by for-profit insurance companies is commonly termed commercial insurance. Individuals may purchase commercial insurance on their own or through a group plan. Group health care insurance is also sponsored by nonprofit organizations (e.g., labor unions or the Blue Cross insurance plans).

Table 6-3 How Will the Individual Mandate Be Enforced?

Year	Penalty for No Insurance
2014	$95 or 1.0% of taxable income (whichever is greater)
2015	$325 or 2% of taxable income (whichever is greater)
2016	$695 or 2.5% of taxable income (whichever is greater)

The individual mandate does not apply to persons whose income is below a tax filing threshold, who are without coverage for < 3 months, demonstrate financial hardship, have religious objections, or are American Indians, undocumented immigrants, or incarcerated persons.

Source: Kaiser Family Foundation. Focus on health reform: Summary of new health reform law (2011). Retrieved from http://www.kff.org/healthreform/upload/8061.pdf (accessed April 9, 2012).

This information was reprinted with permission from the Henry J. Kaiser Family Foundation. The Kaiser Family Foundation, a leader in health policy analysis, health journalism, and communication, is dedicated to filling the need for trusted, independent information on the major health issues facing our nation and its people. The Foundation is a nonprofit private operating foundation, based in Menlo Park, California.

Employer- Based Insurance

About 55 percent of the U.S. population receives health insurance benefits through an employer-sponsored health insurance plan (DeNavas-Walt, Proctor, and Smith 2011). Sixty percent of employers offer health insurance, but only two in three employees are covered by their employer's plans (Kaiser Family Foundation and Health Research and Educational Trust 2011). Reasons for not acquiring employer-sponsored insurance coverage include cost, coverage by an employed spouse, waiting periods, and part-time employment. In 2009, 70 percent of insurance plans in the employer-sponsored insurance market specifically included physical therapy (Department of Labor 2011). These plans often included occupational therapy and speech therapy in the therapy benefit.

Slightly over half of persons with employment-based insurance are covered by employers who self-insure (Fernandez 2008). Self-insurance means that a company or organization chooses not to participate in a risk pool organized by an insurance company (commercial insurance) and instead establishes its own separate insurance fund internally to pay for covered events and benefits. Sponsors usually contract with a health insurance company to administer the plan. Many self-insured companies and organizations supplement this method of insurance by purchasing "stop-loss" coverage to cap their liability for claims that are higher than anticipated.

Self-insurance is most common in businesses or labor unions with at least 100 members (Garfinkel 1995). Fernandez (2008) reported that 65 percent of large firms self-insure, while only 12 percent of small firms do so. This method of insurance enables large organizations to manage health care insurance costs by predicting and dispersing risk in a known risk pool while simultaneously avoiding expensive marketing and administrative costs. Self-insured health care insurance plans are exempt from state regulation (ERISA exemption). As a result, this form of insurance is popular with multistate organizations that would be affected by individual state mandates and regulations.

In the late 1990s, two new forms of financing for medical care services emerged that are in competition with health care insurance: buyer-sponsored organizations and provider-service organizations. Both of these types of contract mechanisms bypass the traditional insurance company actuarial function and incorporate this process into the operations of either employer purchasers or large provider organizations. In this way, direct contracting occurs between employer purchasers of health care and health care providers.

The increasing interest and sophistication of large employers in purchasing medical care insurance products has caused some of them to form cooperatives and directly contract with providers to obtain care for their employees. This type of contracting group is called a buyer-sponsored organization. Lyles et al. (2002) found that this program performed "reasonably well" in restraining cost growth without negatively affecting quality.

Individual Insurance

About 30 million (10%), Americans are covered by health insurance purchased in the individual insurance market (DeNavas-Walt, Proctor, and Smith 2011). Pauly and Herring (2007) have described the individual insurance market as "extraordinarily untidy, variegated, and malleable" because "it has the task of picking up those who do not obtain employer-group coverage." (p. 770). At least half of the individual insurance market in 30 states is controlled by 1 insurance company (Kaiser Family Foundation 2011). Reform of the individual and small employer–based health insurance market was a major emphasis of the PPACA.

American Health Benefit Exchanges

The PPACA instructed the states (or the federal government in the absence of state action) to create a new marketplace (starting in 2014) for individuals (U.S. citizens and legal immigrants) and small employers (< 100 employees) to purchase health insurance— **American Health Benefit Exchanges** (Kaiser Family Foundation 2011). These exchanges will allow persons to view, compare, and purchase health insurance using standardized information about the costs and benefits of each plan. Only privately-sponsored plans that meet **essential health benefits** criteria will be allowed to participate in the exchanges

Table 6-4 Essential Health Benefits Categories in American Health Benefit Exchange Plans

Ambulatory patient services

Emergency services

Hospitalization

Maternity and newborn care

Mental health and substance use disorder services, including behavioral health treatment

Prescription drugs

Rehabilitative and habilitative services and devices

Laboratory services

Preventive and wellness services and chronic disease management

Pediatric services, including oral and vision care

Source: Essential Health Benefits: HHS Informational Bulletin. Retrieved from http://www.healthcare.gov /news/factsheets/2011/12/essential-health-benefits12162011a.html (accessed at April 11, 2012).

(see Table 6-4). The law prescribes that the specific benefits in plans (e.g., visits of occupational or physical therapy) should be consistent with a "typical employer plan" but can vary state by state. (Department of Health and Human Services 2011). At least two "multistate" insurance plans must be offered in each exchange, and the law also created a nonprofit cooperative model (Consumer Operated and Oriented Plan) that can be offered in the exchanges.

Insurance plans in the American Health Benefit Exchange will also vary by costs paid "out of pocket" by the consumer. The PPACA establishes four tiers of benefit packages plus a catastrophic insurance option for persons under age 30 that allow consumer choice of the type of insurance they are required to purchase (see Table 6-5). The tiers have different actuarial values. The actuarial value of an insurance plan is the percentage of the benefits that are covered by the plan's premiums and not by deductibles, co-payments, and co-insurance (Kaiser Family Foundation 2011c). Premiums for benefits packages in the bronze tier will be lower than for packages in the gold or platinum tier but will have higher deductible, co-payment, or co-insurance costs if a person uses the insurance. Total out-of-pocket expenses in these exchange plans are limited by the current health savings account (HSA) limit for high deductible insurance plans ($6,050 for individuals and $12,100 for families in 2012). Catastrophic plans cover expenses only over the health savings account limits except for up to three primary care visits each year.

Table 6-5 Benefit Tiers in American Health Benefit Exchange Plans

Benefit Tier	% of Essential Health Benefits Covered by the Plan (Premium)
Bronze	60%
Silver	70%
Gold	80%
Platinum	90%

Source: Kaiser Family Foundation. Focus on health reform: Summary of new health reform law, (2011). Retrieved from http://www.kff.org/healthreform/upload/8061.pdf.

This information was reprinted with permission from the Henry J. Kaiser Family Foundation. The Kaiser Family Foundation, a leader in health policy analysis, health journalism, and communication, is dedicated to filling the need for trusted, independent information on the major health issues facing our nation and its people. The Foundation is a nonprofit private operating foundation, based in Menlo Park, California.

Table 6-6 Premium Credits and Out-of-Pocket Expense Subsidies in American Health Benefit Exchange Plans

A. Premium Credits

Annual Income	% of Annual Income to Be Spent on Premiums
0–133% FPL	2%
134–150% FPL	3–4%
151–200% FPL	4–6.3%
201–250% FPL	6.3–8.05%
251–300% FPL	8.05–9.0%
301–400% FPL	9.5%

B. Out-of-Pocket Expense Subsidy of a Benefit Tier Plan

Annual Income	Actuarial Value of Benefit Tier Increased to
100–150% FPL	94%
151–200% FPL	87%
201–250% FPL	73%
251–300% FPL	70%

Since cost is a known barrier to obtaining health insurance, the PPACA provides for subsidies and tax credits for certain individuals and businesses who participate in the exchange. Eligibility for subsidies is dependent upon income. All persons with incomes less than 133 percent of the federal poverty level will be eligible for health insurance through Medicaid (see Chapter 9). Uninsured persons with incomes between 133 percent and 400 percent of federal poverty level are eligible for a limit on premiums (premium credit) and/or out-of-pocket expense subsidies that are scaled to their annual income (see Table 6-6).

Regulation of Insurance

Insurance is only useful if it provides contracted benefits when needed at an affordable cost. The failure of insurance to meet these obligations has prompted the intervention of government into the insurance marketplace. States have primary responsibility to regulate insurance. The ability of states to regulate medical care insurance is affected by federal legislation. In this section, we will explore the role of the state and federal governments in regulating the insurance marketplace.

State Regulation

Each state has an insurance department that licenses and regulates the activities of insurance companies doing business in the state. There are two primary purposes of state insurance regulation: maintaining solvency requirements and market regulation (National Association of Insurance Commissioners 2012). Insurance companies are required to be licensed in their state of incorporation and in the states where they sell insurance products. Solvency requirements mandate that insurance companies maintain capital reserves and financial strategies to cover their anticipated losses. This lessens the possibility of an insurance company facing bankruptcy due to a simultaneous increase in claims and inadequate financial reserves. Some states regulate the premiums charged by insurers, and all states monitor the marketing and eligibility determination (underwriting) practices of insurance companies.

Insurance departments also investigate consumer complaints regarding insurance. Examples of these laws include the prohibition of "gag clauses" on providers and state requirements for mandatory benefits in health insurance contracts. The ability of states to regulate health care insurance, however, is significantly limited by federal law, specifically, the Employee Retirement Income Security Act (ERISA) and the Consolidated Omnibus Reconciliation Act of 1985 (COBRA).

Employee Retirement Income Security Act of 1974

The Employee Retirement Income Security Act of 1974 (ERISA) is a federal statute enacted to standardize regulation of pension and employee benefit plans. The law establishes minimal reporting requirements on pensions and prohibits state regulation of health care self-insurance plans. ERISA prevents state regulators from establishing consumer advocacy, minimal solvency, or benefit requirements in this popular form of employment-based insurance (Polzer and Butler 1997). In addition, it protects managed care organizations from state malpractice lawsuits (Hellinger and Young 2005). It does not prevent states from regulating closed provider panels in managed care organizations (see Chapter 7) through "any willing provider" laws (Goodyear 2001). The PPACA does impose many of its reforms on self-funded health plans (i.e., dependent coverage until age twenty-six, ninety-day limit on waiting periods and no lifetime or annual limits on benefits) (Health Reform Source 2011). Self-funded plans, however, will not have to meet the essential benefits or limitations on deductibles requirements of the PPACA.

Continuation Issues

The high cost of medical care insurance has made it increasingly difficult for some people to obtain coverage. This is especially true for those who lose employment-based coverage due to a change in life status or employment. The Consolidated Budget Reconciliation Act of 1985 (COBRA) was enacted to deal with the problem of loss of health care insurance due to change in life status or employment. The Health Insurance Portability and Accountability Act of 1996 limits the ability of insurance companies to deny coverage based on pre-existing conditions.

COBRA mandates that individuals who lose employment-based health care insurance for reasons other than gross misconduct are eligible to continue coverage for eighteen months at full cost to themselves. This law provides that insurance must be also offered to the spouse and dependents of employees who had family-type coverage. In the event of an employee death, a divorce, or a child no longer maintaining eligible-dependent status, the spouse or dependents can purchase coverage for up to three years. Coverage is terminated on the first occurrence of one of the following events: end of the mandated period, the employer discontinues health care insurance for all employees, or the premiums are not paid. The PPACA did not affect the COBRA mandate (DOL 2010).

Conclusion

In this chapter we have discussed the structure of insurance contracts and the insurance market that reimburses for health care services, including occupational therapy and physical therapy. Health care insurance prevents financial disaster for those who are ill or disabled and provides a source of funding for health care providers. Insurance contracts define eligibility, covered events, covered services, and the sharing of the costs of health care insurance. Insurance is offered in both group and individual insurance markets. Problems with moral hazard in insurance markets were addressed by the Patient Protection and Affordable Care Act of 2010. This resulted in new federal requirements for all persons to obtain health insurance (or pay a penalty) and significant reform of the private health insurance market. Oversight of the financial stability of the health care insurance industry is also performed by state government.

Chapter Review Questions

1. Define the purpose of health care insurance.

2. Define and discuss the concept of risk in health care insurance.

3. What are actuarial analysis and actuarial adjustment?

4. Define moral hazard, favorable selection, and adverse selection.

5. Define the basics of an insurance contract:
   a. Eligibility
   b. Covered events
   c. Covered services

d. Cost limits for the beneficiary and the provider
e. Coordination of benefits

6. Explain the organization of health insurance markets.
   a. Employer-Based (group)
   b. Individual
   c. American Health Benefit Exchanges
   d. Guaranteed Issue
   e. Individual Mandate
   f. Essential Health Benefits

7. Define the role of state government in regulating health care insurance.

Discussion/Case Questions

1. The "individual mandate" was a controversial issue that was decided by the U.S. Supreme Court. Discuss the individual mandate as it reflects different understandings of individual and social responsibility.

2. Mr. Smith is receiving therapy services in your outpatient clinic. He has a service benefit plan with a $200 annual deductible, $500 out-of-pocket maximum, 75-25 co-insurance, and a $1 million overall plan limit. To date, he has utilized $100 worth of covered plan benefits. Therapy charges are $500. What is the out-of-pocket cost of therapy services to Mr. Smith?

3. Consider this statement: "Insurance contracts inform the beneficiary and provider about what services and how much of the cost of care will be paid for by the insurance company." Define and discuss the implications of this statement for the practice of occupational therapy and physical therapy.

References

DeNavas-Walt, C., B.D. Proctor, and J.C. Smith. 2011. U.S. Census Bureau, Current Population Reports, P60 239, *Income, Poverty and Health Insurance Coverage in the United States: 2010.* Washington DC: U.S. Government Printing Office.

Department of Labor. 2010. Health care reform and COBRA. Retrieved from http://www.dol.gov/ebsa/faqs/faq-healthcarereform.html (accessed April 13, 2012).

_____. 2011. Selected medical benefits: A report from the Department of Labor to the Department of Health and Human Services, April 15, 2011. Retrieved from http://www.bls.gov/ncs/ebs/sp/selmedbensreport.pdf (accessed April 15, 2012).

_____. 2012 What is the Health Insurance Portability and Accountability Act of 1996 (HIPAA)? Retrieved from http://www.dol.gov/ebsa/faqs/faq_consumer_hipaa.html (accessed April 13, 2012).

Fernandez, B. 2008. CRS Report R41069 Self-insured health insurance coverage. Congressional Research Service, June 25, 2010. Retrieved from http://www.ncsl.org/documents/health/SelfInsuredPlans.pdf (accessed April 11, 2012).

Fisher, T.F. 2003. Perception differences between groups of employees identifying the factors that influence a return to work after a work-related musculoskeletal injury. *Work* 21(3): 211–20.

Gabel, J.R., G.A. Jensen, S. Hawkins. 2003. Self- insurance in times of growing and retreating managed care. *Health Affairs* 22(2): 202–10.

Garfinkel, S.A. 1995. Self-insuring employee health benefits. *Med Care Res Rev* 52(4): 475–91.

Goodyear, J. 2001. What is an employee benefit plan? ERISA preemption of "any willing provider" laws after Pegram. *Columbia Law Review* 101(5): 1107–39.

Health Reform Source. 2011. How does the new law apply to companies with self- funded plans? Kaiser Family Foundation. Retrieved from http://healthreform.kff.org/faq/how-does-new-law-apply-to-companies-with-self-funded-plans.aspx (accessed April 13, 2012).

Hellinger, F.J., and G.J. Young. 2005. Health plan liability and ERISA: The expanding scope of state legislation. *Am J Pub Health* 95(2): 217–223.

Kaiser Family Foundation. 2011a. Focus on Health Reform: Summary of new health reform law. Retrieved from http://www.kff.org/healthreform/upload/8061.pdf (accessed April 11, 2012).

_____. 2011b. Focus on Health Reform: How competitive are state insurance markets? Retrieved from http://www.kff.org/healthreform/upload/8242.pdf (accessed April 11, 2012).

_____. 2011c. Focus on Healthcare Reform: What the actuarial values in the Affordable Care Act mean. Retrieved from http://www.kff.org/healthreform/upload/8177.pdf (accessed April 16, 2012).

Kaiser Family Foundation and Health Research and Educational Trust. 2011. Employer health benefits: 2011 summary of findings. Retrieved from http://ehbs.kff.org/pdf/8226.pdf (accessed April 11, 2012).

Lyles A., J.P. Weiner, A.D. Shore, J. Christianson, L.I. Solberg, P. Drury. 2002. Cost and quality trends in direct contracting arrangements. *Health Affairs* 21(1): 89–102.

National Association of Insurance Commissioners. 2012. State insurance regulation: History, purpose and structure. Retrieved from http://naic.org/index_consumer.htm (accessed April 16, 2012).

National Council on Compensation Insurance, Inc. 2010. *Calendar-accident year underwriting results*. Boca Raton FL: NCCI.

Pauly, M.V., and B. Herring. Risk pooling and regulation: Policy and reality in today's individual health insurance market. *Health Affairs* 26(3): 770–79.

Polzer, K., and P.A. Butler. 1997. Employee health plan restrictions under ERISA: Employee Retirement Income Security Act. *Health Affairs* 16(5): 93–102.

Private Insurance and Therapy Practice

CHAPTER OBJECTIVES

At the conclusion of this chapter, the reader will be able to:

1. Describe various insurance options in the private market.

2. Define and describe the main principles employed by managed care organizations:

   a. Limited access to the entire universe of providers
   b. Payment mechanisms that reward efficiency
   c. Enhanced quality-improvement monitoring

3. Describe the primary features of managed care products (plans):

   a. Managed indemnity
   b. Preferred provider organization
   c. Health maintenance organization
   d. Point-of-service plan

4. Define and discuss different provider-network models that contract with managed care organizations:

   a. Staff model
   b. Group model
   c. Network model
   d. Independent practice association

5. Explain the purpose and structure of long-term-care insurance, workers, compensation, and casualty insurance.

6. Critically discuss some of the advantages and disadvantages of different insurance options in the private market.

7. Explain ways to effectively communicate with representatives from the insurance industry.

KEY WORDS

Aggregation
Benchmarking
Bundled
Case Management
Consumer-Directed
  Health Plan
Credentialing
Gatekeeper
Health Maintenance
  Organization
Health Savings
  Account
High Deductible
  Health Plan
Leverage
Managed Care
Managed Indemnity
Panel
Penetration
Point of Service
Preferred Provider
  Organization
Therapy Benefit
  Manager

CASE EXAMPLE ··

Sheila, a physical therapist, and Marc, an occupational therapist, work at an outpatient therapy clinic in the community. They primarily follow a case load of orthopedic patients. Although they are aware that most of the patient care is reimbursed by managed care organizations (MCOs), they do not pay attention to the day-to-day management of billing and insurance. Two factors, however, increase their awareness of MCOs. One is a denial of continued coverage for a patient they felt would benefit from more therapy. Second, they learn that the therapy clinic lost a major contract with a MCO as another therapy clinic undercut them when negotiating their annual contract. They learn that

the loss of the contract will have major ramifications on staffing. Although Sheila and Marc recognize that they cannot do anything about the loss of the MCO contract, they decide to do something about the denial of care for the patient that they are following. Therefore, they make an effort to find out about the appeal process offered by the MCO and successfully work with the patient and the MCO to get continued therapy.

Case Example Questions:

1. What is the effect of managed care on access, cost, and quality of care?

2. How have you observed therapy practices adapting to the changing insurance environment?

Introduction

Many forces (e.g., employer awareness of the cost of care, the disincentives that make fee-for-service inefficient) came together to change the medical delivery system that was once based on solo providers receiving fee-for-service payments or indemnity insurance. Fee-for-service involves insurance payment to beneficiaries for covered health care expenses regardless of the place of care and without restriction to a network (Pollitz 2006). In lieu of fee-for-service plans, the current private insurance insurance market is now primarily dominated by managed care plans with new emerging payment models, such as consumer-based health care. Most Americans receive insurance coverage from employer-sponsored plans (Pollitz 2006).

In Chapter 6, we introduced the basic purpose and characteristics of health care insurance. In Chapters 8 and 9, we will discuss social insurance: the primary form of government-sponsored health insurance. A "public option" or government-sponsored insurance plan was not included in the Patient Protection and Affordable Care Act of 2010. Therefore, the private health insurance plans offered in the American Health Benefit Exchanges will take one or more forms of managed care that are discussed in this chapter. This chapter addresses many forms of managed care relevant to therapy practice including preferred provider organizations, health maintenance organizations, and consumer-based health care. In addition, we discuss long-term-care insurance, workers' compensation insurance, and casualty insurance. We conclude by describing communication skills to work effectively with any insurer.

Managed Care

Because of years of being sheltered from the rising costs of health care and due to the availability of the latest and greatest medical technology, many working Americans used the health care system without much restriction or awareness of costs. Likewise, hospitals and physicians did not feel constrained to contain costs or hold back on providing services. As concerns rose with rising health care costs in the 1970s, the federal government and employers looked for new ways to reduce health care expenditures. One of their ideas was the use of provider prepayment to encourage cost-conscious, efficient, effective care (Sultz and Young 1999). Though the concept of prepayment for services had been adopted by various employers to care for their employees, it was not until the passage of the **Health Maintenance Organization** (HMO) Act in 1973 that managed care and the concept of prepayment were thrust into the forefront of health insurance policy. Beginning in the late 1980s employer concerns about the costs of health care expedited the growth of **managed care** plans. The growth of managed care was also propelled by the ERISA exemption that prevented states from regulating employer-sponsored, self-insured health insurance plans (Noble and Brennan 1999; see Chapter 6).

It is important to note the difference between managed care and HMOs. Whereas HMOs are organizations that serve beneficiaries for a fixed fee and provide both financing and delivery of health care services, managed care is a broader concept referring to the principles that payment and the provision of service are interdependently linked. All HMOs represent some form of managed care; while most insurance companies apply at least some managed care principles in different forms of their insurance products (see the section on managed care products later in this chapter).

Defining Managed Care

While many people use the term *managed care*, they may have different ideas about what it really means. Thus, managed care may describe one type of system for some people, but a totally different system to someone else. A minimal definition of managed care is "a system that integrates the financing and delivery of health services" (Barton 1999). Because of the widespread disparity in the definitions of "managed care," it has become an umbrella term to describe the many different organizational structures that try to accomplish the goal of linking the delivery and financing of health care services.

Though managed care has many definitions, all managed care organizations (MCOs) have certain features in common (Kongstvedt 1999). Recall that in traditional indemnity insurance, the provider is paid a "reasonable and necessary" fee after delivering a service, without restriction on the number or type of services provided. The insurer acts as a processor of claims and makes no determination on the appropriateness of the care that was provided. Managed care health insurance plans expand the role of the insurer using three principles: 1) limited access to the universe of providers, 2) payment mechanisms that reward efficiency, and 3) enhanced quality-control procedures. The insurer's role in managed care organizations is expanded from claims processing to determining, on some level, the appropriateness of the care and the access by the beneficiary to plan benefits.

How widely and strictly these principles are utilized varies between managed care products. In general, managed care plans that are more restrictive and uniform in their benefits packages (e.g., HMOs) are less expensive than other forms of managed care and traditional indemnity insurance. Other types of managed care organizations (e.g., PPO and POS plans) provide some but not all features of managed care. Open access to care is improved, but these plans are more expensive. Thus, a variety of insurance options at different prices are available to consumers in the marketplace. Before we discuss the specific types of managed care products, let us explore each of these managed care principles in more detail.

Managed Care Principles

The three major managed care principles are presented in Table 7-1. A short description and application of each principle is included in the table. We will consider each principle separately.

LIMITED ACCESS TO THE UNIVERSE OF PROVIDERS   Managed care organizations typically establish a **panel** of health care providers (i.e., a group of physicians, therapists, hospitals, etc.) that are contracted with or employed by the managed care organization to deliver care to plan beneficiaries. The panel should be geographically distributed and be inclusive of all necessary services to serve the population of patients covered by the plan.

Table 7-1 Managed Care Principles

Principle	Description	Application
Limited access to providers	Controlled number of providers	Open/closed panels
		Credentialing
	Controlled patient access	Gatekeeper
Payment rewards efficiency	Discounts	Discounted fee-for-service
	Bundling	Case-based payment
	Capitation	Per member per month
Quality improvement	Data collection	Utilization review
	Peer review	Clinical pathways
		Benchmarking
		Case management

A panel is usually less than the universe of providers in the area. A limit on the number of accepted providers sets up a competitive situation in marketplaces with heavy managed care **penetration**. In such marketplaces the MCO has **leverage** to force providers to accept lower rates to maintain a patient base.

Provider panels may be either open or closed. An open panel allows any provider who agrees to the terms of the contract to join and be part of the panel. A closed panel allows only a finite number of providers to participate, even if there are others who qualify and desire to be part of the panel. When HMOs organize their provider panels, the providers often go through a **credentialing** process that reviews their education, clinical experience, and professional behavior. Regardless of how a panel of providers is put together or how big the panel may be, the extent to which patients view the provider panel as sufficient is highly subjective and depends greatly on whether or not "their" provider is on the list. This situation led to many consumer complaints about closed-panel managed care plans. Later in this chapter, we discuss how providers organize themselves in response to the insurer's initiative to create panels (see the discussion of managed care provider structures).

Most MCOs limit or refuse benefits to members if they receive care from noncontracted providers. In some managed care models, authorization is done through primary care physicians who act as **gatekeepers**. Patients who want to visit a specialist, such as a physical or occupational therapist, must first go to their primary care provider and obtain a referral. The purpose for using some form of authorization is to reduce the number of "unnecessary" visits to more expensive specialists and thus save money. A less strict preauthorization policy may allow patients to visit any physician directly without getting a referral from the primary care physician, but require them to get authorization for the more expensive procedures, such as hospital admissions. While all managed care products utilize a provider panel, authorization schemes vary.

Payment Mechanisms That Reward Efficiency

As stated at the beginning of the chapter, traditional indemnity insurance provides few incentives for patients or providers to be efficient users of health care. The financial risk of health care is borne by the insurer, hence, the importance of actuarial analysis. Also, payment is made retrospectively, that is, after the intervention has occurred. In a managed care environment, providers are reimbursed for their services through a variety of mechanisms that either "bundle" individual services and procedures into one fee category or create new payment mechanisms altogether (e.g., discounted fee-for-service, case-based payment, capitation) (see Chapter 2). Some of these payment models utilize retrospective reimbursement (e.g., discounted fee-for-service), and other schemes utilize prospective payment systems (e.g., case-based payment, capitation). For further discussion of retrospective and prospective payment systems in Medicare, see Chapter 8. With these incentives, the provider assumes either some or all the financial risk associated with patient care. Sharing of financial risk between the provider and the insurer is an important concept in managed care as providers are at risk for losing money for the decisions they make with care and financial resources. Let us consider how this works.

In a discounted fee schedule environment, providers accept a contract that is less than the full charge for certain services. In return for accepting this discounted fee, the provider is assured a set of patients who subscribe to the contracted health plan. The provider is paid per procedure, but at a lower rate than "reasonable and necessary." Most of the financial risk is still borne by the insurer. The insurer must anticipate usage rates for plan benefits and collect enough premium dollars to pay providers. The insurer has little control over the amount of services that are utilized.

Under a **bundled** payment system, the insurer begins to limit financial risk. This is done by paying one fee to the provider for a set of patient services. It may be as simple as an insurer collating several procedures on a fee schedule that are commonly performed together to create one new fee category (while typically discounting the total of individual fees or eliminating certain fees altogether). Or, as in the case of Medicare, the insurer may deny payment for certain procedures that are billed at the same time as another procedure. Bundling occurs when payment is made for an entire visit or day (per diem) or episode of care, inclusive of all individual procedures and services. These payment mechanisms are all examples of case-based payment, which was discussed in Chapter 6.

All of these payment mechanisms share financial risk between the insurer and provider. The more procedures, visits, or days of treatment provided, the greater the cost of delivering services. In the traditional indemnity and discounted fee-for-service systems, these costs are passed on to the insurer. Bundled and case-based payment mechanisms separate reimbursement from procedure incidence. Instead of being paid more money for increased procedures, providers receive fixed fees. The type and incidence of individual procedures is left to the provider, who assumes some of the financial risk of the cost of delivering more procedures. Therefore, an incentive is created for the provider to control costs of care within the reimbursement amount offered by the insurer.

Capitation completely separates payment from treatment incidence. Capitation prospectively pays the provider a predetermined sum for each covered member of the plan on a regular basis (usually monthly). The provider is paid even if the plan member does not access covered services during that month. Conversely, the provider is not paid extra for the cost of delivering services that exceed the capitation payment. Capitation payment systems transfer financial risk almost entirely to the provider. If the provider's expenses are greater than the capitation payment for the plan members for the month, then the provider loses money. However, if the provider can care for that population for less than the capitation reimbursement amount, then profits are realized. Thus, the incentive is to engage in coordinated preventive care and keep patients healthy while avoiding expensive or extensive health care services. These incentives are so powerful that, in some cases, the withholding of necessary services has been alleged against providers and MCOs using capitated payment models.

Enhanced Quality-Improvement Monitoring

Managed care plans intend to integrate the financial and delivery mechanisms of health care. As we discussed, they do this by controlling access to health care services and by creating payment mechanisms that encourage efficiency. True integration of the financing and delivery of health care services requires policy related to quality as well as access and cost. Since quality is clearly in the purview of providers, this has been the most difficult policy principle for MCOs to implement.

To affect the quality of health care, MCOs perform utilization review, clinical pathways, benchmarking, and **case-management** functions. Utilization review and clinical pathways were introduced in Chapter 3 (see also Reynolds 1996). MCOs use these procedures to track the care of plan members. **Benchmarking** is an ongoing process of utilization review implemented by an MCO to improve quality over time. The report cards discussed in Chapter 3 are an application of benchmarking. Case management is used to coordinate care, especially for high-cost care, provided to managed care plan members.

Key health care professionals in the managed care environment are case managers. Case managers coordinate, in a holistic manner, all aspects of a patient's care with an emphasis on the timely administration of necessary care. Case management is defined as "a collaborative process of assessment, planning, facilitation, care coordination, evaluation, and advocacy for options and services to meet an individual's and family's comprehensive health needs through communication and available resources to promote quality cost-effective outcomes" (Commission for Case Management Society of America [CMSA], 2009 as cited by CMSA 2010). Although nurses dominate the case-management field, physical and occupational therapists can assume case-management roles and become certified as case managers through the Commission for Case Management Certification. A more recent innovation is the use of **therapy benefit managers** as an intermediary between the utilizer of therapy services (patient and therapist) and the managed care organization to evaluate the appropriateness of therapy services. Therapy benefit managers are employed by companies that contract with MCOs to track therapy services, evaluate administrative records, and advise the MCO on the utilization and medical necessity of therapy services and the structure of the physical therapy insurance benefit.

In summary, managed care organizations use three principles: controlled access, cost incentives for efficiency, and quality-improvement mechanisms to integrate the financing and delivery of health care. A number of managed care products have been developed that incorporate the principles just discussed. The following section examines some of these managed care products.

Managed Care Products

Several types of managed care products exist that vary in their organizational structure and how they reimburse providers. These managed care plans range from those that are less aggregated (discounted fee-for-service) to those that are more aggregated (i.e., bundle payments either by episode of illness, per day/visit, or per member). **Aggregation** refers to the extent of integration between the financial and delivery components of the form of managed care. This section briefly discusses the following managed care products: managed indemnity, preferred provider organizations, health maintenance organizations, and point-of-service plans. The primary features of these products are described in Table 7-2.

Managed Indemnity

Managed indemnity, the least aggregated form of managed care, is a fee-for-service reimbursement strategy that adds a pre-authorization component along with utilization review. Thus, it is just one step removed from the fee-for-service systems of the past. The beneficiary in this system is required to obtain pre-authorization for inpatient stays and other services. Failure to do so could result in no reimbursement. On a more positive note, beneficiaries in this system have maximum choice in selecting their health care provider, and there are few restrictions on the amount or type of services they can receive.

Preferred Provider Organizations

A **preferred provider organization** (PPO) is a contracted relationship between a panel of providers and the purchaser of health care services (i.e., the managed care organization). The contract is usually an agreed upon discounted fee-for-service for a set of specific services provided to beneficiaries. The plan uses pre-approval, utilization review, and discounted reimbursement to control costs. Health care providers benefit from an increased pool of patients, low financial investment, and more autonomy than in other managed care

Table 7-2 Managed Care Products

Product	Characteristics
Managed indemnity	Open panel
	Discounted fee-for-service
	Pre-authorization
	Utilization review
Preferred provider organization	Open or closed panel
	Discounted fee-for-service and case-based payment
	Pre-authorization/utilization review
Health maintenance organization	Closed panel
	Discounted fee-for-service, case-based payment or capitation
	Gatekeeper authorization
Point-of-service plan	Contains elements of both HMO and PPO plans
	Rules based on which option patient chooses

products. Beneficiaries have a choice of providers within the panel. Limited or no reimbursement is available for providers who are not contracted panel members. Currently, PPOs are the primary employee-based insurance utilized in today's health care environment (Kaiser 2010), and it is estimated by one source that approximately 69 percent of Americans with health insurance have PPOs (AAPPO 2012). PPOs are believed to be popular because they provide more flexibility and choice than other forms of managed care such as HMOs (AAPPO 2012).

Health Maintenance Organizations

A health maintenance organization (HMO) is a highly aggregated form of managed care. HMOs typically utilize gatekeeper physicians, pre-approval, and utilization review to control plan costs. Beneficiaries access plan benefits only upon referral from their primary care physician and only from panel providers. There is no reimbursement for providers who are not on the HMO panel. Provider payment can take various forms, including discounted fee-for-service, case-based, and capitation. Capitation is most common in the HMO form of managed care.

Point of Service (POS)

A hybrid managed care plan is the **point-of-service** (POS) plan. POS products contain both an HMO and PPO form of managed care. In this plan, beneficiaries are able to choose their provider at the time services are needed. Benefits are typically paid at a higher percentage for persons choosing their primary care providers (HMO product) rather than other providers in the panel (PPO product). Thus, patients have more flexibility to choose the provider they think is most appropriate for the current condition.

Consumer-Directed Health Plans

Often used in conjunctions with PPO models, **consumer-directed health plans** allow individuals greater control over their health care utilization and subsequently over their health care spending. This greater control includes when, where, and how they access health care services and how much they spend on services. However, at the same time, these plans discourage over use of health services that raise costs in the system (Starr 2011). One common approach to discourage over use is requiring co-payments associated with various types of health care visits. Alternatively, **health savings accounts** (HSAs), which are usually coupled with **high deductible health plans** (HDHPs), can discourage unnecessary use of the health care system.

Created with amendments to Medicare legislation and signed into law by President George W. Bush in December 2003, health savings accounts (HSAs) consist of accounts that individuals own and subsequently use to pay for their current and future medical expenses. Used in conjunction with HDHPs, these accounts help pay for first-dollar medical expenses not covered in HDHPs. Individuals can have an HSA only if they are covered by a HDHP, they do not have any other health coverage, including Medicare, and cannot be claimed as a dependent on someone else's tax return (DOT 2012).

While the HSA is owned by the individual, contributions can be made by the employer, the individual, or both. HSA contributions made by the employer are not taxed while individual contributions are tax deductible; rules for contributions also include yearly maximums that vary by year. For 2013, this maximum is $3250 for individuals and $6450 for families (Free News Network, Inc. 2010). Those individuals that are 55 years old or older are allowed to make additional contributions to "catch up" as long as they are not enrolled in Medicare. Funds in HSAs account earn interest as well as additional earnings through various investment options, both of which can be used tax-free to pay for qualified medical expenses.

High deductible health plans have a minimal deductible (for 2013) of $1,250 for individual coverage and $2,500 for family coverage. Additionally, the annual out-of-pocket maximum for 2013 cannot exceed $6,250 for individuals or $12,500 for families, respectively (Benson 2012). Both of these limits change annually for inflation. It is also important to recognize that within the HDHPs there is quite a bit of variation in deductibles above the minimum required and out-of-pocket expenses below the required maximum. No first-dollar coverage, or coverage for the entire value without a deductible (Investopedia 2012), is allowed for services other than preventive services. This ban on first-dollar coverage also applies to prescription drugs or therapy services. All prescription drugs are subject to the plan's deductible. Individuals can choose to access their employer's plan's physician panel and take advantage of negotiated rates or go elsewhere for their care.

Using HSAs as part of a HDHP may offer a number of advantages. HDHPs usually have lower health insurance premiums than lower deductible plans. Monies in HSAs are used at the discretion of the individuals to pay for current qualified medical expenses or saved for future health care–related needs. Individuals can decide when to put money into the account and how much, up to the maximum allowed limited. Once funds are in the account, they stay in the account until used to pay for qualified medical expenses. Additionally, HSAs are portable and stay with individuals regardless of job status or geographic locations. As discussed, there is the potential tax savings associated with HSAs including tax-deductible contributions, tax-free investment earnings, and tax-free withdrawals for qualified medical expenses.

There are disadvantages for having an HSA and an HDHP. One disadvantage is that although HSAs and HDHPs work better for healthy individuals who can afford the high deductible, they do not work as well for lower-income individuals or those with chronic conditions (Kulkarni 2011; Mayo Foundation for Medical Education and Research 1998–2012). HDHP/ HSA plans combine two forms of restraint on utilization of services: a high deductible, and a managed care plan (Starr 2011). To access therapy with these plans, consumers must recognize its value. Therapists need to market their services so that consumers will select to spend their HSA money on therapy. Another disadvantage is that money that is withdrawn from an HSA can only be used for medical expenses, or the person will pay a tax penalty (Mayo Foundation for Medical Education and Research 1998–2012).

The use of HSA and HDHP appears to be appealing to employers as positive mechanisms to control the growth of their health care expenditures. As Figure 7-1 and the accompanying table show, there is a growing interest in these types of plans.

Year	Conventional	HMO	PPO	POS	HDHP
2000	8	29	42	21	0
2005	3	21	61	15	0
2006	3	20	60	13	4
2007	3	21	57	13	5
2008	1	20	58	12	8
2009	1	20	60	10	8
2010	1	19	58	8	13
2011	1	17	55	10	17

FIGURE 7-1 Percentage of Plan Type Offerings and Enrollment

Source: Kaiser Family Foundation; Employer Benefits 2011 Annual Survey. http://ehbs.kff.org/pdf/2011/8225.pdf

This information was reprinted with permission from the Henry J. Kaiser Family Foundation. The Kaiser Family Foundation, a leader in health policy analysis, health journalism, and communication, is dedicated to filling the need for trusted, independent information on the major health issues facing our nation and its people. The Foundation is a nonprofit private operating foundation, based in Menlo Park, California.

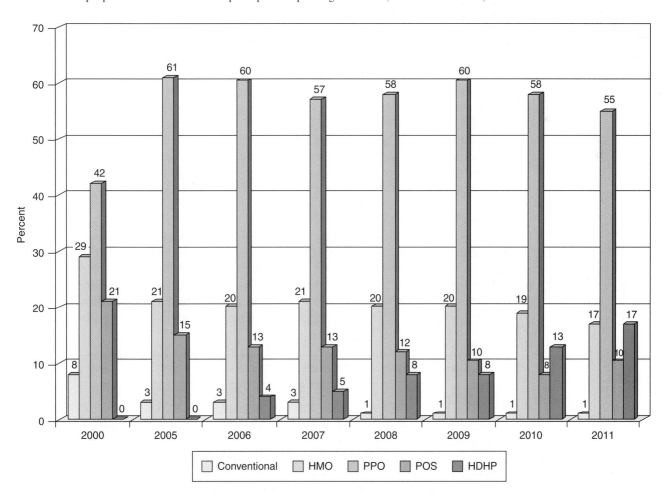

Market Shares of Health Plan Types

As discussed, the PPO health plan is the most common health plan. Figure 7-1 and the accompanying table display the distribution of health plan enrollment for covered workers. As the figure and table show, conventional (i.e., indemnity) plans are almost extinct while PPOs are most popular. It is also interesting to note the rising utilization of high deductible plans.

Managed Care Provider Structures

We introduced and discussed the various types of managed care. As we discussed in the last chapter, insurance is a set of two contracts: one between beneficiary and the insurance company and one contract between the insurance company and providers (e.g., physical therapists and occupational therapists). In order for managed care to work, insurers must develop relationships and contracts with the provider community, including physical therapists and occupational therapists. These relationships take various forms that result in the provider panels discussed in the preceding section. The structure of these panels is the focus of this section.

An MCO is typically looking to create a comprehensive panel of providers that cover a certain geographic region. There are several methods that an MCO utilizes to create a provider panel. In broad terms, MCOs adopt four general model types that describe how provider contracts are established; specifically, a staff model, a group model, a network model, and an independent practice association (IPA) model (see Table 7-3). The more integrated models are characterized by a tightly structured organization that allows increased control of the delivery and cost of health care services. These models typically limit patient choices when it comes to obtaining care. Models that have relatively less integration are less structured and offer more choice to their patients.

Staff Model

In a staff model, individual providers are employed by the HMO and receive a base salary for services. Some HMOs may pay incentives based on performance. The largest example of a staff model HMO is Kaiser of California, which salaries its physicians and therapists, and even owns many of its network hospitals. Other staff model HMOs may not own the hospitals, but salary providers and contract with hospitals. Beneficiaries in a staff model HMO receive coverage for a comprehensive set of conditions for a fixed price per month, but they must be treated within the HMO. This is a highly integrated form of managed care.

Group Model

Group model HMOs deliver health care services to their beneficiaries by contracting with provider group practices. The HMO contracts with just one multispecialty group to provide health care services. Some of these models have exclusive relationships with their provider group practice, referred to as a captive group, in which the provider group only serves patients from one HMO. In a nonexclusive relationship, also known as an independent group, the provider group practice may have contracts to provide services to

Table 7-3 Managed Care Provider Structures

Staff model	Providers are salaried employees of the MCO.
	MCO may own many of the institutional providers (e.g., hospitals).
Group model	MCO contracts with a multispecialty provider group for services.
Network model	MCO contracts with several provider groups for services.
Independent practice association (IPA)	Organization of independent or small group practices that contract with an MCO.

multiple HMOs. The provider group may be paid by various mechanisms, including fee-for-service or capitation. The group model is most commonly seen in large multispecialty physician practices.

Network Model

The network model HMO is similar to the group model, but it contracts with multiple provider group practices, including both primary care and specialty groups. This model may offer greater geographical coverage than the group model. Compared to the staff and group models, the network model is significantly less integrated.

Independent Practice Associations

Independent practice associations (IPAs) are organizations that contract with individual providers or small provider group practices for the purposes of managed care contracting. The HMO then contracts with the IPA to provide health care services to the patients that belong to the HMO. Providers in this model are able to keep their individual or group practices. Thus, they see patients from multiple HMOs as well as patients who do not participate in an HMO. The IPA model is most commonly used by private practice physical therapists and occupational therapists as a contracting organization to negotiate with a MCO.

Active Learning Exercise
PTPN Corporation is a good example of a national independent practice association of physical therapists, occupational therapists, and speech language pathologists. To learn more, go to http://www.ptpn.com/.

OTHER FORMS OF PRIVATE INSURANCE   To this point, we have been discussing the various forms of managed care that comprise the private health insurance system in the United States. In this section, we are going to turn our attention to other forms of insurance that address health problems not specifically covered by private health insurance: long-term-care needs, injuries or illnesses caused in the workplace, and health issues caused by automobile or home accidents.

Long-Term-Care Insurance

The increased risk of expensive long-term care and the limitations of private health care and social insurance plans in sponsoring this coverage have spawned the development of long-term-care insurance. In 2012, the average yearly cost for nursing home care in a double room was $81,030 and assisted living care was $42,600 (MetLife Mature Market Institute 2012). Brown and Finkelstein (2008) estimated that one in three 65-year-old Americans will enter a nursing home and that the usual length of stay is less than one year. However, 12–22 percent of persons entering a nursing home will live more than three years. Private long-term-care insurance is an important source of benefits to pay for nursing home and other supportive services. Private health insurance and Medicare have limited or no benefits for this type of care. As we will see in Chapter 9, Medicaid covers long-term care in certain instances of extreme financial need.

   To date, about 7 million (or 10% of older adult) Americans purchased long-term-care insurance policies (Sengupta, Reno, and Burton 2011). Long-term-care insurance is primarily purchased in the individual insurance market. An advantage of a long-term-care insurance policy is to protect personal assets in the event of the need for long-term-care. Medicare has only a short-term nursing home/home health benefit (see Chapter 8), and Medicaid (the largest payer of long-term care in the United States) requires persons to "spend down" their savings to qualify for long-term-care reimbursement (see Chapter 9). Long-term-care policies typically have a waiting period (e.g., 100 days) that serves as a form of a deductible and a plan limit on the amount of benefits—usually a cap on the length of the benefit period.

Long-term-care insurance provides benefits to people with physical illness, cognitive impairments, and other chronic diseases that result in impairments and functional limitations. Eligibility for benefits is based on loss of function in activities of daily living (ADL) or the onset of a significant cognitive impairment. Six ADLs are commonly examined to determine eligibility: bathing, continence, dressing, eating, toileting, and transferring. An inability to perform at least two of these tasks without assistance usually initiates benefits (NAIC 2008). Some plans require physician certification of benefit needs (Ali 2005).

Long-term-care insurance benefits may cover services at home, or in skilled nursing facilities, assisted living facilities, and adult day care centers. Some plans will limit coverage to home-based or skilled nursing facility care. Other plans will cover services across a continuum of post-acute care, such as home health, assisted living, and skilled nursing facilities. Services can include room and board, personal assistance, and professional care (e.g., occupational therapy, physical therapy). Typically, cost limits on benefits are established as a per diem or per-episode rate. Case management to determine eligibility and coordinate benefits is used in long-term-care insurance plans (Scharlach et al. 2003). Costs for benefits are more reasonable if a person gets a plan earlier in life.

Although there are many positive aspects about obtaining long-term-care insurance, there are some concerns. These concerns include the high cost of insurance and the deductible time period for which the person pays out of pocket. Currently with most plans people wait 90 days to receive the insurance, and by then may not need the services. Additionally premiums continue to rise with a low default rate, which puts more demand on the insurer. Policies are also very complicated, so it is suggested that people thinking of purchasing one consult with an advisor (Mayer 2012). Long-term-care insurance has been found to be effective in preventing institutionalization, reducing stress in informal caregivers (Cohen et al. 2001), and protecting assets (Praeger as cited by Mayer 2012).

Workers' Compensation Insurance

Workers' compensation insurance originated in the early part of the 20th century. It was precipitated by the increasing incidence of industrial workplace injuries, lost worker wages, worker disabilities, and workplace litigation. Workers' compensation remains a strong program in today's health care market. The purpose of workers' compensation insurance is to protect workers, free employers from excessive litigation, and decrease the incidence of occupational injuries (Clayton 2004). In 2010, 4,547 persons died in workplace accidents, and there were 3.1 million workplace injuries of which 1.2 million injuries or illnesses required time off from work (median length is eight days) for recovery (Department of Labor 2011a). Farming, forestry, and fishing are the industries with highest incidence of workplace injury, and executives and managers have the lowest incidence of need for workers' compensation (Leigh et al. 2006). Stressful jobs, lack of job control, and environmentally hazardous conditions are associated with higher incidence of workers' compensation claims in men (Crimmins and Hayward 2004). The prevalence of musculoskeletal injury in the population makes workers' compensation insurance a program of importance to physical therapists and occupational therapists. Sprains and strains account for 42 percent of injuries (Department of Labor 2011a). Back pain accounts for 11 percent and carpal tunnel syndrome for 1 percent of workers' compensation claims.

Workers' compensation insurance is an example of no-fault insurance (Kiselica et al. 2004). Employers are liable for damages due to workplace-related illness and injury regardless of the circumstances surrounding the event. To be eligible for workers' compensation, an individual must be injured or acquire an illness while performing employment activities or functions (Calfee 1998). The source or severity of the injury, however, can be disputed (Hirsch 1997).

Workers' compensation laws establish statutorily determined benefits for workers and protect employers from lawsuits over expenses related to workplace injuries. Workers' compensation laws are state-specific within broad guidelines established in federal law (Occupational Safety and Health Act of 1970). Some states require employers to participate in state-operated programs. Other states permit employers to purchase workers' compensation insurance in the private market. Employers pay the full premium for workers' compensation insurance. Workers' compensation currently covers about 125 million American workers and paid out $58.3 billion in benefits at a cost to employers of nearly $74 billion in 2009 (Sengupta, Reno, and Burton 2011).

Workers' compensation insurance consists of three benefit programs: health care insurance, disability income replacement, and vocational rehabilitation. The medical benefits start immediately after the injury and are unlimited. Medical benefits are provided until "maximal medical improvement" or a return to employment occurs (Durbin 1997). Income replacement begins after a three- to seven-day waiting period (Sengupta, Reno, and Burton 2011). Most claims are medical only, but the most expensive cases include health insurance and income replacement (Sengupta, Reno, and Burton 2011).

The cash benefits may be temporary or permanent depending on the injury or illness. About 60 percent of claims are temporary in nature, but the most expensive claims are due to permanent disability (Sengupta, Reno, and Burton 2011). Outpatient services are the dominant mode of medical care delivery in workers' compensation programs (Himmelstein et al. 1999). Medical benefits are paid without deductible or co-insurance to the injured employee.

Choice of physician and provider is a source of contention in workers' compensation law (Himmelstein et al. 1999; LaDou 2005). Since eligibility for benefits is based on a determination that an injury or illness is work-related, the choice of provider to make the determination is important. Some states allow open choice of provider by the injured employee. Other states permit the employer to select the physician to determine eligibility for benefits.

Durbin (1997) reviewed the process that determines the amount of income replacement for a workers' compensation claim. Disability is classified using five categories:

1. Fatal
2. Permanent total
3. Permanent partial
4. Temporary total
5. Temporary partial

Disability benefits are paid as income replacement payments (typically 66 percent of pre-injury income) while the worker is not employable. Temporary benefits are paid after a three to seven-day waiting period until maximal medical improvement is reached or the worker has a medical release to return to work (Hirsch 1997).

Permanent benefits are provided after maximal medical improvement has been attained. A significant variability in rating permanent disability across the country has been found (Barth 2004; Patel et al. 2003). Permanent partial disability payments are determined based on a schedule of benefits. Scheduled injuries include impairments of the limbs, eyes, and ears. Each of these body parts is assigned a statutory length of time in weeks of disablement based on the schedule and a physical impairment rating. Impairment of function is rated using the American Medical Association Guides to the Evaluation of Permanent Impairment (AMA 2008). This percentage rating is multiplied by the schedule of weeks for benefits to determine the degree of permanent disability. This figure is multiplied by the pre-injury wage to determine the total disability.

Certain types of permanent partial disabilities are nonscheduled (e.g., injury to the visceral organs, trunk, or neck and head, claims of psychological disability). The National Academy of Social Insurance (2011) outlines four methods that states use to determine a permanent disability income replacement for unscheduled conditions:

1. Impairment-based approach
2. Loss of earning capacity approach
3. Wage loss approach
4. Bifurcated approach

An impairment-based approach is used in 19 states and provides a benefit based on the severity of impairment not considering future lost earnings. The loss of earning capacity approach is used in 13 states and provides a benefit based on an estimate of lost future earnings. The bifurcated approach uses an impairment approach for workers who return to the workforce and a loss-of-earnings approach for persons who cannot return to work.

Workers' compensation insurance costs in recent years have stabilized and actually declined. Employer costs of the program as a ratio to wages are currently at their lowest since 1980 (Sengupta, Reno, and Burton 2011). Recent trends in workers' compensation include the use of managed care and self-insurance programs to restrain the growth in costs (D'Andrea and Meyer 2004). In 2004, California passed a major workers' compensation reform bill intended to increase the use of evidence-based practice in their state plan (Guidotti 2006). As a result, the size of disability ratings and cash benefits has fallen by one third (Leigh and McCurdy 2006). Disability case management and utilization review are now in widespread use. Contracted-provider networks that limit open choice of providers are used. A newer trend is for the development of integrated primary, secondary, and tertiary care networks in plans that can provide 24-hour coverage. Costs are lower in these types of systems (Baldwin et al. 2002; Green-McKenzie et al. 2002). Injured workers may become frustrated with the workers' compensation system when their case lasts for a long time or when providers are not readily available. Other reasons for frustration are a lack of understanding of the workers' compensation system, obtaining conflicting medical opinions, and not being able to identify decision makers. (Kosny et al. 2011).

Fraud and abuse in the workers' compensation system is commonly alleged (Durbin 1997; Hirsch 1997). Several types of moral hazard have been described in the workers' compensation program (Durbin 1997; Hirsch 1997). First, the generous benefit packages in workers' compensation plans provide incentives for employees to file false claims or to exaggerate symptoms. Second, the high costs of the program have incentivized employers to aggressively manage these costs and jeopardize the medical care of persons with legitimate injury or illness. Third, the presence of insurance tends to make employers more safety conscious and employees less safety conscious. Fourth, the fee-for-service reimbursement mechanism of some workers' compensation plans incentivizes providers to overtreat conditions.

Casualty Insurance

Automobile or homeowner's insurance includes a medical care benefit. A person must have been injured in an automobile accident or home accident to be eligible for covered medical benefits. Depending on the state, determination of fault in the accident situation will establish responsibility of claims. In these cases, a legal judgment is sometimes necessary to determine who pays for therapy services. Casualty insurance is most commonly provided using a fee-for-service reimbursement structure, although managed care principles are sometimes used to reimburse providers. These products utilize case management, utilization reviews, contracted-provider networks, and discounted fee mechanisms to control costs.

Working with Insurance Companies: Importance of Good Communication

Good communication skills are crucial therapist competencies across the health care system. Several of the strategies we discuss are summarized in Table 7-4. It is important to develop rapport with key people in the health care system, such as case managers, utilization review coordinators, and primary care providers. Regular communication helps increase the awareness of other health care providers about the benefits of therapy.

Table 7-4 Good Communication Skills with Insurers

1. Develop and strengthen rapport with key players (e.g., primary care practitioners, case managers, utilization review coordinators, gatekeepers).
2. Learn the language of business to better communicate with the key players.
3. Communicate intervention to key players, use evidenced-based assessments, and share evidenced-based data supporting practice.
4. Be aware of the mission and goals of the insurer that you are working with.
5. Educate the insurer about the benefits and value of therapy.
6. Understand the needs and values of all customers (e.g. patients, employers, primary care practitioners, physicians, insurers).
7. Advocate for patients and profession.

Communication and demonstrating treatment effectiveness enhances respect for therapy. Furthermore, effective communication keeps therapists aware of the insurer's goals, such as achieving quality care in a cost-effective, timely manner. Although the following section specifies ways for therapists to effectively communicate with case managers, the principles can be applied with others in the health system.

Case managers regardless of having a nonmedical or medical background may not have an in-depth understanding of therapy. Therefore, good communication makes a difference in the ability for patients to access and benefit from therapy services. One suggestion is to think like a case manager when monitoring internal cases. Therapists who consider the perspective of the case manager look at discharge planning from the initiation of therapy and communicate with the case manager from the initiation of treatment. Having regular communication and contact keeps communication open. Another suggestion is to demonstrate the value of therapy by providing effective intervention resulting in patient satisfaction and cost savings (Fosnought 1996; Foto 1997). Doing in-house case management by collecting and communicating outcome data to the insurer about length of stay (LOS), functional status at discharge as compared to entry, costs of providing care, and patient satisfaction enhances respect for the therapist (Foto 1996). Additionally, therapists can educate case managers from other disciplines about the rehabilitation aspects of patient care (Lohman 1998).

Therapists need to carefully analyze their customers and what they value. For example, with managed care, the key customers are MCOs, primary care physicians, patient employers, and patients. Each may have a different perspective on what is expected from the therapist. MCOs usually value the most economical, streamlined, quality care (Foto 1997). Therefore, a therapy clinic that offers diversified care has an edge in getting contracts over one that specializes in one type of care. Additionally, belonging to a therapy network or a larger hospital network helps market to insurers (Lansey 1996), especially with changes occurring in the marketplace with health care reform. Producing outcomes that are functional and sustainable enhances marketing efforts (Foto 1996). Practitioners from therapy clinics should market to get coverage from several insurers so that if a contract is lost they still have adequate coverage.

Finally, patients are the main customers therapists regularly see. Patients value caring health care provision, clear and courteous communication, and an overall satisfactory experience from therapy (Foto 1997). One way to demonstrate care so as to improve patient satisfaction is to advocate for the patient. Advocacy is done by pre-authorizing an adequate treatment amount and by communicating regularly about patient status. Advocacy also means being assertive about the patient's rights if there are problems with the insurer. Insurers offer appeal processes, which can be accessed if there is a perception of unfair coverage or other problem. If the appeals process is accessed, it is important to have clear, objective documentation. In addition, providing effective treatment through careful planning in the time-restricted health care world is an important marketing tool for both the patient and the provider (Miller 1999).

Active Learning Exercise

Objective: Determine the case manager's role in managing patients.

Network with a case manager and ask for her perspective on how she reviews patients who are receiving rehabilitation. Ask the case manager what she likes to see in documentation from therapists.

If possible, spend the day with this person and reflect about the experience.

Answer the following questions:

Comment on how her perspective correlates or differs from your perceptive as a therapist following a patient.

Reflect about what you learned.

This exercise can also be completed with any appropriate insurance representative.

Conclusion

This chapter describes the philosophy and organization of many types of private insurance approaches in the United States. Managed care, and specifically the PPO type, is the dominant form of private health insurance. However, other types of private insurance such as workers' compensation and long-term-care insurance, provide health benefits for specific populations. Regardless of the type of private insurance, insurers are interested in cost control and quality management. Newer payment approaches such as health savings accounts continue to emerge and grow in the marketplace. Therapists need to keep abreast of the macro picture of trends in the marketplace as well as the micro picture of how to work effectively with the insurance companies. Knowledge about the focus of the insurance industry and the health care marketplace as well as good communication skills are necessary to work effectively in the private insurance market.

Chapter Review Questions

1. Define managed care.

2. Identify and describe three principles used by managed care organizations to influence the delivery of health care.

3. Compare and contrast the four types of managed care products.

4. Compare and contrast the four types of managed care provider structures.

5. Describe consumer-based health care and discuss how therapy can be successfully accessed by patients in that system.

6. Define and explain the purpose and structure of long-term-care insurance, workers' compensation insurance, and casualty insurance.

7. Describe effective communication skills with insurers.

Chapter Discussion Questions

1. You are working as a manager in a department that contracted for the past two years with Happy HMO. Although its payment rates are on the low side, your department has been able to meet budget. This year, when you renegotiate the contract with Happy HMO, even lower payment rates are requested. You know that with the lower rates your department will not be able to meet budget. What will you do?

2. You are starting a clinic in an area that is highly infiltrated by MCOs. Other therapy clinics currently have all the contracts. Provide a minimum of three suggestions for how you might negotiate a contract that is financially feasible.

3. You are following a patient with a cerebral vascular accident (CVA) sustained one month previously. The case manager discharged the patient and will not authorize any additional time. What will you do?

4. Research the appeal process for therapy patients from a local MCO.

5. Research the set up of workers' compensation in your state.

6. Review your own health insurance plan for therapy coverage.

7. Meet with a manager of a therapy department and discuss how he/she works effectively with insurers.

References

Ali, N.S. 2005. Long-term care insurance: buy it or not! *Geriatr Nurs* 26(4): 237–40.

American Association of Preferred Provider Organizations (AAPPO). 2012. PPO Advocacy. Retrieved from http://aappo.interactivemedialab.com/Resources /PPOAdvocacy.aspx http://www.aappo.org/index .cfm?pageid=10.

American Medical Association (AMA). 2008. Clarifications and corrections: Guides to the evaluation of permanent impairment, 6th ed. Retrieved from http://www.ama-assn .org/resources/doc/bookstore/guidesclarifications.pdf.

Baldwin, M.L., W.G. Johnson, and S.C. Marcus. 2002. Effects of provider networks on health care costs for workers with short-term injuries. *Med Care* 40(8): 686–695.

Barth, P.S. 2004. Compensating workers for permanent partial disabilities. *Soc Sec Bull* 65(4): 16–23.

Barton, P.L. 1999. *Understanding the U.S. health services systems.* Chicago: Health Administration Press.

Benson, C. 2012. 2013 Health savings contribution limits, high-deductible health plan minimum deductibles and out-of-pocket minimums announced. Retrieved from http://hlbtr.com/about-us/whats-new/5-10-2012/2013 -health-savings-contribution-limits-high-deductible-health -plan-minimum-deductibles-and-out-of-pocket-minimums -announced.aspx.

Brown, J.R., and A. Finkelstein. 2008. The interaction of public and private insurance: Medicaid and the long-term-care insurance market. *Am Econ Rev* 98(3): 1083–1102.

Calfee, B.E. 1997. Workers' compensation litigation review: Part I. *AAOHN J* 45(11): 609–11.

_____. 1998. Workers' compensation litigation review: Part II. *AAOHN J* 46(1): 45–46.

Case Management Society of America (CMSA). 2010. Standards of practice for case management. Retrieved from http://www.cmsa.org/portals/0/pdf/memberonly /StandardsOfPractice.pdf.

Clayton, A. 2004. Workers' compensation: A background for Social Security professionals. *Soc Sec Bull* 65(4): 7–15.

Claxton, G., I. Gil, B. Finder, B. DiJulio, S. Hawkins, J. Pickreign, H. Whitmore, and J. Gabel. 2006. *Employ health benefits 2006 annual report.* Menlo Park, CA: Henry J. Kaiser Family Foundation; Chicago, IL: Health Research and Educational Trust. Retrieved from http://kaiserfamilyfoundation.files .wordpress.com/2013/04/7527.pdf (accessed September 2007).

Cohen, M.A., J. Miller, and M. Weinrobe. 2001. Patterns of informal and formal caregiving among elders with private long-term care insurance. *Gerontologist* 41(2): 180–187.

Crimmins, E.M., and M.D. Hayward. 2004. Workplace characteristics and work disability onset for men and women. *Sozial und Präventivmedizin* 49(2): 122–131.

D'Andrea, D.C., and J.D. Meyer. 2004. Workers' compensation reform. *Clin Occup Environ Med* 4(2): 259–271

Dembe, A.E. 2001. Access to medical care for occupational disorders: Difficulties and disparities. *J Health Pol Soc Policy* 12(4): 19–33.

Department of Labor. 2011a. Bureau of Labor Statistics. 2010 census of fatal occupational injuries. Preliminary data. Retrieved from http://www.bls.gov/iif/oshwc/cfoi/cftb0250 .pdf (accessed April 12, 2012).

_____. 2011b. Bureau of Labor Statistics. Workplace injury and illness summary. Economic News Release. Retrieved from http://www.bls.gov/news.release/osh.nr0.htm (accessed April 12, 2012).

Durbin, D. 1997. Workplace injuries and the role of insurance: Claims costs, outcomes, and incentives. *Clin Orthop* 336: 18–32.

Eddy, D.M. 1997. Balancing cost and quality in fee-for-service versus managed care, *Health Affairs* 16(3):162–173.

Fosnought, M. 1996. PTs as case managers: An evolving role. *PT: Magazine of Physical Therapy* 4: 46–53.

Foto, M. 1996. Excelling in a managed care environment. *OT Practice* 1(1): 20–22.

_____. 1997. Preparing occupational therapists for the year 2000: The impact of managed care on education and training. *Am J Occup Ther* 51: 88–90.

Free News Network Inc. 2010. HSA Contribution Limits 2013. Retrieved from http://healthsavingsaccountrules.com/2013 -HSA-Contribution-Limits-Changes.html.

Green-McKenzie, J., S. Rainer, A. Behrman, and E. Emmett. 2002. The effect of a health care management initiative on reducing workers' compensation costs. *J Occup Environ Med* 44(12): 1100–05.

Guidotti, T.L. 2006. The big bang? An eventful year in workers' compensation. *Ann Rev Publ Health* 27: 153–66.

Himmelstein, J., J.L. Buchanan, A.E. Dembe, and B. Stevens. 1999. Health services research in workers' compensation medical care: Policy issues and research opportunities. *Health Serv Res* 34(1 pt. 2): 427–37.

Hirsch, B.T. 1997. Incentive effects of workers' compensation. *Clin Orthop* 336: 33–41

Investopedia. 2012. First-dollar coverage. Retrieved from http:// www.investopedia.com/terms/f/first_dollar_coverage .asp#axzz1wlKoU8Ls.

Kaiser Family Foundation. 2010. Employer health benefits: 2010 summary of findings, 1–8. Retrieved from http://www.dickersonbenefits.com/uploads/file/KFF _SummaryOfFindings.pdf.

_____. 2011. Employer benefits 2011 annual survey. Retrieved from http://ehbs.kff.org/?page=charts&id=2&sn=20&ch =2134 (accessed June 2012).

Kiselica D., B. Sibson, and J. Green-McKenzie. 2004. Workers' compensation: A historical review and description of a legal and social insurance system. *Clin Occup Environ Med* 4(2): 237–47.

Kongstvedt, P.R. 1999. Managed health care. In L.F. Wolper, ed., *Health care administration: Planning, implementing, and managing organizational delivery systems,* 3rd ed. (522–44). Gaithersburg MD: Aspen.

Kosny A., E. MacEachen, S. Ferrier, and L. Chambers. 2011. The role of health care providers in long term and complicated workers' compensation claims. *J Occup Med* 21(4): 582–90.

Kulkarni, S. 2011. FAQ On HSAs: The basics of Health Savings Accounts. Retrieved from http://www.kaiserhealthnews.org /stories/2011/november/04/frequently-asked-questions-on -health-savings-accounts.aspx.

LaDou, J. 2005. Occupational medicine: The case for reform. *Am J Prev Med* 28(4): 396–402.

Lansey, D. 1996. Reimbursement: Keeping track of managed care. *PT Magazine of Physical Therapy* 4(12): 22–23.

Leigh, J.P. 2011. Economic burden of occupational injury and illness in the United States. *Milbank Q* 89(4): 728–72.

Leigh, J.P., and S.A. McCurdy. 2006. Differences in workers' compensation disability and impairment ratings under old and new California law. *J Occup Environ Med* 48(4): 419–25.

_____, G. Waehrer, T.R. Miller, and S.A. McCurdy. 2006. Costs differences across demographic groups and types of occupational injuries and illnesses. *Am J Ind Med* 49(10): 545–853.

Lohman, H. 1998. Occupational therapists as case managers. *Occup Ther in Health Care* 11: 65–76.

Mayer, C.E. 2012. Long-term-care insurance offers protection, but it's not right for everyone. *Washington Post*. Retrieved from http://www.washingtonpost.com/national/health-science /long-term-care-insurance-offers-protection-but-its-not-right -for-everyone/2012/01/09/gIQAyySmLQ_story.html.

Mayo Foundation for Medical Education and Research. 1998–2012. Health savings accounts: Is an HSA right for you? Retrieved from http://www.mayoclinic.com/health /health-savings-accounts/GA00053.

Mechanic, D. 1994. Managed care: Rhetoric and realities. *Inquiry* 31(2): 124–28.

MetLife Mature Market Institute. 2011. Market survey of long-term care costs. Retrieved from http://www.metlife.com /mmi/research/2011-market-survey-long-term-care-costs .html#graphic (accessed April 12, 2012).

Miller, R.E. 1999. Hands in the new millennium: Therapist commentary. *J Hand Ther* 12: 182–83.

_____, and H.S. Luft. 1994. Managed care plan performance since 1980. *JAMA* 271(19): 1512–19.

National Academy of Social Insurance. 2012. Workers' compensation: Benefits, coverage, and costs, 2010. Retrieved from http://www.nasi.org/sites/default/files/research/NASI _Workers_Comp_2010.pdf (accessed April 18, 2013).

National Association of Insurance Commissioners. 2008. Consumer alert: Long term care insurance fact sheet. Kansas City MO: NAIC.

Noble, A.A., and T.A. Brennan. 1999. The stages of managed care regulation: Developing better rules. *Journal of Health Politics, Policy and Law* 24(6): 1275–1305. doi:10.1215/03616878-24-6-1275.

Nugent, J. 1996. Reimbursement: Planning for managed-care. *PT Magazine* 4: 32–34.

Patel B., R. Buschbacher, and J. Crawford. 2003. National variability in permanent partial impairment ratings. *Am J Phys Med Rehabil* 82(4): 302–06.

Pollitz, K. 2006. Private insurance 101. Retrieved from http://www.kaiseredu.org/Tutorials-and-Presentations /Private-Health-Insurance.aspx.

Reynolds, J.P. 1996. LOS: SOS? *PT Magazine* 4(2): 38–47.

Scharlach A.E., N. Giunta, B. Robinson, and T.S. Dal Santo. 2003. Care management in long-term care insurance: Meeting the needs of policyholders? *Care Manage J* 4(2): 73–81.

Sengupta, I., V. Reno, and J.F. Burton. 2011. Workers' compensation: Benefits, coverage, and costs. National Academy of Social Insurance, Washington DC, August 2011. Retrieved from http://www.nasi.org/sites/default/files /research/Workers_Comp_Report_2009.pdf (accessed April 13, 2012).

Starr, P. 2011. *Remedy and reaction: The peculiar American struggle over health care reform*. New Haven: Yale University Press.

Sultz, H.A., and K.M. Young. 1999. *Health care USA: Understanding its organization and delivery*. Gaithersburg MD: Aspen.

U.S. Department of the Treasury (DOT). 2012. Health Saving Accounts and other tax-favored health plans. Retrieved from http://www.irs.gov/pub/irs-pdf/p969.pdf.

8

Medicare

CHAPTER OBJECTIVES

At the conclusion of this chapter, the reader will be able to:

1. Explain the history of the Medicare program.

2. Describe the organization and scope of the Medicare program.

3. Relate the eligibility criteria and benefits in the Medicare Part A program:

   a. Hospital inpatient program
   b. Skilled nursing facility
   c. Hospice
   d. Home health care

4. Discuss the mechanisms of provider reimbursement under Medicare Part A:

   a. Cost-based reimbursement
   b. Prospective payment:

      1. Hospitals: Medical Severity Diagnosis-Related Groups
      2. Skilled nursing facilities: Resource Utilization Groups
      3. Inpatient rehabilitation facilities: Case Mix Groups
      4. Home health agencies: Home Health Resource Groups

5. Relate the eligibility criteria and benefits in the Medicare Part B program:

   a. Outpatient hospital programs
   b. Comprehensive Outpatient Rehabilitation Facilities (CORFs)
   c. Physical Therapist in Private Practice/Occupational Therapist in Private Practice

6. Discuss the structure of fee schedules as a method of provider reimbursement in the Medicare Part B program.

7. Relate the eligibility criteria and benefits in the Medicare Part C program.

8. Describe the quality-control procedures employed in the Medicare program:

   a. Recognize fraud and abuse in Medicare

9. Define the structure and interaction of private health insurance plans with Medicare.

10. Relate the proposals for reform of the Medicare program.

KEY WORDS

Benefit Period
Case Mix Adjustment
Certification
Cost-Based Reimbursement
Coverage Determinations
Entitlement
Fee Schedule
Functional G Codes
Medically Necessary
Medicare Administrative Contractor
Medicare Advantage
Medicare Assignment
Medicare Physician Fee Schedule
Medigap
Multiple Procedure Payment Reduction
Physician Quality Reporting System
Prospective Payment
Social Insurance
Sustainable Growth Rate
Therapy Cap
Vested

CASE EXAMPLE ·

Mrs. Miller is a 76-year-old widow who has health insurance coverage through Parts A and B of traditional Medicare. She worked for 15 years as a bookkeeper and made regular payroll contributions into the Hospital Insurance Trust Fund. She is **vested** in the Medicare program. When she became eligible for Medicare at age 65, she purchased the Part B program to help pay for her physician visits and a Part D Medicare plan to help pay for her outpatient prescription drug costs.

Mrs. Miller has been experiencing pain and limited mobility in her left hip for many years. It has reached the point where she has elected to receive a total hip replacement to relieve the pain and disablement. She understands that Medicare will help pay for her hospital and post-hospital care. Mrs. Miller has her surgery in the local community hospital and stays for four days. She receives good nursing care as well as visits from the occupational therapist and physical therapist. Her stay will cost her $1,156, and the government will pay the hospital a flat rate payment for her surgery. Mrs. Miller then is transferred to a skilled nursing facility (SNF) to get stronger before she can return home. At the SNF, she is evaluated by the team using the Minimum Data Set and her needs are identified. She stays 20 days and receives therapy each day. The facility is paid a flat rate for each day of her

care by the government based on the initial assessment and the amount of therapy time Mrs. Miller received. Mrs. Miller then goes home and receives a visit from a physical therapist and occupational therapist to help adjust to her home environment and continue her recovery. This care lasts for one month, and the home health agency is paid a flat fee for the episode based on her needs identified in a comprehensive initial evaluation. Mrs. Miller does not pay anything out-of-pocket for her SNF or home health care.

Two months after her total hip replacement surgery, Mrs. Miller is still experiencing some hip pain and weakness. Her surgeon sends her to a physical therapist for an evaluation. The standard **fee schedule** amount for this examination is $69.44. Mrs. Miller pays her physical therapist out-of-pocket for this examination, with the fee applied to her annual $140 deductible. Her course of therapy lasts one month, and her pain is relieved and strength is improved. The total cost of the therapy was $800. After her $140 deductible is paid, Mrs. Miller is responsible for 20 percent of the remaining amount set in the Medicare fee schedule.

Case Example Question:

1. Describe the strengths and limitations of the benefits in the Medicare program.

Introduction

Medicare is the most influential insurance program affecting the United States health care system. This is for two reasons. First, Medicare is the largest single payer of health care services in the United States. Second, it is organized and managed by the federal government, which has enormous statutory and regulatory authority over many activities performed by health care providers, including occupational therapists and physical therapists. It is important, then, for therapists and all health care providers to understand this program. Changes in the program affect the daily delivery of health care in the United States.

We will open this chapter by briefly reviewing the history of how Medicare came to be such a large and influential program. Second, we will introduce how Medicare is organized and administered. Third, we will explore the major components, or "parts," of Medicare that provide services to many Americans. We will then pay close attention to the methods by which providers, including therapists, are paid for services. These payment systems have powerful effects on the organization of the health care delivery system, especially how Medicare defines and regulates therapy services. Next, we will review the organization of quality-control programs in Medicare with special attention to fraud and abuse detection. Finally, we will examine efforts to reform Medicare, including proposals to increase private insurance participation in the delivery of Medicare services.

History of Medicare

The origin of Medicare needs to be considered in the context of the movement to provide universal national health insurance to all Americans (Ball 1995; Friedman 1995). Prior to 1965, Americans who needed institutional health care services had two broad choices: pay privately or receive services in public health care facilities (Blaisdell 1992). This two-tiered system developed in the first half of the century as medical care began to rely increasingly on technology (Blaisdell 1994). Medical care was not delivered primarily in the patient's home by a private physician. Hospitals became institutions where a person could receive the latest technology applied to the treatment of disease and illness. At the same time, social movements began to call for improved access to medical care for people with limited financial resources. Beginning in the late 19th century and into the 20th century, many European countries began to institute universal health insurance for their citizens. American efforts at universal coverage (still incomplete) can be traced back to 1912 and have continued to the current date.

Medicare has been identified as an interim step in the development of universal health insurance for all Americans. By the early 1960s, one in two elderly Americans lacked health care insurance to pay for hospital care (Davis and Burner 1995). Elderly Americans were known to have an increased need for hospital services, and they had fewer resources to pay for this care. Legislative attempts to enact an insurance program for older Americans commenced in 1957, and after the landslide election of Lyndon Johnson as president in 1964, proponents of public health insurance for older Americans had firm control of the Congress and the executive branch. Medicare was vigorously opposed by organized medicine, which had defeated all previous attempts at federal health insurance. The final proposals for Medicare included government subsidies for private health insurance, government payments for medical care for low-income elderly persons, and a health insurance program administered through Social Security (Corning 1969). In July 1965, Medicare was passed by Congress, and shortly thereafter, it was signed into law by President Johnson.

Hospital insurance for elderly Americans was enacted as part of a package of benefits. This package is sometimes referred to as a "three-level cake" (Friedman 1995). Two of the final three proposals were included in the legislation. Parts A and B were created to provide health insurance through the Social Security program. Hospital Insurance (HI), or Part A Medicare, provided coverage for inpatient hospital stays and short-term residential care for rehabilitation in other facilities. Supplementary Medical Insurance (SMI), or Part B Medicare, was intended to provide coverage for professional services (e.g., physicians, occupational therapists, physical therapists). Medicaid, the third tier of the cake, was enacted as an extension of the 1960 Kerr-Mills legislation that provided funds to states to care for the poor. We will discuss Medicaid in Chapter 9.

Until 2003, most major changes in the Medicare program were reforms to the payment systems. These reforms will be discussed later in this chapter. In 2003 (to some extent in 1997), Congress enacted changes that have increased the private insurance company role in designing competitive Medicare. The Part D outpatient prescription drug benefit (2003), the most significant benefit upgrade since 1965, uses private insurance contractors to develop and market competing prescription drug coverage products. In 2010, the Congress made several changes to Medicare in the Patient Protection and Affordable Care Act.

Medicare and Medicaid have been effective in increasing access to health care services for people who are older, people with a disability, people with low incomes (Medicaid), and people with end-stage renal disease and amyotrophic lateral sclerosis (Medicare). These are populations that often do not have access to affordable, private health insurance. As can be seen, Medicare is a very important and influential program. In this next section, we will introduce the Medicare program by reviewing how it is organized and the size of its various components. We will follow this discussion with an explanation of its parts.

Scope and Organization of Medicare

Table 8-1 describes the basic characteristics of the Medicare program. Medicare provides health insurance to about one in six Americans. Medicare consists of two programs: original Medicare and Medicare Advantage. Original Medicare, the most popular program, consists of Part A and, for most persons, Part B Medicare. Part A Medicare, the Hospital Insurance benefit, provides for hospital, short-stay skilled nursing facility, inpatient rehabilitation facility, and home health care/hospice for eligible beneficiaries. Part B Medicare, or Supplementary Medical Insurance, provides coverage for outpatient hospital, office visits to therapists and physicians, and durable medical equipment needs. The Medicare Advantage program was enacted by Congress in 2003 as a redesign of the 1997 Medicare Part C program. Unlike original Medicare, Medicare Advantage programs utilize private insurers to organize a benefit package that is comparable to original Medicare within a managed care framework. A fourth program, Medicare Part D, is the prescription drug benefit that is either a privately sponsored, stand-alone program or included in a Medicare Advantage plan.

Medicare is the largest payer of health care services in the United States. In 2010, the Medicare program spent $513 billion on health care for 48.6 million beneficiaries. It is the dominant form of insurance for persons over age 65 (aged) and persons with long-term

Table 8-1 Characteristics of the Medicare Program

A. Enrollment: 48.6 million (2011)
   1. Aged: 40.2 million
   2. Disabled: 8.3 million
   3. Part A only: 3.8 million
   4. Part B only: 0.4 million
   5. Parts A and B: 44.4 million
B. Expenditures: $513.6 billion (2010)
   1. Part A: $245.2 billion
   2. Part B: $268.4 billion
C. Persons Served (2011):
   1. Hospital: 7.5 million
   2. Skilled Nursing Facility: 1.8 million
   3. Home Health Agency: 1.8 million
   4. Hospice: 1.2 million
   5. OP Physician: 32 million
D. Number of Providers Receiving Medicare Payments (2011):
   1. Hospital: 6,177
   2. Skilled Nursing Facility: 15,716
   3. Home Health Agency: 10,914
   4. OP Physical Therapy: 2,536
   5. Comprehensive OP Rehabilitation Facility: 354
E. Program Administrative Costs: 1.3 percent

Source: Centers for Medicare and Medicaid Services. Data Compendium, 2011. Accessed at http://www.cms.gov/DataCompendium/13_2011_Data_Compendium.asp#TopOfPage on February 16, 2012.

disabilities. Two in three dollars of Medicare expenditures are paid out of the Hospital Insurance Trust Fund (Part A) to hospitals, home health agencies, and skilled nursing facility providers. Medicare operates in all states and territories and affects all providers. It operates at less than a 2 percent administrative cost (Kaiser Family Foundation 2011a). Almost since its inception, concerns have arisen about the cost of the Medicare program (Russell and Burke 1978). In its first year, Medicare cost less than $2 billion. It was funded by a 0.35 percent payroll tax on the first $6,600 of a worker's earnings (Davis and Burner 1995). Today, the government collects a 2.9 percent (1.45% from the employee and 1.45% from the employer) payroll tax on all earnings to fund Medicare Part A and primarily uses general revenues and beneficiary out-of-pocket costs (premiums and co-insurance) to fund the other parts of the program. As the "baby boom" population ages and more people are eligible for Medicare and the beneficiary-worker ratio increases, there are concerns about the long-term financial viability of the program. Revenue to support the Medicare program is placed in a trust fund. Currently, the trust fund is projected to be solvent until 2024 (Board of Trustees 2011). The Board of Trustees advises the Congress about the fiscal status of the program each year.

Medicare is a good example of a federal **entitlement** program. In an entitlement program, eligible persons have a guarantee to a defined set of benefits identified in the law. Once in place, entitlement benefits are difficult to change (see the discussion of public vs. private policy in Chapter 1). To control cost growth, the usual strategy has been to control the growth in reimbursement to providers. We will discuss several examples of payment strategies that have been developed in Medicare to incentivize more efficient care. Medicare (and Medicaid) is also an example of **social insurance**. Social insurance means that economic resources are transferred from one group to another group to meet a defined social need, in this case health care. Taxes are paid by working Americans to provide health care benefits to nonworking Americans: the elderly and the permanently disabled. Unlike private health care insurance, those who pay the premiums (in this case, taxes) are not typically eligible for program benefits.

Medicare policy (e.g., eligibility and program benefits) is established by congressional legislation. Changes in the policy structure of Medicare require changes in the statute and cannot be made administratively. However, many procedures that implement the policy are developed administratively. As an entitlement program, Medicare differs from Medicaid in one important aspect. Everyone who meets the eligibility requirements, regardless of income, can participate in Medicare. In contrast, Medicaid is a means-tested program that limits benefits to people who often have not made regular contributions to the program (e.g., low-income persons, children). The popularity of Medicare as the "third rail" of American politics can be tied to its structure as a "pay as you go" program with guaranteed benefits to those who have made regular contributions to the program over many years.

Medicare procedures (e.g., eligibility, reimbursement), are developed and implemented by the Centers for Medicare and Medicaid Services (CMS). This agency is part of the Department of Health and Human Services. Claims review and processing of eligibility and benefits are performed by private organizations, usually insurance companies, that each provide this service to a defined region of the country. Historically, intermediaries were claims contractors that processed Part A claims, and carriers did the same for Part B claims. CMS is combining these functions into claims review organizations called **Medicare Administrative Contractors** (MACs) (see Figure 8-1) The country is divided into 15 jurisdictions or areas for the purpose of processing Medicare claims. Contractors serve an area, and all therapy claims are processed by the appropriate MAC. MACs also advise therapists about the latest interpretations of the appropriateness and eligibility of therapy services (local coverage decisions).

We are now ready to explore the Medicare program in detail. First, we will explore the eligibility criteria for Medicare. Then, we will examine the benefit packages for Parts A and B. To help us understand the benefits and payment structure of the Medicare program, we will introduce and follow a patient case: Mrs. Miller, a 76-year-old Medicare beneficiary who needs a total hip replacement.

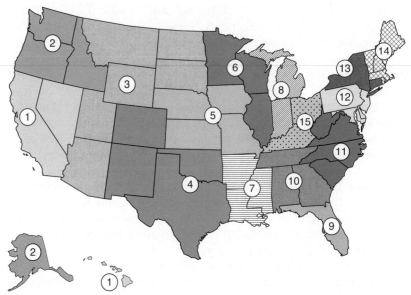

FIGURE 8-1 Medicare Part A and B Medicare Administrative Contractor Jurisdictions

Source: http://www.cms.gov/MedicareContractingReform/Downloads/Primary_AB_MAC_Jurisdictions_MAP.pdf. Accessed on February 16, 2012.

Medicare Eligibility

Program eligibility is primarily determined by meeting the criteria of Medicare Part A. Persons participating in both Parts A and B are also eligible to choose a Medicare Advantage plan in place of their Parts A and B traditional benefits. The Part D prescription drug benefit is available to original Medicare or Medicare Advantage beneficiaries through the purchase of a stand-alone plan or through a Medicare Advantage plan that includes a prescription drug benefit.

Part A Eligibility

Eligibility for Medicare Part A benefits is based on a record of payroll or premium contributions, age, marital status, or the presence of permanent disability. Most individuals qualify based on age (currently age 65) and a record of payroll contributions into the program for forty quarters (10 years). After paying into the program for 10 years, an individual is vested and eligible for benefits after reaching the minimum eligibility age. Spouses of vested Medicare beneficiaries are also eligible for Medicare at age 65. No monthly premium is required of vested beneficiaries or their spouses for participation in the Part A program.

Persons who are not vested in the program can receive Medicare benefits after reaching age 65 and agreeing to pay a monthly premium (see Table 8-3). Individuals younger than age 65 are eligible for Medicare benefits if they have been declared permanently disabled by the Social Security Administration for 24 months (see Chapter 4), have end-stage renal disease, or have amyotrophic lateral sclerosis.

Part B Eligibility

Persons who are eligible for premium-free Medicare Part A (vested persons over age 65, spouses of vested beneficiaries, persons with permanent disabilities, and persons younger than age 65 with end-stage renal disease) are automatically eligible for Part B Medicare.

Part B Medicare is an optional benefit package. Most people enroll in Medicare Part B when they become eligible for Medicare Part A (see Table 8-1). A person who declines Medicare Part B is eligible to enroll at a later date during special enrollment periods at a higher cost. About 25 percent of Medicare Part B program costs are paid by enrollees. Monthly Medicare Part B premiums vary by annual income and by the addition

Table 8-2 2012 Medicare Part B Monthly Premiums

If annual income is:			
Individual Tax Return	Joint Tax Return	Monthly Premium	Premium with Prescription Drug
<$85,000	<170,000	$99.90	$99.90
$85,000–$107,000	$170,000–$214,000	$139.90	$151.50
$107,001–$160,000	$214,001–$320,000	$199.80	$229.70
$160,001–$214,000	$320,001–$428,000	$259.70	$307.80
>$214,001	>$428,000	$319.70	$286.20

Source: Monthly Medicare Premiums for 2012. Retrieved from http://www.socialsecurity.gov/pubs/10536.html (accessed February 17, 2012).

of a prescription drug benefit (see Table 8-2). This is usually deducted automatically from Social Security checks. There is a $140 annual Part B deductible and a 20 percent co-insurance rate on Part B benefits beginning each January 1.

ORIGINAL MEDICARE

Part A: Hospital Insurance

Benefits

Table 8-3 outlines the three basic benefits included in Medicare Part A: inpatient hospital care, short-term skilled nursing facility care, and home health care/hospice. These benefits include room and board (hospital and skilled nursing facility) and **medically necessary**

Table 8-3 2012 Medicare Part A Benefits/Beneficiary Costs

A. Monthly Premiums: $0 for vested individuals
 $248 for persons with 30–39 quarters of payroll contributions
 $451 for persons with < 30 quarters of payroll contributions
B. Hospital Inpatient Coverage
 1. Deductible: $1,156
 2. Ninety days of "medically necessary" care per benefit period
  a. Co-insurance
   1. First 60 days: $0
   2. Day 61–90: $289 per day
 3. Sixty lifetime reserve days
  a. Co-insurance: $578 per day
C. Skilled Nursing Facility Coverage
 1. Deductible: $0
 2. One hundred days of post-hospital care
  a. Co-insurance
   1. First 20 days: $0
   2. Day 21 to 100: $144.50 per day
D. Home Health Care/Hospice
 1. No deductible or co-payment

Source: Medicare Premium and Co-Insurance Rates for 2012. Accessed at https://questions.medicare.gov/app/answers/detail/a_id/2309/~/medicare-premiums-and-coinsurance-rates-for-2012 on February 17, 2012.

professional services provided by the institution. Medically necessary services, including physical therapy and occupational therapy, must meet program requirements (see the Medicare and Therapy Services section) and be authorized by a provider with physician status (e.g., a medical or osteopathic physician). Although vested beneficiaries do not pay a monthly premium, the most commonly used Part A benefits are not free. Beneficiary out-of-pocket costs include a deductible (hospital care) and daily co-insurance fee (after 60 days of hospital care and 20 days of skilled nursing facility care).

Benefit Period

The Part A deductible and co-insurance is calculated using a **benefit period**. Unlike most forms of private health insurance, Medicare does not determine deductibles and co-insurance payments for Part A benefits based on an annual period. Instead, a single episode of Part A benefits (and its associated deductible and benefits) is defined as the time from admission to the hospital until the patient is out of a hospital or skilled nursing facility for 60 days. All Part A benefits during this period are covered by one deductible and co-insurance fee (including the case of a readmission). Conversely, a beneficiary who needs 2 episodes of Part A benefits in the same calendar year that are more than sixty days apart owes 2 deductibles and the appropriate co-insurance fee for each episode of care. This scenario would typically not occur in the private health insurance market.

In our hypothetical example, consider the implications of the benefit period on the potential cost of care to be paid by Mrs. Miller. She enters the hospital for a total hip replacement. She pays the initial $1,156 in charges as her deductible. Scenarios A and B in Case 8-1 illustrate the effect of the benefit period in calculating Medicare Part A benefits. Both scenarios describe another hospital admission for a complication related to her total hip replacement. In scenario A, Mrs. Miller owes nothing for the care because it occurred within 60 days of the discharge from the skilled nursing facility (i.e., the same benefit period). In scenario B, Mrs. Miller is required to pay another deductible expense for the care because it occurred after the first benefit period expired. Even though this problem may have occurred within the same calendar year, Mrs. Miller needs to pay an additional $1,156 deductible for this hospital stay.

Case Example 8-1 Medicare Part A Benefit Period

Mrs. Miller is admitted to the hospital for a total hip replacement. She spends 4 days in the hospital and another 20 days in a skilled nursing facility receiving nursing care, physical therapy, and occupational therapy services.

Out-of-Pocket Cost to Mrs. Miller

Deductible:	$1,156
Co-Insurance:	$0
Total:	$1,156

Ten days after returning home, Mrs. Miller develops hip pain due to a dislocation and reenters the hospital for a five-day inpatient stay. She returns home after being discharged from the hospital.

Out-of-Pocket Cost to Mrs. Miller

Deductible:	$0
Co-Insurance:	$0
Total:	$0

OR

Three months after returning home, Mrs. Miller falls and dislocates her hip joint. She reenters the hospital for a five-day inpatient stay. She returns home after being discharged from the hospital.

Out-of-Pocket Cost to Mrs. Miller

Deductible:	$1,156
Co-Insurance:	$0
Total:	$1,156

Part A Payment Structures

From the time Medicare was established until 1983, Part A providers were paid based on the costs they could reasonably justify when caring for Medicare beneficiaries. The intent was to reimburse providers a fee for each service received by a beneficiary based on "reasonable and necessary" charges in their region. This method of payment, common to private insurance plans at the time, was known as **cost-based reimbursement**. Every provider was required to produce a detailed cost report to Medicare on the direct and indirect costs of caring for beneficiaries for the year. This retrospective system of payment provided few incentives for providers to be efficient when delivering services. As long as costs could be documented and were allowed by Medicare, providers had every incentive to provide as much care as possible and expect government payment.

Beginning with hospitals in 1983 and now applied to all Part A providers, Medicare has phased out cost-based reimbursement in favor of various forms of **prospective payment**. Cost reports are still required as an accounting report, but payment is determined based on sets of predetermined criteria. Prospective payment identifies payment amounts up-front based on sets of patient characteristics, service needs, and facility characteristics determined at the time of admission to, during, or at discharge from a Part A service. These mechanisms are all examples of case-based payment systems. Instead of being paid for each individual service (e.g., nursing, physical therapy) and procedure (e.g., ADL training) based on individual facility costs, providers are paid an all-inclusive rate for a day or multiple days (an episode) of care. We discussed the incentives of these systems in Chapter 5. Occupational therapists and physical therapists continue to record individual patient visits and units of service for cost reports and for internal management purposes. Each payment system does differ by the unit of service, (e.g., per day or per episode). Let's now explore the four Part A benefits: acute and long-term care hospital, skilled nursing facility, home health, and inpatient rehabilitation hospital.

Acute and Long-Term Care Hospital Benefit

Medicare Part A provides a short-stay, acute hospitalization benefit to care for acute illnesses, diseases, or for surgical care. In most cases, the length of stay for a beneficiary in a hospital is not more than a few days. Recovery after a Part A hospitalization stay typically occurs in a skilled nursing facility, at home with services provided through a home health agency, or in an inpatient rehabilitation facility. Medicare Part A beneficiaries with complex medical conditions who require longer-term (on average more than 25 days) recovery periods using inpatient hospitalization services such as respiratory therapy, physical therapy, or occupational therapy can receive services in a special class of hospital—the long-term care hospital (LTACH). Typically, these patients have cardiovascular and pulmonary diseases and are not infrequently discharged from an acute hospital intensive or critical care unit directly to a LTACH. If the discharge is directly from an acute hospital or within 60 days of an inpatient hospital stay, no new deductible is charged for that benefit period (co-insurance charges for the benefit period related to the acute hospital stay may apply).

Hospital Prospective Payment

In 1983, the federal government initiated prospective payment for inpatient hospital stays by classifying patients into groups that could predict resource utilization. This system of patient classification is called **case mix adjustment**. Several patient characteristics are used to determine which group a patient should be assigned to: diagnosis, surgery, patient age, patient sex, and discharge destination. Using these criteria, the Centers for Medicare and Medicaid Services has established 751 Medical Severity Diagnosis-Related Groups, or MS-DRGs, in order to classify patients at discharge from the hospital into payment groups (Centers for Medicare and Medicaid Services 2011a). Classification into an MS-DRG is based on the primary diagnosis, up to eight comorbid conditions, and up to six procedures received by the patient during the acute hospital stay. A different (but similar methodology) system is used for long-term care hospitals: the Medical Severity–Long–Term Care–Diagnosis-Related Groups or MS-LTC-DRGs. The top ten DRGs for hospitals in 2010 are listed in Table 8-4. Reimbursement amounts for each group are

Table 8-4 Top Ten Medical Severity Diagnosis-Related Groups in the United States (2010)

1. Major Lower Limb Joint Replacement
2. Major Sepsis
3. Psychoses
4. Esophagitis, Gastritis, and Digestive Diseases
5. Heart Failure with Major Complications
6. Heart Failure without Major Complications
7. Kidney and Urinary Tract Infections
8. Pneumonia
9. Syncope
10. Chest Pain

Source: Medicare Short Stay Hospital DRGs by Discharges. Fiscal Year 2010. Accessed at http://www.cms.gov /DataCompendium/13_2011_Data_Compendium.asp#TopOfPage on February 28, 2012.

established based on cost reporting and billing information collected by CMS. DRG payments are intended to be inclusive of all direct and indirect hospital costs. Hospitals can receive other payments for patients who justifiably exceed day or cost limits and if the hospital treats a "disproportionate share" of low-income Medicare beneficiaries.

Payment to a hospital for a Part A stay is determined by multiplying a national standardized rate (approximately $5,200 for an MS-DRG and $40,000 for an MS-LTC-DRG in 2012) by a DRG relative weight that accounts for the severity of the condition and the cost of care. For example, the surgical MS-DRG 470-Major Joint Replacement or Reattachment of Lower Extremity is listed with a relative weight of 2.0866. The actual payment is further modified by adjusting the labor portion of the standardized rate for local conditions and any "add-on" payments for treating a large number of poor Medicare beneficiaries or if the facility is a teaching hospital. The average Part A hospital payment in 2010 was $10,737 ($9,466 covered by Medicare, $576 covered by another third-party payer, and $746 by the beneficiary).

When introduced in the 1980s, the effect of hospital prospective payments on the health care system was dramatic. The DRG cost-control mechanism resulted in a sharp reduction in inpatient hospital utilization (Menke et al. 1998; Takemura and Beck 1999; Whetsell 1999). Patients spent fewer days in the hospital and received fewer services than in the previous cost-based reimbursement environment. The effect of the DRG system on occupational therapists and physical therapists, however, was positive. Patients needed rehabilitation services to move out of inpatient hospitals. In addition, need for rehabilitation qualified patients for a recuperative stay in a skilled nursing facility, inpatient rehabilitation facility, or at home. More care that was originally provided in hospitals was transferred to skilled nursing facilities and home health agencies. The demand for therapists increased.

The reorganization of care from inpatient hospital care to subacute or SNF care caused Congress to act to limit the ability of providers to unfairly profit from an early patient discharge from the hospital to an SNF or home health care. In 1997, Congress established a "transfer rule" that reduces the DRG payment to the acute hospital for patients who are discharged more than 1 day earlier than the average for the 10 DRGS with the highest rate of acute hospital transfers to post-acute care (Gilman et al. 2000).

SKILLED NURSING FACILITY BENEFIT   The skilled nursing facility (SNF) benefit under Medicare Part A provides short-term nursing and skilled rehabilitation services (up to 100 days) in a Medicare-certified unit per benefit period that is related to the recovery from an acute hospital stay. Medicare does not pay for long-term institutionalization, nor can beneficiaries access the SNF directly without a hospital stay. Medicare-certified skilled nursing facility units are located both in free standing nursing homes and in hospitals. Hospital units are commonly referred to as subacute, swing bed, transitional care, or restorative care units (see Chapter 11). Although they are physically within an acute care hospital, these units are licensed as skilled nursing facility beds, and Medicare patients receiving unit services are covered by the SNF benefit. Prior to admission to a SNF unit, a patient must have had at least a 3-day stay in a hospital during the preceding 30 days and be certified for admission to the SNF by a physician.

Each Medicare beneficiary who receives services in a skilled nursing facility is assessed and reassessed using a standardized examination set called the *Resident Assessment Instrument,* or RAI (Centers for Medicare and Medicaid Services 2011c). The RAI consists of three parts: the Minimum Data Set (MDS), the Care Areas Assessment, and the RAI utilization guidelines (Centers for Medicare and Medicaid Services 2011c). The MDS provides a comprehensive description of the status and problems being experienced by the nursing home resident. Identified problems or changes in patient function trigger a process called Care Areas Assessment or CAAs. CAAs are a structured process for the care team to identify, analyze, address, and follow up on patient problems. They are most commonly implemented when patients are long-term residents of a skilled nursing facility, and they will be explained in Chapter 9 with Medicaid. The Utilization Guidelines provide information about the implementation of the RAI. The Resident Assessment Instrument represents a significant improvement in the coordination and planning of care for Medicare beneficiaries in skilled nursing facilities and has been applied internationally. Occupational and physical therapists will be involved with the RAI on a daily basis. In this next section, we will introduce the Minimum Data Set, which is used for both patient care planning and Part A reimbursement.

MINIMUM DATA SET (MDS)   The Minimum Data Set is a "core set of screening, clinical and functional status elements, including common definitions and coding categories, which forms the foundation of the comprehensive assessment for all residents of long-term care facilities certified to participate in Medicare or Medicaid." (Centers for Medicare and Medicaid Services 2011c). The MDS is required for any resident staying in a facility greater than 14 days. MDS assessment is coordinated by a registered nurse with input from a variety of professionals, including physical and occupational therapists. A list of the major sections of the MDS can be found in Table 8-5. In order to conduct the assessment, the resident must be observed, communicated with, and examined by staff over several days.

The schedule of MDS assessment depends on the anticipated length of stay and reason for the beneficiary's stay. Persons in the facility for a short-term stay related to a hospital admission (Part A benefit) such as rehabilitation for a total hip replacement, are

---

Table 8-5 Major Data Sections for Minimum Data Set Version 3.0

A. Identification Information
B. Hearing, Speech, and Vision
C. Cognitive Patterns
D. Mood
E. Behavior
F. Preferences for Customary Routine and Activities
G. Functional Status
H. Bladder and Bowel
I. Active Disease Diagnoses
J. Health Conditions
K. Swallowing/Nutritional Status
L. Oral/Dental status
M. Skin Condition
N. Medications
O. Special Treatments and Procedures
P. Restraints
Q. Participation in Assessment and Goal Setting
R. Care Area Assessment Summary

Source: Center for Medicare and Medicaid Services. 2011. RAI Version 3.0 Manual. Accessed at https://www .cms.gov/NursingHomeQualityInits/20_MDS30RAIManual.asp#TopOfPage on February 22, 2012.

assessed by day 5, 14, 30, 60, and 90 of the stay. This information is used to set reimbursement rates for their stay (see Resource Utilization Group payment). For persons entering an SNF not under Medicare Part A (OBRA admission; see Chapter 9 on Medicaid), the MDS is administered at admission, quarterly, annually, and when a significant change in patient status occurs during a skilled nursing facility stay.

OTHER MEDICARE REQUIRED ASSESSMENTS (OMRA)   There are three other types of assessments related to therapy services that are components of the RAI. These therapy-intensity assessments are used to gather information for proper placement of patients into payment groups (RUGS) when their therapy needs change outside the period of the standard assessments. The Start of Therapy Other Medicare Required Assessment (SOT-OMRA) is an optional assessment that is used to capture the intensity of therapy services to assure the appropriate payment rate in the SNF payment system. The End of Therapy Other Medicare Required Assessments (EOT-OMRA) is a required report for patients who have been classified into the rehabilitation services payment groups in order to determine a new payment category. The Change of Therapy Other Medicare Required Assessment (COT-OMRA) is used to document a change in the number or intensity of therapy services that require a reclassification of a continuing therapy patient into a new payment category. OMRAs are shorter assessments than the standard assessments.

SKILLED NURSING FACILITY PROSPECTIVE PAYMENT   Skilled nursing facility (SNF) prospective payment is based on the classification of persons residing in nursing homes into Resource Utilization Groups (RUGs-IV) (Centers for Medicare and Medicaid Services 2011b). The determination of the RUGs class for a person is based on the results of the MDS assessment, the medical diagnosis, documented therapist contact time, nursing restorative interventions, and certain behavioral observations. MDS assessment for a Part A beneficiary is regularly completed by SNF staff for a 5-day, 14-day, 30-day, 60-day, and 90-day report on patient status. The 5-day assessment will set the daily payment rate for days 1–14, the day-14 assessment will set the per diem rate for days 15–30, and so on. Prospective payment for skilled nursing facility care is based on the calculation of a *per diem* amount based on a federal standard base rate that is adjusted by a conversion factor based on Resource Utilization Group classification and a cost of living factor for local wage conditions. An example is provided later in this chapter. These payments are updated each year for inflation and to control cost growth of the program. The intent of the RUGs system is to identify the service needs of persons in skilled nursing facilities and to pay an all-inclusive payment to providers for this care. There are 66 Resource Utilization Groups in 1 Resource Utilization Groups in 1 of of 8 categories: rehabilitation plus extensive services, rehabilitation, extensive services, special care, clinically complex, impaired cognition, behavior problems, and reduced physical function. The rehabilitation categories are of most interest to occupational and physical therapists working in skilled nursing facilities. Table 8-6 describes the rehabilitation subcategories of the RUGs-III classification system. Assignment into specific RUGs payment groups within these categories is performed using an ADL index based on patient need for assistance with bed mobility, transfers, eating, and toilet use. The calculation of therapy intensity is important to an accurate classification of the patient into an appropriate rehabilitation RUGs subcategory. Therapy intensity is determined by examining a "look-back period" of the prior five to seven days of stay in the skilled nursing facility and recording the number of therapy services (e.g., PT, OT, or speech) and the minutes of therapy that the patient received. The number of therapy minutes assigned to a patient is also affected by the mode of therapy delivery: individual, concurrent, or group. All minutes of individual therapy are assigned to the patient. Concurrent therapy is the simultaneous treatment by the therapist of two patients who are not performing the same activities. In this case, the number of minutes assigned to each patient for the session is halved. Group therapy is four patients performing the same therapy activity. In this case, the number of minutes is divided by four and assigned to each patient equally for the session. Group therapy minutes cannot exceed 25 percent of all patient minutes reported for RUGs classification. Therapy minutes do not include the initial evaluation, documentation time, or nonskilled services. Patient rest time is not counted, but aide set-up time is counted toward the therapy minutes.

Table 8-6 Resource Utilization Groups: Rehabilitation Subcategories

Ultra High Rehabilitation Plus Extensive Services	Ultra High Rehabilitation
Very High Rehabilitation Plus Extensive Services	Very High Rehabilitation
High Rehabilitation Plus Extensive Services	High Rehabilitation
Medium Rehabilitation Plus Extensive Services	Medium Rehabilitation
Low Rehabilitation Plus Extensive Services	Low Rehabilitation

Extensive services include tracheostomy care, ventilator, or respirator use; isolation for infectious organisms; and an ADL score of at least 2.

Ultra High rehabilitation services is a minimum of 720 minutes of therapy each week that includes at least 2 disciplines, one of which is at least 5 days per week and the other discipline is at least 3 days per week.

Very High rehabilitation services are at least 500 minutes of therapy each week that includes services from 1 discipline for 5 days per week.

High rehabilitation is at least 325 minutes of therapy each week that includes 1 discipline for 5 days per week.

Medium rehabilitation is at least 150 minutes of therapy each week on 5 days from any combination of physical therapy, occupational therapy, and speech/language pathology.

Low rehabilitation is 45 minutes per week of skilled therapy services on 3 days from any combination of 3 disciplines and 6 days per week of restorative nursing.

Source: Final Rule for Medicare PPS and Consolidated Billing for SNFs for FY 2010 and MDS 3.0. Federal Register, August 11, 2009. Accessed at http://edocket.access.gpo.gov/2009/pdf/E9-18662.pdf on February 28, 2012.

Since the intensity of services such as rehabilitation therapy can change based on the patient's status and response to treatment, the RUGs system is designed to change payment groups consistent with these changes during the Part A stay. This requires the therapists to document interventions and the time of therapy closely in order to accurately determine the appropriate daily payment rate.

Home Health Care Benefit

Patients qualify for the Part A home health care benefit based on home confinement and the need for skilled nursing and/or rehabilitation services, including physical therapy and occupational therapy, in order to recover after an acute hospital stay. Home health care therapy is provided in the patient's residence, which need not be an institutional setting. Physician certification of home confinement after a face-to-face visit is necessary. In general, patients may not leave the home except for necessary medical treatments (e.g., a physician visit) or occasional, community outings (e.g., attending a church service). Home health care services are ordered by a physician, who is required to recertify the continued need for skilled care every 62 days.

Patients may qualify for Medicare reimbursement of home health care as a Part A benefit or a Part B benefit. Those who are enrolled in both Part A and Part B Medicare are entitled to 100 visits of home health care if they meet the general eligibility criteria and have had a 3-day hospital stay within the prior 14 days. If they no longer qualify for Part A home health (e.g., exceed the 100-visit limit or are no longer homebound), a beneficiary is able to continue necessary home health care though Part B Medicare financing.

Everyone receiving home care services is evaluated using a tool called the Outcome and Assessment Information Set, or OASIS-C (Centers for Medicare and Medicaid Services 2011e). OASIS assesses and describes the care needs of persons receiving home health care and serves as the primary data set used to determine home health prospective payment. The OASIS can be completed by a physical therapist or occupational therapist. The initial assessment must be completed within five days of referral for care and can only be completed by a physical therapist. An updated or discharge OASIS can be completed by an occupational therapist or physical therapist. There are several forms of the

Table 8-7 Outcome Assessment and Information Set (OASIS-C) Major Sections

A. Patient History and Diagnosis
B. Living Arrangements
C. Sensory Status
D. Integumentary Status
E. Respiratory Status
F. Cardiac Status
G. Elimination Status
H. Neuro/Emotional/Behavioral Status
I. ADL/IADLs
J. Medications
K. Care Management
L. Therapy Need and Plan of Care
M. Emergent Care

Source: Center for Medicare and Medicaid Services. 2011 OASIS-C Manual. Outcome Assessment and Information Set. Start of Care Version. Accessed at http://www.cms.hhs.gov/HomeHealthQualityInits/12 _HHQIOASISDataSet.asp#TopOfPage on February 16, 2012.

OASIS survey: start of care and resumption of care, follow up, transfer to inpatient facility, discharge, and death at home. OASIS collects information in a checklist format about patient demographics, history, diagnosis, living arrangements, social support, patient attributes (e.g., sensation and integument), activities of daily living performance, medications, equipment, and therapy need (see Table 8-7). Therapy need in OASIS-C is the anticipated number of combined therapy visits that are expected to be completed for the proper care of the patient in consultation with the physician. OASIS is to be completed within 5 days of the start of a home health care episode, between day 55 and 60 of a continuing episode, and within 2 days of the completion of a home health care episode. Data are reported to the Centers for Medicare and Medicaid Services through state contacts on a monthly basis.

In addition to the OASIS-C, Medicare requires additional patient assessments for therapist services. A functional assessment of basic activities of daily living (ADLs), such as bathing, walking, and use of assistive devices, needs to be documented in the clinical record at admission and at least every 30 days of treatment. A functional assessment is also required on the 13th and 19th visits of any therapy discipline by all involved therapists to compare the results of a functional assessment to prior assessments and note the progress or lack of progress toward goals. The plan of care should be reviewed at this point, adjusted, and a new plan of care certified as indicated. The purpose of these assessments is to document the rehabilitation potential and progress toward goals of the patient as a result of the therapy intervention. Failure to complete the assessments as defined would result in a denial of payment. A patient who does not meet the definition of skilled therapy services (see Medicare and Therapy Services section) would not qualify for therapy services under the Part A home health benefit.

Hospice Benefit

Hospice services are provided to Medicare beneficiaries who select this treatment option and have been diagnosed with a terminal illness. Core hospice services identified by Medicare for coverage are nursing, social services, medicine, and counseling. Physical therapy and occupational therapy are among the optional hospice benefits.

Home Health Agency Prospective Payment

Home health agency prospective payment was implemented in 2000 (Centers for Medicare and Medicaid Services 2007d). Unlike skilled nursing facilities, home health agencies are paid using a 60-day episode of care. This payment is intended to cover all home health services (including physical therapy and occupational therapy) received by the beneficiary during this period of care. Durable medical equipment is excluded from this payment mechanism and is paid using a fee schedule (see Part B reimbursement). Using historical claims and cost report data, CMS determines a "standardized prospective payment rate" for each episode of care annually. In 2012, this rate was $2,138.52 per episode of care (Centers for Medicare and Medicaid Services 2011). Similar to the SNF prospective payment formula, this rate is adjusted for individual patient needs and the geographic differences in costs of care delivery.

The effect of individual patient needs on provider reimbursement is based on the determination of a Home Health Resource Group (HHRG) classification. Data for HHRG classification are generated from the OASIS completed at admission and a record of the number of therapy visits received by the beneficiary. These data determine three domains used to classify the patient into 1 of 153 HHRGs. These domains are clinical severity factors, functional severity factors, and services utilization factors. Similar to RUGs, each HHRG is assigned a case mix weight factor that reflects the intensity of services or health problems experienced by the beneficiary. This case mix factor is used in combination with a local wage condition factor to determine the prospective payment rate. In 2011, CMS promulgated new regulations and payment incentives for reimbursement of therapy services. The regulations included requirements for therapist evaluations and assessments (discussed earlier in this chapter). Case mix weights were adjusted to incentivize episodes of care with fewer therapist visits.

Inpatient Rehabilitation Facility Benefit

The inpatient rehabilitation facility (IRF) benefit provides for intensive and coordinated therapy services in a rehabilitation hospital setting. Patients must require at least three hours of therapy for at least five days per week to qualify for this benefit. This requirement is termed the "three-hour rule." The facility must also meet the "60 percent rule" to participate in this benefit. The 60 percent rule states that at least 60 percent of the facility's patients must be from certain patient diagnosis categories (Medicare Payment Advisory Commission 2009). The intent of the rule is to prevent overutilization of therapy for cases that do not require this level of therapy. A list of the diagnoses can be found in Table 8-8. A review of this list will provide the reader with a good sense of the patient problems seen in this setting.

Each Medicare beneficiary is evaluated using a standard assessment tool called the Inpatient Rehabilitation Facility–Patient Assessment Instrument (IRF-PAI) (Centers for Medicare and Medcaid Services, 2011) (see Table 8-9). The instrument should be completed within three days of admission and seven days of discharge from inpatient rehabilitation. All sections of the instrument are required to be completed except the Medical Needs and Quality Indicator sections. The central evaluation piece of the IRF-PAI is the Functional Independence Measure (the FIM™). This tool was widely used by inpatient rehabilitation facilities prior to the development of the IRF-PAI.

Table 8-8 Patient Diagnoses That Comprise the 60 percent Rule for Inpatient Rehabilitation Facilities

Stroke
Spinal Cord Injury
Congenital Deformity
Amputation
Major Multiple Trauma
Fracture of the Femur
Brain Injury
Polyarthritis, Including Rheumatoid Arthritis
Neurological Disorders Including Multiple Sclerosis, Motor Neuron Disease, Polyneuropathy, Muscular Dystrophy, and Parkinson's Disease
Burns

Source: Medicare Payment Advisory Commission. Rehabilitation facilities (inpatient) payment system. 2008. Retrieved from http://www.medpac.gov/documents/MedPAC_Payment_Basics_08_IRF.pdf (accessed February 28, 2012).

Table 8-9 Inpatient Rehabilitation Facility–Patient Assessment Instrument Major Sections

Background and Demographic Information

Medical Information

Medical Needs

Functional Modifiers

Functional Independence Measure Score

Discharge Information

Quality Indicators: Respiratory Status, Pain, Pressure Sores, Safety

Source: Center for Medicare and Medicaid Services. Inpatient Rehabilitation Facility-Patient Assessment Instrument. Accessed at http://www.cms.hhs.gov/InpatientRehabFacPPS/downloads/CMS-100036.pdf on February 28, 2012.

Inpatient Rehabilitation Facility Prospective Payment

The third Part A prospective payment system is for inpatient rehabilitation facilities. The structure of the system is similar to that used for hospitals and home health agencies. Each patient is evaluated using the Inpatient Rehabilitation Facility–Patient Assessment Instrument (IRF-PAI) (Centers for Medicare and Medicaid Services 2011e). Information from the IRF-PAI, the medical diagnosis, and comorbidities is used to classify patients into 95 Case Mix Groups (CMGs) that are used for payment purposes (Centers for Medicare and Medicaid Services 2011f). Each Case Mix Group is assigned a weight that is multiplied by a national standard payment conversion factor. In 2012, this amount was $14,109. The actual weight is tiered by the presence or absence of patient comorbid conditions. Like hospitals and home health agencies, this is a per-episode payment. As in the examples of hospitals, skilled nursing facilities, and home health agencies, final facility payment is adjusted for local wage conditions and certain outlier characteristics.

Case Example of a Part A Prospective Payment System Calculation

Each of the Part A prospective payment systems utilizes a common method to derive a payment to a provider for beneficiary services. The payment systems share the following characteristics:

- Use of a standardized patient assessment instrument
- Classification of patients into homogeneous groups based on the results of the assessment (case mix adjustment)
- Adjusting a standardized payment amount by a case mix adjustment weight factor and certain other factors (e.g., local wage conditions)
- Consolidated or all-service inclusive billing

The results of most of these systems is a per-episode payment to the facility. The skilled nursing facility payment is a per-day, not per-episode payment. The SNF RUGs system provides a common and useful example to see the application of these systems. Table 8-10 illustrates an example from the SNF PPS.

In this example, the RUX Resource Utilization Group has been selected. The RUX group is in the Rehabilitation Plus Extensive Services category and would be used for a beneficiary requiring one of the extensive services and the most intensive therapy services in a skilled nursing facility. The baseline for the per diem rate is an unadjusted federal rate, either for an urban facility or a rural facility. In this example, an urban facility has been selected. Four components of the base rate are identified: nursing case mix, therapy case mix, therapy non-case mix, and non–case mix. The case mix costs vary by RUGs group. No therapy case-mix or non-case-mix cost is included in RUGs that do not include a rehabilitation service. The unadjusted per diem federal rate is $335.62. As can be seen in the example, the unadjusted rates are then updated in a two-step process. First, the RUGs conversion rate is applied to the case mix value. In this example, the RUX conversion factor is 1.9 for nursing case mix and 2.25 for therapy case mix. This changes the per diem rate to $675.31.

Table 8-10 SNF Prospective Payment: Federal Per Diem Rate Calculations for RUX

Unadjusted Federal Per Diem Rate (Urban)- $335.62	
Nursing case mix: $160.62	Therapy case mix: $120.99
Therapy non-case mix: $15.94	Non-case mix: $81.97

RUX Conversion
Nursing case mix (1.9): $305.18
Therapy case mix (2.25): $272.23
Non-case mix: $97.91
Total per diem rate: $675.31

Wage Conditions Adjustment
Total labor-related component: $472.72
Adjusted for Omaha: $446.91 (× 0.9454)
Adjusted for San Francisco: $734.09 (× 1.5529)
Total non-labor-related component: $202.59
Total per diem rate in Omaha: $649.50
Total per diem rate in San Francisco: $936.68

Source: Center for Medicare and Medicaid Services. Medicare Program. Prospective Payment System and Consolidated Billing for Skilled Nursing Facilities-Final Rule (73 FR 46415). Federal Register. CMS-1534-F. Accessed at http://edocket.access.gpo.gov/2008/e8-17948.htm on March 2, 2012.

This higher payment reflects the greater service needs of these beneficiaries. The second step is to adjust the rate for local cost of living conditions, specifically labor costs. To do so, the labor portion (about 70%) of the per diem rate is multiplied by a conversion factor. In this example, the Omaha conversion factor is .9454 and the San Francisco conversion factor is 1.5529. As can be seen, this results in a final per diem rate that is lower in Omaha than in San Francisco. This difference reflects the cost of living in these two communities.

Part B: Supplementary Medical Insurance (SMI)

Benefits

Medicare Part B pays for most of the costs of health-related professional services, outpatient care, home health care, durable medical equipment, prosthetics, and orthotics. Each beneficiary is responsible for a $140 annual Part B deductible before receiving program benefits and is responsible for a 20 percent co-insurance rate (see Medicare Part B reimbursement). Medicare Part B will pay for therapy services provided in outpatient departments, homes, residential facilities, and, in certain circumstances, other inpatient environments (e.g., skilled nursing facilities).

Provider Types

Medicare Part B regulations define different types of therapy providers. All Medicare Part B provider types are reimbursed using a fee schedule (see Part B reimbursement). Therapy services must meet program requirements (see Medicare and Therapy section), but some of these settings where therapists work have slightly different rules.

OUTPATIENT HOSPITAL PROGRAMS   Hospital outpatient programs (e.g., radiology, rehabilitation, laboratory services) provide a wide range of medically necessary, skilled services to community-dwelling Medicare beneficiaries.

COMPREHENSIVE OUTPATIENT REHABILITATION FACILITY   A comprehensive outpatient rehabilitation facility (CORF) is a multidisciplinary provider that allows a beneficiary to receive multiple rehabilitation services at one location (Centers for Medicare and Medicaid Services 2011h). A CORF consists of at least the following services: physician care, physical therapy, and social services. In addition, occupational therapy, speech/language therapy, respiratory therapy, nursing, prosthetics, and orthotics services can be offered through a CORF.

PHYSICAL THERAPISTS AND OCCUPATIONAL THERAPISTS IN PRIVATE PRACTICE Physical therapists in private practice (PTPP) and occupational therapists in private practice (OTPP) are two other recognized Medicare Part B provider types (Centers for Medicare and Medicaid Services 2011i). In this arrangement, physical and occupational therapists in solo practices, unincorporated partnerships, unincorporated group practices, and physician/nonphysician group practices can be recognized as therapists in private practice. Physical therapists employed in institutional (Part A) environments are not eligible for this classification. They must maintain an independent office with sufficient equipment to practice in order to qualify as a Medicare provider. These therapists apply for Medicare reimbursement through their regional Medicare Administrative Contractor. Certification by Medicare includes a licensure review and an on-site visit of the therapist's office.

Part B Payment Structures

Earlier in this chapter, we reviewed the criteria for the Part B Medicare therapy benefit. Physical therapists and occupational therapists who bill for these services use the Physician Fee Schedule. This is the same billing system used by physicians in outpatient practice. Unlike physician services, a financial limitation has been placed on this benefit. We will discuss the "therapy cap" in this section. The intent of this section is to introduce and discuss the fee schedule and therapy caps.

FEE SCHEDULE The Medicare Part B payment methodology for physical and occupational therapy services is the **Medicare Physician Fee Schedule** (MPFS). A fee schedule is a list of procedures with associated payments. This list of procedures is coded using Current Procedural Terminology, or CPT (American Medical Association 2010). In the case of the MPFS, the payments are determined by a formula that accounts for the costs of providing the service. These costs are determined using a method called the Resource-Based Relative Value Scale, or RBRVS. The fee schedule payment for each procedure can be calculated by the following formula (National Health Policy Forum 2011):

$$Payment = Relative\ Value\ Unit \times Geographic\ Adjustment \times$$
$$Standardized\ Conversion\ Factor$$

Each year, CMS calculates a relative value unit for each procedure. A relative value unit has three components: work value, practice expense, and malpractice expense. Work value represents the technical ability, knowledge, and skill to perform the procedure. Relative value units also include information about the overhead costs necessary to perform the

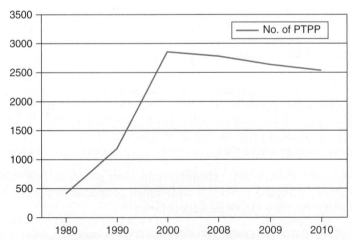

FIGURE 8-2 Number of Outpatient Physical Therapists Participating in Medicare, 1980–2010.

Source: Centers for Medicare and Medicaid Services Data Compendium, 2011 Edition, Table VI.3. Accessed at http://www.cms.gov/DataCompendium/13_2011_Data_Compendium.asp#TopOfPage on February 12, 2012.

Table 8-11 Medicare Part B Reimbursement: Fee Schedule for a Private Practice Therapist

Physical Therapy Evaluation: CPT 97001
2011 National Conversion Factor: $36.08
Work-related RVU: 1.20
 Geographic practice cost index adjustment
  Omaha ($\times$ 1.0) = 1.2
  San Francisco ($\times$ 1.07) = 1.28

Practice expense RVU: 0.91
 Geographic practice cost index adjustment
  Omaha ($\times$ 0.9) = 0.74
  San Francisco ($\times$ 1.36) = 1.24

Malpractice expense RVU: 0.05
 Geographic practice cost index adjustment
  Omaha ($\times$ 0.32) = 0.02
  San Francisco ($\times$ 0.51) = 0.2

Total relative value units (RVU) = 2.16
 Adjusted total for Omaha = 1.96
 Adjusted total for San Francisco = 2.72

Fee schedule payment for 97001
 Standard amount (2.16 $\times$ 36.08) = $77.93
 In Omaha (1.96 $\times$ 36.08) = $70.72
 In San Francisco (2.72 $\times$ 36.08) = $98.14

Source: Physician Fee Schedule Search. Retrieved from http://www.cms.gov/apps/physician-fee-schedule/search/search-criteria.aspx (accessed March 2, 2012).

procedure (practice expense and malpractice). Each of these three components of the RBRVS is adjusted for differences in local costs of providing the procedure to beneficiaries. The sum of the adjusted factors is multiplied by a standard conversion factor or national payment amount to determine the fee schedule payment.

Consider the example in Table 8-11. We will use the Physical Therapy Evaluation CPT code 97001 to illustrate how a fee schedule payment amount is determined. The occupational therapy evaluation CPT Code 97003 has very similar resource value units. In our example, we will consider a non-facility-employed therapist. CMS does set different practice expense RVUs for some facility and non-facility-based procedures. Each relative value unit (RVU) has a factor applied to it that accounts for the work-related and practice-overhead costs associated with the procedure. Each RVU is further adjusted by a local cost index (the GPCI). As can be seen, this adjustment increases the RVU factor in San Francisco as compared to Omaha. The sum total of the adjusted RVUs is multiplied by the standardized conversion factor to determine the fee schedule amount for this CPT code. The fee schedule payment in San Francisco is about one-third more than a physical therapist in Omaha would expect.

Physical therapists and occupational therapists commonly, but not exclusively, use codes in the 97000 series, or Physical Medicine and Rehabilitation section of the CPT system. Some of the therapy codes are procedure-only and some codes are timed codes. For example, evaluation codes are one unit procedure-only codes, irrespective of time spent on the evaluation. Many procedures, (e.g., therapeutic exercise) are timed codes. Timed codes are based on a 15-minute procedure length called a unit of therapy. CMS has further defined treatment units (see Table 8-12). Therapists are to use this table to accurately report units of timed procedure codes.

Table 8-12 Counting Minutes for Timed Codes in 15-Minute Units

< 8 minutes	0 Units
> = 8 minutes through 22 minutes	1 Unit
> = 23 minutes through 37 minutes	2 Units
> = 38 minutes through 52 minutes	3 Units
> = 53 minutes through 67 minutes	4 Units
> = 68 minutes through 82 minutes	5 Units
> = 83 minutes through 97 minutes	6 Units
> = 98 minutes through 112 minutes	7 Units
> = 113 minutes through 127 minutes	8 Units

Source: Center for Medicare and Medicaid Services. Medicare Claims Processing Manual. Chapter 5. Part B Outpatient Rehabilitation and CORF/OPT Services. Accessed at http://www.cms.hhs.gov/manuals/downloads /clm104c05.pdf on May 22, 2007.

Financial Limitations on Medicare Part B Therapy Services

Financial limitations on Part B reimbursement for therapy services have been proposed or have occurred in recent years using three mechanisms: the sustainable growth rate, multiple procedure payment reduction, and the therapy cap. Let's briefly explore each mechanism.

Over the last several years, the proposed new standardized conversion factor for determining MPFS payment has been presented at a much lower payment amount than in the previous year. This is due to a congressional policy called the **sustainable growth rate** or SGR. The sustainable growth rate is a complex formula that examines factors associated with growth in the Medicare Part B program and attempts to adjust for this growth by limiting the overall costs of the Medicare Part B benefit. For example, in 2011, the standardized conversion factor for the MPFS was $36.08. The proposed amount for 2012 was $24.67. As can be seen, if implemented, the effect of this change on the revenue generated by a therapist practice would be considerable. Except for one year in the early 2000s, the SGR has not been implemented, as Congress annually has placed a moratorium on its use.

In 2011, CMS implemented another method to limit reimbursement under Medicare Part B to occupational and physical therapists. This method is called **multiple procedure payment reduction** or MPPR. The full practice expense portion of the fee schedule amount is paid on the highest practice expense procedure on multiple procedure visit days. The MPPR reduces the practice expense portion of subsequent procedures during the same visit by 20–25 percent. The net effect is to reduce the fee schedule payment amount by approximately 7 percent.

For over a decade, there has been a financial limit on the responsibility of Medicare to pay for therapy services provided by physical therapists or occupational therapists in private practice (**therapy cap**) (Centers for Medicare and Medicaid Services 2012). In 2011, the limit was set at $1,880 per beneficiary per year. The $1,880 limit applies separately to occupational therapy but is a combined limit for speech/language pathology and physical therapy. Beneficiaries receiving services in outpatient clinics, at home, and in skilled nursing facilities are affected. In 2012, beneficiaries receiving services in outpatient hospital environments will be subject to the therapy cap. However, the authority to apply the cap to these beneficiaries expires in 2013 so the long-term effect of cap is uncertain.

For some beneficiaries, this "therapy cap" has been burdensome, so Congress has acted periodically to place a moratorium on the therapy caps for most of the period since 2000. More recently, Congress has acted by providing an exceptions process for medically necessary therapy that exceeds the cap. If beneficiaries require medically necessary services beyond the cap, an automatic exception is possible for services costing up to $3,750. Services exceeding that amount require a manual review and exceptions process (pre-authorization).

FUTURE OF MEDICARE PART B THERAPY REIMBURSEMENT The "therapy cap" has been complicated and difficult to administer. On several occasions, a moratorium or an exceptions process has been instituted. The Centers for Medicare and Medicaid Services is currently evaluating the development of a prospective payment system for Medicare B reimbursement of therapy services. If adopted, the basis of a prospective payment system will be similar to the Part A systems: standardized evaluation information, case mix categorization of patients into payment groups, and a form of case rate payment that will include pay-for-performance incentives (RTI International 2011).

Provider Participation

Medicare Part B providers, including physical therapists and occupational therapists in private practice, can elect to accept or not accept the fee schedule amount as payment in full. This is called accepting or declining **Medicare assignment**. A provider that accepts the Medicare assignment agrees to the fee schedule amount as payment in full for the procedure less the deductible and 20 percent co-insurance that is the responsibility of the beneficiary. A provider who does not accept Medicare assignment can still obtain Part B reimbursement but agrees to accept a 5 percent payment reduction from the Medicare fee schedule reimbursement. This provider can charge the beneficiary the full charge for the procedure up to 15 percent limit over the fee schedule amount. The difference between the fee schedule amount and the provider charge along with the deductible and co-insurance is the responsibility of the beneficiary.

Medicare and Therapy Services

Need for rehabilitation is a major criterion that qualifies an individual for a Medicare-funded stay in a skilled nursing facility, services at home through a home health agency, or therapy as an outpatient in a clinic environment. The intent of the benefit is to continue the process of recovery after an acute illness and hospital stay. The Medicare program defines certain requirements for outpatient therapy services that will qualify as meeting a Medicare benefit (Centers for Medicare and Medicaid Services 2011i). These requirements include:

- Therapy services were required by the condition of the beneficiary.
- The beneficiary must be under the care of a physician or nonphysician practitioner.
- A plan of care exists that was designed by the therapist or physician/nonphysician practitioner and is periodically approved by the physician or nonphysician practitioner.
- Services must be provided on an outpatient basis (outpatient benefit only).
- All of the above requirements are certified by a physician or nonphysician practitioner as being met.

Let's explore each of these requirements in detail.

Therapy Services

The Medicare program defines therapy services as physical therapy, occupational therapy, and speech/language pathology. Other professions including recreational therapy, athletic training, kinesiotherapy, and massage therapy are not eligible to participate in the therapy benefit. Therapy services must be provided by licensed providers (not students or aides). Physical therapists, occupational therapists, speech/language pathologists, physical therapist assistants, and occupational therapy assistants can participate in the Medicare program under the therapy benefit. If care is provided by the assistant, then "general supervision" must be provided by the therapist except in the physical therapist in private practice where "direct supervision" is required. Physicians and, if allowed by state law, nonphysician providers, may also participate under the therapy benefit "incident to" services provided in their practice as long as they meet the other program requirements (e.g., documentation).

Table 8-13 Medicare Definition of Skilled Therapy Services

1. The services must be of a level of complexity and sophistication, or the condition of the patient must be of a nature that requires an occupational or physical therapist.
   a. Or the supervision of a therapist, i.e., the services of a physical therapist assistant or occupational therapy assistant.
      1. Services must be provided with proper supervision.
   b. The diagnosis or prognosis of the beneficiary is not enough to demonstrate the need for skilled therapy services.
2. The services must be provided with the expectation that the condition of the patient will improve in a reasonable and generally predictable period of time, the services must be necessary for the establishment of a safe and effective maintenance program or, in the case of a progressive degenerative disease, periodic visits are permitted to make equipment changes or provide services to maximize function.

Source: Center for Medicare and Medicaid Services. Sec. 220.01 Conditions of Coverage for Outpatient Physical Therapy, Occupational Therapy, and Speech-Language Pathology Services. Retrieved from www.cms .hhs.gov/manuals/Downloads/bp102c15.pdf (accessed February 28, 2012).

THERAPY SERVICES ARE REQUIRED BY THE CONDITION OF THE PATIENT Implicit to the purpose of the therapy benefit is the assumption that the care is "reasonable and necessary" based on the needs and condition of the beneficiary. The determination of reasonable and necessary care is based on the plan of care (see below) and a definition of "skilled" physical therapy and occupational therapy. Table 8-13 summarizes the components of the Medicare definition of skilled therapy services. Table 8-14 provides some examples of skilled therapy services. This definition is important since most private insurance companies and the review of Part A claims will utilize this definition in determining the appropriateness of therapy services for reimbursement.

Care that does not meet this definition is nonskilled therapy and is not reimbursed by the Medicare program. Maintenance therapy is one example of nonskilled care. For example, general exercise and routine assistance with activities of daily living and ambulation are not covered by the Medicare benefit. However, a therapist is providing a skilled service if he develops a maintenance therapy program. In addition, therapy services are skilled when provided to a beneficiary with a progressively degenerative condition who needs periodic services to improve or maintain function. A 2012 out-of-court settlement of a lawsuit brought by patients against CMS reinforces that coverage "does not turn on the presence or absence of a beneficiary's potential for improvement from therapy but rather on the beneficiary's need for skilled care" (Lieber 2012).

The condition of the patient is another important determinant of the need for therapy services. For example, diagnosis, age, comorbidities, social status, acuity/stability of the condition, risk to the patient if unskilled care is provided (e.g., a recent fracture), and

Table 8-14 Selected Examples of Medicare Definitions of Skilled Rehabilitation Services

Physical Therapy
1. Evaluation and reevaluations
2. Designing a plan of care
3. Regular assessment of the patient's condition
4. Patient and family instruction
5. Selection of adaptive equipment

Source: Center for Medicare and Medicaid Services. Sec. 220 and 230 Conditions of Coverage for Outpatient Physical Therapy, Occupational Therapy, and Speech-Language Pathology Services. Retrieved from www.cms .hhs.gov/manuals/Downloads/bp102c15.pdf (accessed February 28, 2012).

prognosis are all determinants of the need for therapy services. It is important that the status of these issues be included in the patient record.

COVERAGE DETERMINATIONS   Medicare promulgates specific rules and guidelines on determining the medical necessity and claims procedures for occupational therapy and physical therapy through **coverage determinations**. Coverage determinations may apply to all MAC jurisdictions (national) or may just apply to a specific region (local). CMS maintains a medical coverage database at http://www.cms.gov/center/coverage.asp which provides a searchable forum for providers to locate the rules and guidelines that apply to their practice.

BENEFICIARY MUST BE UNDER THE CARE OF A PHYSICIAN OR NONPHYSICIAN PRACTITIONER   The Medicare program will reimburse for therapy services only if provided with a referral and certification (see below) of a physician or nonphysician provider. This requirement persists irrespective of state law, which may permit a form of direct access to therapy services. A physician is defined as an allopathic physician (M.D.), an osteopathic physician (D.O.), a podiatrist, or an optometrist (low-vision services only). Dentists and chiropractors are not able to refer or certify Medicare beneficiaries for therapy services. A nonphysician practitioner is a physician assistant, nurse practitioner, or clinical nurse specialist. Typically, these providers practice with a practice agreement with a medical physician.

A PLAN OF CARE EXISTS THAT WAS DESIGNED BY THE THERAPIST OR PHYSICIAN/ NONPHYSICIAN PRACTITIONER   A written, active plan of care must be developed and maintained for each Medicare beneficiary. Most commonly, these plans are developed by the therapist upon referral of the physician or nonphysician practitioner. Each plan of care must be signed by the person who developed it and include their professional designation (e.g., PT or OTR). At a minimum, each plan must contain the following elements:

- Patient diagnosis
- Long-term treatment goals
- Type, amount, frequency, and duration of therapy services

The type of therapy includes the procedures to be used. The amount of therapy is the number of procedures or visits per day. The frequency of therapy is the number of visits or encounters per week. The duration of therapy is the number of weeks or sessions over time. Therapists can make minor changes in the plan of care independently (e.g., decreasing the frequency or duration of therapy). Major changes in the plan of care require certification. A change in long-term goals is an example of a major change.

CERTIFICATION   Occupational therapy and physical therapy services under the Medicare program must be periodically reviewed and approved by a physician or nonphysician practitioner as meeting program requirements. Initial certification should occur as soon as possible and within 30 days of the start of the intervention. Therapy services need to be certified at no less than 90-day intervals. Certifications should occur on or before the 90-day period expires (e.g., a change in long-term goals or a change in the patient's condition). If certifications are not present on a timely basis, this is a justification for denial of payment unless extenuating circumstances preventing such certification can be explained with the billing.

SERVICES MUST BE PROVIDED ON AN OUTPATIENT BASIS   This requirement applies only to the Part B benefit. Beneficiaries receiving therapy services under Part A—in the hospital, skilled nursing facility, or home health agency—are not subject to these rules. The Medicare outpatient therapy benefit defines four groups of persons as eligible for therapy services:

1. A provider to outpatients in the patient's home
2. A provider to outpatients who come to the outpatient clinic
3. A provider to inpatients of other institutions
4. A supplier to outpatients in the patient's home or in an outpatient clinic

Therapy services at home and in an outpatient clinic are covered by the Part B therapy benefit. A supplier is a therapist employed by a physician/nonphysician group practice.

Therapy Documentation

The Centers for Medicare and Medicaid Services have identified several reports, with specific expectations for each report, that need to be submitted with a Part B Medicare claim. Documentation rules are important policies to understand since noncompliance will delay or prevent reimbursement for care. There are three types of therapy documentation: evaluation/reevaluation, progress reports, and treatment notes.

EVALUATION/REEVALUATION Therapist evaluation/reevaluation of the Medicare patient should demonstrate the need for therapy services and outline the plan of care. The criteria for need for therapy services and the plan of care have already been discussed. Three comprehensive patient examination tools will provide a comprehensive documentation format needed for physical therapists and occupational therapists:

1. Patient Inquiry by Focus on Therapeutic Outcomes (FOTO)
2. Activity Measure for Post Acute Care (AM-PAC)
3. OPTIMAL by Cedaron by the American Physical Therapy Association

Reevaluations are typically done by therapists when the goals change (may require new certification) or when the patient is nearing discharge from therapy.

PROGRESS REPORTS/TREATMENT NOTES/DISCHARGE SUMMARY Progress reports are required each 30 days or 10 visits, whichever is less. These reports justify the continuing need for therapy care and should also demonstrate improvement in the patient's condition. Physical therapist assistants and occupational therapy assistants may contribute to the progress report for the patient.

Treatment notes are the daily or per-visit records of the patient's condition, the intervention, and responsiveness to therapy. Each treatment note needs to be dated, including the interventions the patient received and the treatment time in minutes for any timed procedure codes and the total treatment time.

A discharge summary is required for each Medicare Part B beneficiary receiving therapy services. At a minimum, the discharge summary should cover the period from the last progress report to discharge, but it could review the progress of the patient over the entire episode of care.

"Incident To" Therapy Procedures

Therapy services are also a Medicare benefit when provided by a physician or nonphysician practitioner who, within the scope of their state practice act, provides care that meets all of the preceding program requirements (see also the "in-office ancillary exception" for physician self-referral). Providers prohibited from participating in the therapy benefit such as athletic trainers, massage therapists, or kinesiotherapists are also prohibited from providing services incident to the physician or nonphysician practitioner care. A therapy assistant may not provide incident-to therapy services in a physician or nonphysician practitioner office.

Medicare Managed Care

Medicare Advantage Plans

The Balanced Budget Act of 1997 created a new part of the program: Part C. Part C reorganized and expanded the Medicare managed care programs and choices for beneficiaries. In 2003, Congress reformed Medicare again by enactment of the Medicare Prescription Drug Improvement and Modernization Act of 2003 (Scully and Roskey 2004). This act represented a shift in policy towards increasing competition by encouraging private companies to contract with the government and providers to provide Medicare benefits vs. the traditional policy of government contracting directly with providers (Gold 2005). The Part C plans were included into what are termed **Medicare Advantage** plans.

Currently, about 25 percent of beneficiaries choose to receive their Medicare benefits through a Medicare Advantage (MA) plan. Beneficiaries pay their Part B premium to the managed care company. Other out-of-pocket costs (e.g., a premium for prescription drugs or co-payments for therapy visits or hospital services) can be imposed. The out-of-pocket costs can be different from traditional Medicare (e.g., co-payments for all hospital days or outpatient therapy services). In return, a Medicare Advantage plan may offer benefits not provided in traditional Medicare (e.g., wellness visits, vision, or dental care). Cooper and Trivedi (2012) report that 11 MA plans offered fitness club memberships. A Medicare Advantage plan beneficiary can also receive an outpatient prescription drug benefit (an MA beneficiary cannot have a Part D prescription drug plan).

There are four types of Medicare Advantage plans (Centers for Medicare and Medicaid Services, 2007):

1. Medicare health maintenance organizations (HMOs)
2. Medicare preferred provider organizations (PPOs)
3. Private fee-for-service plans
4. Medicare Special Needs Plans

Medicare health maintenance organizations are similar in structure to HMOs discussed in Chapter 6. The HMO is the most common form of Medicare Advantage plan (Kaiser Family Foundation 2011b). Like HMOs in the private insurance market, benefits are available only within the plan network. There are two types of Medicare PPOs (Kaiser Family Foundation 2011). A regional PPO uses a statewide or multistate network. A local PPO has a smaller network of providers within a county or several counties within a locality. A beneficiary may access care outside the network at higher out-of-pocket costs. Private fee-for-service plans are offered by private insurance companies but, unlike the HMO option, the provider is paid on a per-service basis (Centers for Medicare and Medicaid Services 2011j). These plans can have higher out-of-pocket costs and providers may bill the beneficiary up to 15 percent more than the fee schedule amount (see Medicare assignment). Medicare Special Needs Plans are new and provide a managed care option for persons who have certain chronic diseases or disabling conditions, live in institutional environments (e.g., a nursing home), or are Medicare-Medicaid dual eligible (see Chapter 9) (Piper 2006).

MA plans are paid a capitated rate by the government based on average costs to care for beneficiaries in the county of residence. Cost savings to the Medicare program for patients using managed care options have not materialized (Gold 2012; McGuire, Newhouse, and Sinaiko 2011). Medicare HMOs typically cost less than traditional Medicare, but Medicare PPOs are more costly to the program (MEDPAC 2011). Medicare Advantage plans are attractive to beneficiaries looking for lowering the out-of-pocket costs of traditional Medicare (Gold 2012).

MEDICARE OUTPATIENT PRESCRIPTION DRUG BENEFIT

Medicare Part D

The Medicare Part D program was added in 2003 with the enactment of the Medicare Modernization Act (Centers for Medicare and Medicaid Services 2007). Medicare Part D establishes an outpatient prescription drug benefit for beneficiaries. The Medicare Part D program is a continuation of the policy to increase private health plan activity in the Medicare program. Rather than a government-sponsored standard benefit, the Medicare Part D benefit uses competing private pharmacy benefit plans. There are two mechanisms to participate in Medicare Part D: a stand-alone prescription drug plan or a plan integrated into a Medicare Advantage plan.

To participate in Medicare Part D, a beneficiary pays a monthly premium and other co-payments (Kaiser Family Foundation 2011c). The amount of these out-of-pocket costs varies by the type of plan. Payment of these fees provides the beneficiary with access to outpatient prescription drugs at reduced cost. The types of drugs are limited by the formulary developed by the plan and, in certain cases, prior approval of the health plan. A formulary is a list of drugs that are covered by the plan. The government requires at least two drugs per class to be included in the formulary. In addition, the Part D benefit has a coverage gap for annual costs between $2,400 to $3,850. This means that if a person's drug costs are greater between these two amounts, there is no insurance coverage. The standard plan covers most costs under $2,400 or over $3,850 per year. Low-income beneficiaries are eligible for assistance with out-of-pocket costs.

Private Health Insurance and Medicare

As was explained above, the traditional Medicare program provides many insurance benefits for beneficiaries but also has significant deductibles and co-payments. In addition, the benefit package does not cover foreign medical care services or some preventive health care services. As a result, some private insurance companies offer a Medicare supplemental, or **Medigap**, policy that beneficiaries can purchase to cover these other expenses (Centers for Medicare and Medicaid Services 2011k). Medigap plans cannot be used to pay for out-of-pocket Medicare Advantage plan costs.

Ten Medicare supplemental plans are defined in Medicare law. An insurance company will decide which type of plan it will offer and in which states. All Medigap plans cover Part A hospital co-insurance costs and 365 extra days of care after Medicare ends, Part B co-insurance costs, and the cost of the first three pints of blood each year. Other plans include skilled nursing facility costs, foreign medical insurance, and certain preventive services not covered by Medicare.

Quality and Medicare

The Medicare program ensures quality health care services through three primary processes: provider certification, utilization review, and oversight by quality improvement organizations (QIOs). Providers must submit an application to CMS in order to participate in the Medicare program. **Certification** ensures that providers are licensed and meet other minimum requirements for participation. For hospitals, accreditation by the Joint Commission on Accreditation of Healthcare Organizations (JCAHO) is evidence of certification. CMS independently surveys a small percentage of JCAHO-accredited hospitals each year. Besides providers, CMS also certifies managed care organizations. Occupational and physical therapists in private practice require an on-site visit to a clinic for certification of their practice.

Utilization review is a process of internal audit and review of the processes of care received by beneficiaries, primarily in hospitals. Health care professionals audit patient records, discuss the plan of care with the health care team, and make recommendations regarding the appropriateness of the level of care. Utilization review committees regularly review the quality and appropriateness of care. Utilization review is also performed by external organizations, including quality improvement organization contractors (QIOs). Administrative contractors routinely monitor Medicare claims and investigate possible fraud (see below). QIOs independently contract with CMS to conduct beneficiary protection and education functions (e.g., utilization review, investigation of providers, beneficiary complaint hotlines).

Public reporting of provider quality information is now available for hospitals, skilled nursing facilities, and home health agencies. Information about the quality of Medicare providers is found on the Medicare consumer website (http://www.medicare.gov). This website provides information to consumers allowing them to compare facilities in their region on several quality measures, primarily patient satisfaction. Physicians, occupational therapists, and physical therapists report quality measure data using the **Physician Quality Reporting System** (PQRS) (Centers for Medicare and Medicaid Services 2011l). Currently, therapists receive a small bonus payment for reporting quality data but will be required to participate by 2015 or receive a reduction in Medicare Part B payments. Public data about therapist quality is not currently available on the Medicare consumer website. In 2013, CMS implemented a separate system of reporting patient function on the physical therapy claim form: **functional G codes** (Centers for Medicare and Medicaid Services 2011i). "G" codes are to report initial, anticipated discharge and actual discharge patient functional status at set intervals during the episode of care.

Fraud and Abuse

Medicare fraud and abuse is a multibillion-dollar problem. Much of this fraud and abuse can be attributed to illegal beneficiary activity and unethical and illegal provider behavior. The False Claims Act of 1986, the Health Insurance Portability and Accountability

Act of 1996, and the Patient Protection and Accountable Care Act of 2010 have strengthened the ability of the government to find and prosecute fraud and abuse.

Fiscal intermediaries, carriers, and "program safeguard contractors" perform routine and special audits of many types of provider activities, including practice patterns. Utilization review by these organizations has three levels. Level I reviews the utilization pattern against an "edit" (i.e., a defined number of visits or days of treatment used to initially screen claims for appropriateness). A Level II review is a focused review by a health professional (e.g., a nurse or therapist) who reviews the documentation to determine whether the care meets Medicare guidelines for appropriateness (e.g., a skilled vs. nonskilled service, presence of physician certification). A Level II review may result in a denial of payment on a Medicare claim or referral to a Level III review. A Level III review is an on-site review of patient care documentation and Medicare billing records. In response to the increased efforts of the government to reduce Medicare fraud and abuse, compliance programs are being established by providers in order to avoid allegations of fraud. These programs emphasize timely and accurate documentation and the avoidance of improper business relationships between Medicare providers and contractors.

Fraud is defined as "making false statements or representations of material facts to obtain some benefit or payment for which no entitlement would otherwise exist." (Centers for Medicare and Medicaid Services 2012b, p. 1) Examples of Medicare fraud include billing for services that are not provided or falsely representing the nature of services provided. In addition to these types of fraud, provider waivers of beneficiary payment of the Medicare deductible or co-insurance are another form of Medicare fraud. Abuse is "any practice that is not consistent with the goals of providing patients with services that are medically necessary, meet professionally recognized standards and are fairly priced." (Centers for Medicare and Medicaid Services 2012b, p. 2) Examples of Medicare abuse include misusing codes on a claim or providing unnecessary services.

It is important for therapists to understand the definitions and common causes of Medicare fraud and abuse. A conviction of Medicare fraud can result in expulsion from participation in the program, financial penalties, and/or prison time. A finding of Medicare abuse risks a fraud investigation and also will result in denial of payment for the claim. Therapists who hire therapists who have been excluded from participation in Medicare are also susceptible to penalties under federal law.

Active Learning Exercise

The Office of the Inspector General of the Department of Health and Human Services is responsible for combating fraud and abuse in the Medicare and Medicaid programs. Go to http://www.oig.hhs.gov and learn more about the activities of this office. Examine the List of Excluded Individuals and Entities to see the public listing of persons or organizations who are suspended from participation in Medicare or Medicaid.

PHYSICIAN SELF-REFERRAL RESTRICTIONS   Section 1877 of the Social Security Act prevents physicians from making referrals to certain health care providers or organizations in which they or their family owns or for which they receive a financial compensation. The intent of this law is to prevent unnecessary utilization of Medicare benefits. Therapy services are one of the provider types that are restricted by this law. This restriction is subject to an "in-office ancillary exception." An in-office ancillary exception allows a physician or another person in the physician's office who is under direct supervision to provide therapy procedures. The procedures must be applied in an identified building and use the physician's or group's billing number to file the claim (Centers for Medicare and Medicaid Services 2011m).

Medicare Reform

Reform of Medicare has been ongoing since the program's inception. The first 15 years of the program were marked by an expansion of eligibility (e.g., persons with disabilities or end-stage renal disease) and program benefits (the program has funded numerous medical innovations, such as joint replacements). Since 1983, the Medicare program has implemented multiple cost-restraint initiatives (e.g., prospective payment systems). During its existence, Medicare has become the largest funder of the health care system. Bruce Vladeck (1999), a former Medicare administrator, described the relationship between the growth of the Medicare program and the U.S. medical care system in the last quarter-century as the development of a "Medicare-industrial complex." For many communities, hospitals and health care are as valuable for their economic effect as for their effect on health. The strength of Medicare, then, has a direct effect on the viability of the economic and medical care systems.

Wilensky and Newhouse (1999) outline several major challenges for Medicare in the future. First, the current system of controlled pricing is inefficient and difficult to administer. This adds significant indirect costs to the system. Second, the benefits package has not been comprehensively updated since the program's inception and is out of date. This has created a large market for Medigap plans that are often too expensive for the poor and other vulnerable populations. Persons without Medigap coverage face significant out-of-pocket expense and, as a result, probably do not have access to necessary services. Third, the aging of the baby boom generation will put additional strain on the program to deliver benefits while the number of Americans paying into the system in relation to those receiving benefits declines.

To face these challenges, Congress has so far primarily employed provider payment restrictions to slow the growth in the cost of the program. These are politically acceptable because they affect few beneficiaries, but they are bureaucratic, do not address beneficiary utilization rates, and reinforce interest group politics. Other proposals for reform include means-testing the program, similar in principle to Medicaid, raising the age of eligibility, and expanding the private managed care options in Medicare. Medicare reform is likely to continue into the next decades as Congress and the president struggle with the rising demand for health care by elderly and disabled Americans as the numbers of workers who pay into the program declines. As we finish this edition, the Congress and president are considering a change in eligibility age or means-testing of certain program benefits. Physical therapy and occupational therapy will be affected by whatever changes are enacted in the future.

Conclusion

Medicare is the largest single source of funding for medical care in the United States. It was established in 1965 as a federal entitlement program, Title XVIII of the Social Security Act. It has four parts: Hospital Insurance, Supplementary Medical Insurance, managed care plans, and an outpatient prescription drug benefit. Medicare Part A covers inpatient hospital stays and services, home health care/hospice, and short-term skilled nursing facility care. Medicare Part B covers outpatient services, including physical therapy and occupational therapy. Medicare Advantage provides a range of managed care options for beneficiaries. Medicare Part D provides an outpatient prescription drug benefit either as part of a managed care plan or as a stand-alone benefit. Medicare has been effective in improving the quality of life for persons over age 65 and for persons with permanent disability or end-stage renal disease. It has revolutionized reimbursement systems for providers by defining provider types and implementing cost-based reimbursement models, prospective payment systems, and the fee schedule. As the population ages, Medicare will continue to grow in importance as a major influence on the health care system.

Chapter Review Questions

1. Describe the social and political reasons for the development of Medicare.

2. Define the four parts of Med.

3. Who is eligible for Medicare Part A?

4. Define and describe the services of Medicare Part A.

5. What is cost-based reimbursement? Prospective payment?

6. Identify the patient classification systems used for
   a. Inpatient hospital care
   b. Skilled nursing facility care
   c. Home health care
   d. Inpatient rehabilitation hospital care

7. What three factors determine a prospective payment rate?

8. Who is eligible for Medicare Part B?

9. Define and describe the services of Medicare Part B.

10. Define the types of therapy providers in Medicare Part B.

11. Identify the criteria and describe how Medicare defines therapy services.

12. What is a fee schedule, and how are fee schedule payments determined?

13. Who is eligible for Medicare Part C plans, and what are the benefits offered?

14. Describe how the Medicare program assures the quality of its health plans.

15. Define the most common forms of Medicare fraud and abuse.

16. Review the challenges that will confront the Medicare program in the next decade.

Chapter Discussion Questions

1. Medicare's founders have stated that the Medicare program is one step toward national health insurance. From your understanding of the program, what would be the advantages/disadvantages of using the Medicare model as a template for national health insurance?

2. Discuss how the Medicare definition of the therapy benefit promotes and inhibits the development of occupational therapy and physical therapy as autonomous professions.

3. Consider the examples of Medicare fraud and abuse. Discuss how you can practice so as to avoid committing Medicare fraud.

References

American Medical Association. 2010. *Current procedural terminology: CPT*. Chicago: American Medical Association.

Ball, R.M. 1995. What Medicare's architects had in mind. *Health Affairs* 14(4): 62–72.

Blaisdell, F.W. 1992. The pre-Medicare role of city/county hospitals in education and health care. *J Trauma* 32(2): 217–28.

_____. 1994. Development of the city/county (public) hospital. *Arch Surg* 129(7): 760–64.

Board of Trustees. 2011. 2011 Annual report of the boards of trustees of the Federal Hospital Insurance and Federal Supplementary Medical Insurance Trust Funds. Retrieved from http://www.cms.gov/ReportsTrustFunds/downloads /tr2011.pdf (accessed February 16, 2012).

Centers for Medicare and Medicaid Services. 2007. Medicare Advantage plans. Retrieved from http://www.medicare.gov /Choices/Advantage.asp (accessed May 10, 2007).

_____. 2011a. Acute inpatient PPS. Retrieved from http://www .cms.gov/AcuteInpatientPPS/01_overview.asp (accessed February 28, 2012).

_____. 2011b. Skilled nursing facility PPS. Retrieved from http:// www.cms.gov/SNFPPS/ (accessed February 28, 2012).

_____. 2011c. MDS 3.0 RAI manual. Retrieved from https://www.cms.gov/NursingHomeQualityInits/20 _MDS30RAIManual.asp#TopOfPage (accessed February 22, 2012).

_____. 2011d. Home health PPS. Retrieved from http://www .cms.gov/HomeHealthPPS/ (accessed February 27, 2012).

_____. 2011e. OASIS C. Retrieved from http://www.cms.gov /HomeHealthQualityInits/06_OASISC.asp (accessed February 16, 2012).

_____. 2011f. Inpatient rehabilitation facility PPS. Retrieved from http://www.cms.gov/InpatientRehabFacPPS/ (accessed February 27, 2012).

_____. 2011g. Inpatient rehabilitation Facility–Patient Assessment Instrument. Retrieved from http://www .cms.gov/Medicare/Medicare-Fee-for-Service-Payment /InpatientRehabFacPPS/IRFPAI.html (accessed April 5, 2013).

_____. 2011h. Comprehensive outpatient rehabilitation facility: Fact sheet. Retrieved from http://www.cms.gov /Outreach-and-Education/Medicare-Learning-Network -MLN/MLNProducts/downloads/Comprehensive _Outpatient_Rehabilitation_Facility_Fact_Sheet _ICN904085.pdf (accessed January 2, 2013).

_____. 2011i. Therapy services. Retrieved from http://www.cms .gov/TherapyServices/ (accessed February 22, 2012).

_____. 2011j. Private fee-for-service plans. Retrieved from https://www.cms.gov/PrivateFeeforServicePlans/ (accessed March 12, 2012).

_____. 2011k. Medicare Supplemental Health Insurance (Medigap). Retrieved from http://www.cms.gov/medigap/ (accessed March 12, 2012).

_____. 2011l. Physician self referral. Retrieved from http://www.cms.gov/PhysicianSelfReferral/ (accessed February 29, 2012).

_____. 2011m. Physician Quality Reporting System. Retrieved from http://www.cms.gov/pqrs/ (accessed March 13, 2012).

_____. 2012a. Medicare limits on therapy services. CMS Product 10988. Retrieved from http://www.medicare.gov /Pubs/pdf/10988.pdf (accessed January 2, 2013).

_____. 2012b. Medicare fraud and abuse: Prevention, detection and reporting. Retrieved from https://www.cms.gov /Outreach-and-Education/Medicare-Learning-Network -MLN/MLNProducts/downloads/Fraud_and_Abuse.pdf (accessed April 4, 2013)

Cooper, A.L., A.N. Trivedi. 2012. Fitness memberships and favorable selection in Medicare Advantage plans. *N Engl J Med* 366(2): 150–57.

Corning, P.A. Chapter 5. What makes social welfare policy? In *The history of Medicare.* Retrieved from http://www.ssa.gov /history/corning.html (accessed February 16, 2012).

Davis, M.H., and S.T. Burner. 1995. Three decades of Medicare: What the numbers tell us. *Health Affairs* 14(4): 231–43.

Friedman, E. 1995. The compromise and the afterthought. Medicare and Medicaid after 30 years. *JAMA* 274(3): 278–82.

Gilman, B.H., J. Cromwell, K. Adamache, and S. Donoghue. 2000. *Study of the effect of implementing the post-acute care transfer policy under the inpatient prospective payment system.* Waltham MA: Health Economics Research Institute.

Gold, M. 2005. Private plans in Medicare: Another look. Even if regional plans are not widespread, MMA is likely to dramatically expand the private-sector role in Medicare. *Health Affairs* 24(5): 1302–10.

_____. 2012. Medicare Advantage: Lessons for Medicare's future. *N Engl J Med*, February 22 ePub.

Kaiser Family Foundation. 2011a. Medicare spending and financing: A primer. Retrieved from http://www.kff.org /medicare/upload/7731-03.pdf (accessed April 2, 2013).

_____. 2011b. Medicare Advantage fact sheet. Retrieved from http://www.kff.org/medicare/upload/2052-15.pdf (accessed March 12, 2012).

_____. 2011c. The Medicare prescription drug benefit. Retrieved from http://www.kff.org/medicare/upload /7044-12.pdf (accessed March 1, 2012).

Lieber, R. 2012, October 26. What Medicare will cover even if you're likely not to get better. *NY Times.* Retrieved from http://www.nytimes.com/2012/10/27/your-money/health -insurance/medicare-expected-to-pay-more-costs-of -chronic-conditions.html?pagewanted=all (accessed December 5, 2012).

McGuire, T.G., J.P. Newhouse, and A.D. Sinaiko, 2011. An economic history of Medicare Part C. *Milbank Q* 89(2): 289–332.

Medicare Payment Advisory Commission (MEDPAC). 2008, October. Rehabilitation facilities (inpatient) payment system. Retrieved from http://www.medpac.gov/documents /MedPAC_Payment_Basics_08_IRF.pdf (accessed February 28, 2012).

_____. 2011. Medicare Advantage program payment system. Retrieved from http://www.medpac.gov/documents /MedPAC_Payment_Basics_11_MA.pdf (accessed March 1, 2012).

Menke, T.J., C.M. Ashton, N.J. Petersen, and F.D. Wolinsky. 1998. Impact of an all-inclusive diagnosis-related group payment system on inpatient utilization. *Med Care* 36(8): 1126–37.

National Health Policy Forum. 2011. Medicare's sustainable growth rate: The basics. Retrieved from http://www.nhpf .org/library/the-basics/Basics_SGR_06-21-11.pdf (accessed March 2, 2012).

Piper, K.B. 2006. Medicare Advantage: Understanding special needs plans. *Manag Care* 15(7 Suppl 3): 25–27.

RTI International. 2011. Developing outpatient therapy payment alternatives. Project information. Retrieved from http://optherapy.rti.org/ProjectInfo.aspx#PaymentModels (accessed April 26, 2012).

Russell, L.B., and C.S. Burke. 1978. The political economy of federal health programs in the United States: A historical review. *Int J Health Serv* 8(1): 55–77.

Scully T.A., and C.T. Roskey. 2004. New directions in Medicare managed care. *Healthc Financ Manage* 58(5): 64–68.

Takemura, Y., and J.R. Beck. 1999. The effects of a fixed-fee reimbursement system introduced by the federal government on laboratory testing in the United States. *Rinsho-byori* 47(1): 1–10.

Vladeck, B. 1999. The political economy of Medicare. *Health Affairs* 18(1): 22–36

Whetsell, G.W. 1999. The history and evolution of hospital payment systems: How did we get here? *Nurs Adm Q* 23(4): 1–15.

Wilensky, G., and J.P. Newhouse. 1999. Medicare: What's right? What's wrong? What's next? *Health Affairs* 18(1): 92–106.

9

Medicaid, Military/Veterans Medical Insurance, and Indian Health Service

CHAPTER OBJECTIVES

At the conclusion of this chapter, the reader will be able to:

1 Describe the statutory authorization, size, and purpose of the Medicaid program.

2 Explain the characteristics of persons who receive Medicaid and describe the percentage of the program that is spent on major eligibility groups.

3 Identify and relate the criteria for eligibility for Medicaid benefits.

4 Describe the services covered by the Medicaid program:

    a. Explain optional vs. mandatory benefits as they relate to therapy services.

5 Describe the organization of service delivery in the Medicaid program:

    a. Medicaid managed care

    b. Medicaid waiver programs

6 Relate the eligibility criteria and health insurance benefits for military and veterans health benefit programs.

7 Describe the purpose and organization of the Indian Health Service.

KEY WORDS

Categorical Eligibility

Children's Health Insurance Program

Federal Poverty Level

Home- and Community-Based Waiver

Means-Tested

Medicaid

Medicare-Medicaid Dual Eligibility

Medically Needy Eligibility

Personal Care Services

Safety-Net Provider

Spend Down

Spousal Impoverishment Protection

Tribal Self-Determination

TRICARE

CASE EXAMPLE ···

Sophia is a physical therapist, and Courtney is an occupational therapist working in a United States Public Health Service hospital for the Indian Health Service. In their roles, these therapists provide treatment and consultation services for community members seeking services. They are often asked by physicians and physician's assistants to provide consultation on cases regarding whether to refer a patient to a medical specialist. They work actively in the community to provide prevention and wellness services to address diabetes mellitus, which is endemic to this population. Very few of their patients have private health insurance. It is funding from the Indian Health Service and Medicaid that provides resources for them to work in this community.

Case Example Question:

1. Reflect on how practice in this community is different from practice in the private insurance system. What skills and abilities do therapists need to have to be effective?

Introduction

The preceding three chapters introduced and described several large insurance mechanisms that finance much of the health care system. In Chapter 6, we discussed the purpose of insurance and introduced several ways that health insurance products are organized. In Chapter 7, we learned about private insurance including managed care, long-term care insurance, and workers, compensation. In Chapter 8, we considered Medicare, an example of social insurance and the largest insurance program in the world in terms of dollars spent. In this chapter, we turn our attention to other governmental health care insurance programs: **Medicaid** (including the **Children's Health Insurance Program**) and insurance for military personnel, veterans, and American Indians/Alaska Natives. These programs provide funding support for populations served by occupational therapists and physical therapists.

These insurance programs target populations that either have historically not been able to obtain private health care insurance or, as in the case of the military, veterans, and American Indians/Alaska Natives, for whom the government has a direct responsibility for the health care of plan members. Medicaid serves a large and vulnerable component of our society—the poor, persons with disabilities, low-income women, and children. Like Medicare beneficiaries, these persons often find it difficult to purchase health care in the private health insurance market. The structure of Medicaid displays the societal tension concerning the roles of government and the private sector in providing solutions to the dilemma of access to health care insurance for everyone in the country. Medicaid is a state–federal partnership. Eligibility requirements are sophisticated and limited to certain groups. Benefit packages are generous and rely on managed care and, in many cases, private insurance contracting to deliver the services. The federal responsibility to provide health care to military personnel, veterans, and American Indians/Alaska Natives is clear. The global budgeting process used by these programs, however, is unique to the U.S. health care system.

First, we will consider Medicaid, the largest health care insurance plan in the United States in terms of persons served. The increasing number of uninsured children spawned the State Children's Health Insurance Plan (SCHIP) in 1997 that has been a successful effort to improve health care for low-income children in the United States who do not qualify for traditional Medicaid. We will then explore the Veterans Health Plan and TRICARE, a major source of funding for active and retired military beneficiaries. Finally, we will introduce the Indian Health Service.

Medicaid

What Is Medicaid?

Medicaid is a joint federal–state medical insurance program designed to meet the health care needs of people who meet certain low-income requirements, have high medical costs, or are in certain defined, disadvantaged populations (e.g., low-income pregnant women and children). Medicaid is a **means-tested** program. Unlike Medicare, a beneficiary must qualify by demonstrating a level of need usually based on low income and personal assets or excessive medical expenses. Medicaid insures more Americans, about 49 million persons, than any other health care insurance program in the country.

Medicaid was established in 1965 as Title XIX of the Social Security Act. It replaced the small medical insurance programs for indigent persons that were offered by several states with one large national program. Medicaid was one of the cornerstones of President Lyndon Johnson's Great Society program. Medicaid insurance provides access to medical care for many poor families. However, there are many uninsured persons and families that do not have access to private insurance and do not qualify for Medicaid (see Chapter 2). A significant expansion of Medicaid eligibility by the Patient Protection and Affordable Care Act of 2010 to include more low-income persons is an important method for reducing the rate of uninsurance in the U.S. population. In this chapter, we will explore the complex eligibility requirements of Medicaid and also how Medicaid is being used in health care reform to expand insurance coverage.

All 50 states and the District of Columbia participate in the Medicaid program. Each state has its own Medicaid plan that sets eligibility criteria and benefits within federal guidelines. The program, therefore, varies from state to state. The federal government shares with the states the cost of providing a defined package of medical care benefits to Medicaid beneficiaries. The federal share of a state's program ranges from at least 50 percent up to 74 percent of the total program cost. Poor states pay less than wealthy states. For many states and territories, these shared payments for the Medicaid program are the largest grant they receive from the federal government, and the cost of the program is one of the largest annual expenditures of state funds.

The total cost of the Medicaid program in 2011 was $412 billion (Centers for Medicare and Medicaid Services 2011a) Of this amount, $260 billion was paid by the federal government (63%), and $152 billion was paid by state governments (37%). Unlike Medicare Part A, there is no separate payroll tax for Medicaid. Instead, the source of Medicaid funds is general federal and state revenues. At the state level, Medicaid is a major expense in every budget. States use flexibility in eligibility requirements and benefits to try to meet the complex and sometimes conflicting demands.

Who Receives Medicaid?

As can be seen in Table 9-1, children comprise about 50 percent of the Medicaid beneficiary population but account for about one in five dollars in Medicaid expenditures. Medicaid or SCHIP covers two of five of the 13.5 million children with disabilities in the United States (Tu and Cunningham 2005). While often associated with public assistance programs, it is important to recognize that Medicaid is actually a vital program providing insurance coverage for persons with complex medical needs in need of formal, long-term care services. The populations served by Medicaid include persons with severe intellectual and physical disabilities, and elderly persons who are poor (Kaiser Commission on Medicaid and the Uninsured 2013). The Kaiser Family Foundation found that 5 percent of Medicaid enrollees account for about half of program expenditures (Kaiser Commission on Medicaid and the Uninsured 2013). About two in three Medicaid dollars are spent on the elderly and persons with disabilities (see Table 9-2). Medicaid is the largest purchaser of long-term care in the United States and a critical component for

Table 9-1 Who Receives Medicaid?

Eligibility Category	No. of Enrollees (2011)	% of Medicaid Population (2011)
Total Number of Enrollees	56.1 million	
Number of Children Enrolled	28.3 million	50%
Number of Adults Enrolled	12.2 million	22%
Number of Persons Who Are Blind or Disabled Enrolled	9.6 million	17%
Number of Elderly Persons Enrolled	4.9 million	11%
Number of CHIP Enrolled	5.7 million	

Source: Medicaid Enrollment and Beneficiaries, Selected Fiscal Years (2011). Accessed at http://cms.gov /Research-Statistics-Data-and-Systems/Statistics-Trends-and-Reports/DataCompendium/2011_Data _Compendium.html on April 17, 2012.

funding the "**safety-net**" for the U.S. health care system (Ng, Harrington, and Kitchener 2010). Medicaid funds intermediate and skilled nursing facility care for about 1.6 million Americans (see Table 9-3).

Who Is Eligible for Medicaid?

Eligibility for the Medicaid program is a complicated process that is determined by meeting two sets of criteria: **categorical eligibility** (includes **Medicare-Medicaid dual eligibility**) and **medically needy eligibility**. The complexity of Medicaid eligibility criteria reflects the tension between political understandings of health care insurance as an individual responsibility (libertarian perspective) or a societal responsibility (egalitarian perspective). Like Medicare, Medicaid is a social insurance program, so many persons who pay for the program are not eligible for program benefits. Unlike Medicare, however, Medicaid is a means-tested government program. Nearly all Americans will qualify for Medicare at age 65. Many Americans will not ever qualify for Medicaid. Medicaid participants must demonstrate that they meet limited-income/assets criteria in order to receive benefits.

Table 9-2 Percent of Medicaid Expenditures by Eligibility Category and Type of Service (2008)

Eligibility Category	Total Payment	Inpatient Hospital	Long-Term Care	Other
Elderly	21	1	13	7
Persons with Disabilities	44	5	9	29
Children	19	3	0	17
Adults	14	2	0	11
Unclassified	4	2	0	2

Source: Medicaid Payments by Type of Service and Basis of Eligibility, Fiscal Year 2008. Accessed at http://cms.gov/Research-Statistics-Data-and-Systems/Statistics-Trends-and-Reports/DataCompendium /2011_Data_Compendium.html on April 17, 2012.

Table 9-3 Utilization of Selected Medicaid Services by Number of Persons (2008)

Service	Number of Persons Utilizing
General Hospitals	5.26 million
Intermediate and Skilled Nursing Facilities	1.62 million
Physicians	21.7 million
Dentists	9.8 million
Other Practitioners	5.2 million
Prescription Drugs	24.6 million
Home Health Care	1.2 million
Personal Care Support	1.1 million

Source: Medicaid Eligibles by Type of Service, Fiscal Years 2004–2008. Accessed at http://cms.gov/Research
-Statistics-Data-and-Systems/Statistics-Trends-and-Reports/DataCompendium/2011_Data_Compendium.html
on April 18, 2012.

Income is usually assessed as a percent of the **federal poverty level** or FPL. Federal poverty level income amounts are set annually and are based on family size. For example, the 2011 FPL for a family of four was $22,350. Assets are personal investments or savings that again must be very low in order to qualify for Medicaid.

Table 9-4 identifies the basic groups that qualify for Medicaid benefits. All states are required to cover persons whose circumstances fit into one or more of these categories. Categorically eligible persons are low income and have few assets. They are also

Table 9-4 Medicaid Eligibility

Mandatory Categories

1. Children
   a. Up to age 6 in families with income < 133% federal poverty level
   b. Age 6–28 in families with incomes < 100% federal poverty level
   c. Income levels increased to 200%−300% FPL by CHIP participation
2. Pregnant women in households < 185% FPL
3. Recipients of Supplemental Security Income payments
4. Very low-income caretakers or parents of low-income children under age 18
5. Medicare-Medicaid Dual Eligibles
   a. Qualified Medicare Beneficiary
   b. Specified Low-Income Beneficiary
   c. Qualified Individuals

Medically Needy"Spend Down" Program

1. Institutionalized persons
2. Home-based care

Source: Center for Medicare and Medicaid Services. Medicaid At-A-Glance. 2005. Accessed online at
http://www.cms.hhs.gov/MedicaidGenInfo/ on June 18, 2007.

primarily children. In some instances, children qualify for Medicaid benefits through expanded eligibility offered by the Children's Health Insurance Program (CHIP). While the minimum federal requirement is that states cover children in homes with incomes at or slightly above FPL, all states have increased minimum income eligibility to less than 200 percent (in some states, 300%) FPL. The method for the expansion of publicly funded health insurance coverage to children has been the Children's Health Insurance Program. States have used the CHIP program to expand their Medicaid program, set up a separate children's health insurance program, or establish some combination of Medicaid/children's health insurance program. As a result, many more (8 million) children are covered by health insurance. The CHIP program has been successful in decreasing rates of uninsurance and improving access to health care for low-income children and children with special needs (Duderstadt et al. 2006; Kempe et al. 2005; Kenney and Yee 2007; Seid et al. 2006).

Adults may be eligible for Medicaid if they are pregnant women, persons with disabilities, or low-income persons over age 65. In 2014, Medicaid eligibility is expanding (in states that choose to expand program eligibility) to include all adults with incomes less than 133 percent FPL. For example, a single adult with an income less than $14,483.70 (not currently eligible) will be covered by Medicaid in all states. Currently, pregnant women in families with incomes up to 185 percent FPL are covered by Medicaid (in some states with services limited only to the pregnancy) for the duration of the pregnancy and up to 60 days after delivery. Parents with children in extremely low-income (about 40% FPL) households are currently eligible.

Persons receiving Supplemental Security Income (SSI) (e.g., some persons with disabilities) qualify for Medicaid. Supplemental Security Income was established by Congress in 1972 to provide a monthly cash benefit to low-income (annual income < 75% FPL) citizens with disabilities (including persons who are blind) and persons over age 65. In addition, individuals may not have assets exceeding $2,000 (or $3,000 for couples). The 2012 federal monthly cash benefit is $698 for individuals and $1,048 per couple. This benefit is increased by some state payments and is reduced by income the person earns.

Low-income Medicare beneficiaries qualify for Medicaid coverage of some or all Medicare out-of-pocket costs (see Chapter 8). These persons must meet both income and asset (e.g., personal savings) limits to qualify. A person with an income not exceeding 100 percent FPL and with assets less than $6,600 will qualify for Medicare Part B premium, deductible, and co-insurance payments by Medicaid as a Qualified Medicare Beneficiary. Specified Low-Income Beneficiaries have incomes between 100 percent and 120 percent FPL and receive Medicaid payment for their Medicare B premiums only. Qualified individuals (income > 120% and < 135% FPL) can receive assistance with Medicare B premiums. Dual eligible individuals "are among the sickest and poorest individuals covered by either Medicare or Medicaid" (Kaiser Commission on Medicaid and the Uninsured 2012c, p.2)

Some persons who are categorically eligible but exceed the income and asset limits can qualify for Medicaid as the result of a catastrophic medical event that results in expensive and long-term home or skilled nursing care. These "medically needy" Medicaid beneficiaries qualify by having to "**spend down**" their assets to meet the Medicaid eligibility criteria (Kaiser Commission on Medicaid and the Uninsured 2012b). The medically needy eligibility criteria are a state option that can be included or excluded in each state's Medicaid program. The "spend down" program permits Medicaid coverage for a serious injury of an uninsured child in a household that exceeds the Medicaid income/asset criteria after expenses for treatment reduce the household income or assets to qualification levels.

The medically needy option is used in all states to provide a route for payment of a portion of the long-term nursing home costs for elderly residents or persons with disabilities. Let's consider an example of a typical American over age 65 who requires care in a skilled nursing facility. To do so, we must consider the person's assets (i.e., personal savings), monthly income, and the costs of care. Without long-term care insurance (see Chapter 7), a person is required to first pay for nursing home care from her own savings until these resources are depleted to a personal asset limit before Medicaid will pay for these costs. In order to qualify for Medicaid, personal assets (e.g., savings) are typically limited to a few thousand dollars. The median nonhousing wealth of Americans over age 65 is $216,000 for couples, $44,000 for widows and $23,000 for individuals (2010 dollars; Banerjee 2012). These dollars are spent first before qualifying for Medicaid. Second, we must consider monthly income (e.g., Social Security or pension income). Median monthly household income for retired persons in the United States is $2,540 (2010 dollars; Banerjee 2012). Finally, we need to consider the long-term care costs. In 2011, the monthly expense of an average semiprivate nursing home room is $6,510 (MetLife Mature Market Institute). As can be seen, long-term care costs exceed the typical monthly income of retired Americans by 250 percent and can quickly deplete the assets of many persons. In this situation, without Medicaid, the burden for paying for long-term care for these persons would fall on family or private charity.

The Medicaid program provides an important safety net for indigent persons who require long-term care. After personal assets are depleted ("spent down"), an analysis of income is completed to determine qualifications for Medicaid payment. Most commonly, a person in a nursing home with a monthly income after medical expenses less than 300 percent ($2,094 in 2012) of the SSI limit qualifies for Medicaid. Considering our example, all of this person's income would be spent on long-term nursing home care (except for a small personal allowance of about $50) and the balance ($4,020) would be paid by Medicaid.

The medically needy "spend down" provision creates a unique situation for married couples who often jointly hold assets like investments or bank savings. High long-term care costs for one spouse could bankrupt the community dwelling spouse. A **spousal impoverishment protection** provision in the Medicaid spend down program prevents this situation. A portion of jointly held assets (in Nebraska, $21,912) is protected for the community dwelling spouse. A higher limit ($109,560 in Nebraska) is set for equal sharing between the community dwelling and institution dwelling spouse. Jointly held assets above the high limit are to be spent down for care of the person in the institution until the high limit is reached. Half of the resources between the low limit and high limit are then used to pay for the nursing home care. At this point, the nursing home residing spouse can qualify for Medicaid. In addition, the law states that all of the community dwelling spouse's income is protected, and if it is low, a portion of the nursing home resident's monthly income is also protected to provide for at least $1,825 in monthly income for the community dwelling spouse. States are able to prevent the transfer of assets to children, recover some previously transferred assets, and recover expenses by applying a lien on the assets of an estate in probate if a couple attempts to hide resources that could be used to pay for nursing home care.

In summary, Medicaid eligibility is a complex system of policy trade-offs to both provide a safety net for persons while also reinforcing personal responsibility for providing health insurance. The PPACA of 2010 expanded Medicaid eligibility to all persons up to 133 percent of federal poverty level. This change would make single men and childless couples (who have not been eligible to date) eligible for Medicaid. The United States Supreme Court ruled in June 2012 that states could not be compelled to increase eligibility. While current federal law provides all or nearly all funding for Medicaid eligibility expansion, it is not clear how states will or will not act to increase Medicaid eligibility to the PPACA standard. Medicaid is an excellent example of an egalitarian government program (see Chapter 1). Medicaid is also a very important program for the health care industry since it provides payment for care to persons who are uninsured and have very limited income and resources to pay for care.

Medicaid Services

State agreement to participate in Medicaid and acceptance of matching federal funds mandates the provision of a basic set of benefits in state Medicaid programs. The Medicaid program offers a three-tier package of benefits. A basic benefit package is established for states that only offer Medicaid benefits to categorically eligible populations. An additional benefit package is established for states that offer a medically needy program. Finally, states are able to include several optional benefits at their discretion. Table 9-5 lists the benefit packages offered in Medicaid.

Table 9-5 Medicaid Benefits

A. Mandatory benefits
    1. Inpatient and outpatient hospital services
    2. Laboratory and radiology services
    3. Certified pediatric and family nurse practitioners
    4. Nursing facility services for age 21 or over
    5. Early and periodic screening, diagnosis, and treatment (EPSDT) services under age 21
    6. Family planning services and supplies
    7. Physicians' services
    8. Home health care for persons eligible for nursing facility services
    9. Pregnancy-related services (e.g., nurse-midwife services 60 days post partum care)
    10. Transportation to medical care
    11. Tobacco cessation programs
B. Optional services (partial list)
    1. Prescription drugs
    2. Rehabilitation therapies including occupational therapy and physical therapy
    3. Prosthetics and orthotics
    4. Personal care attendants

Source: Center for Medicare and Medicaid Services. Medicaid Benefits. 2011. Retrieved from http://medicaid.gov/Medicaid-CHIP-Program-Information/By-Topics/Benefits/Medicaid-Benefits.html (accessed April 24, 2012).

Like other health insurance programs, Medicaid provides insurance coverage for inpatient and outpatient hospital care and physician services. Unlike most private health insurance plans, states are required to provide coverage for skilled nursing facilities for everyone over age 21 (categorical eligibility). Many state Medicaid programs provide a prescription drug benefit. Medically necessary physical therapy and occupational therapy are optional services in the Medicaid program. In reality, all states must cover necessary therapy services provided to children in the early and periodic screening, diagnosis, and treatment (EPSDT) program and to categorically eligible persons over age 21 who reside in skilled nursing facilities. These are federally mandated benefits. Some therapy services are commonly covered in the hospital benefit package, but the type and intensity of the covered therapy vary. States may or may not pay for outpatient or home health physical therapy or occupational therapy services (see Table 9-6). Thirty-six states include physical therapy and 32 states include occupational therapy as a benefit for their categorically Medicaid-eligible population. About half of the states offer occupational therapy and physical therapy to their medically needy Medicaid-eligible population.

The high cost of institutionalization has encouraged the development of alternatives to expensive skilled nursing facility care. The **home- and community-based waiver program** is a comprehensive state plan to provide a benefit package to persons with disabilities to support living in community settings rather than in skilled nursing facilities. There are about 300 home and community-based Medicaid waiver programs across the country. A number of these programs provide funding for therapy services to keep Medicaid beneficiaries functional in their communities. **Personal care services** are an optional Medicaid benefit that provides for payment of a nonrelative to assist with activities of daily living or, in some cases, instrumental activities of daily living in the patient's residence. This service can allow persons with disabilities to live in their homes and be employed or enjoy other community activities.

Medicaid is an important part of the financing of the United States health care system. It is the largest insurance program in terms of persons served in the United States. It provides access to health care insurance for many groups of Americans who would otherwise have impaired access to health care due to a lack of employment-based private insurance. Its existence supports safety-net providers who serve individuals in these communities. It provides a package of medical care benefits and certain social benefits that are not covered

Table 9-6 **Access to Therapy Services in Medicaid by Eligibility Group (2010)**

State	PT–Categorical Eligibility	PT–Medically Needy	OT–Categorical Eligibility	OT–Medically Needy
Alabama	No	No	No	No
Alaska	Yes	No	Yes	No
Arizona	Yes	Yes	Yes	Yes
Arkansas	No	No	No	No
California	Yes	Yes	Yes	Yes
Colorado	Yes	No	Yes	No
Connecticut	No	No	No	No
Delaware	Yes	No	Yes	No
District of Columbia	Yes	Yes	No	No
Florida	Yes	Yes	Yes	Yes
Georgia	No	No	No	No
Hawaii	Yes	Yes	Yes	Yes
Idaho	Yes	No	Yes	No
Illinois	Yes	Yes	Yes	Yes
Indiana	Yes	No	Yes	No
Iowa	Yes	Yes	No	No
Kansas	Yes	Yes	Yes	Yes
Kentucky	No	No	No	No
Louisiana	No	No	No	No
Maine	Yes	Yes	Yes	Yes
Maryland	Yes	Yes	No	No
Massachusetts	Yes	Yes	Yes	Yes
Michigan	No	No	No	No
Minnesota	Yes	NA	Yes	NA
Nebraska	Yes	Yes	Yes	Yes
Nevada	Yes	No	Yes	No
New Hampshire	Yes	No	Yes	Yes

(continued)

Table 9-6 *Continued*

State	PT–Categorical Eligibility	PT–Medically Needy	OT–Categorical Eligibility	OT–Medically Needy
New Jersey	No	No	No	No
New Mexico	Yes	No	Yes	No
New York	Yes	Yes	Yes	Yes
North Carolina	No	No	No	No
North Dakota	Yes	Yes	Yes	Yes
Ohio	Yes	No	Yes	No
Oklahoma	No	No	No	No
Oregon	Yes	NA	Yes	NA
Pennsylvania	No	No	No	No
Rhode Island	No	No	No	No
South Carolina	No	No	No	No
South Dakota	Yes	No	No	No
Tennessee	Yes	NA	Yes	NA
Texas	Yes	Yes	Yes	Yes
Utah	Yes	NA	Yes	No
Vermont	Yes	NA	Yes	No
Virginia	No	No	No	No
Washington	Yes	No	Yes	No
West Virginia	Yes	Yes	Yes	Yes
Wisconsin	Yes	Yes	Yes	Yes
Wyoming	Yes	No	Yes	No

Source: Based on data from Kaiser Family Foundation 2010. Medicaid Benefits: Online Database. Benefits By Service: Physical therapy services. Accessed at http://medicaidbenefits.kff.org/service.jsp?yr=5&so=0&cat=4&sv=29&gr=off&x=91&y=17 on April 24, 2012.

in traditional health care insurance plans (e.g., personal care services, long-term skilled nursing facility care). Access to occupational therapy and physical therapy services is generally available but is not consistent between states. Medicaid is also the best example of the utilization of managed care principles in a public health care insurance program.

Medicaid Managed Care

Unlike Medicare, managed care is the dominant form of health care delivery in state Medicaid programs. About 70 percent of Medicaid beneficiaries are enrolled in a managed care plan (Centers for Medicare and Medicaid Services 2011b). In South Carolina and

Tennessee, all Medicaid beneficiaries are enrolled in a managed care plan. Only Alaska, New Hampshire, and Wyoming do not encourage or require managed care enrollment for their Medicaid population.

Medicaid managed care takes two forms: primary care case management and capitation (Regenstein and Anthony 1998). Primary care case management is a fee-for-service managed care program that contracts with physicians who provide routine care and coordinate the referral and utilization of specialty care services. Capitation forms contracts with managed care organizations to provide all the services needed by the beneficiary at a predetermined monthly rate. It is not uncommon for states to have multiple managed care plans in their overall Medicaid program. For example, Arizona has 30 managed care programs that provide Medicaid managed care options statewide or just to certain counties (Centers for Medicare and Medicaid Services 2011c).

The effect of managed care in the Medicaid program has been positive on reducing health disparities, improving access to primary care, and decreasing unnecessary hospitalizations. There is some conflicting data over whether the program reduces costs. Cook (2007) found that participation in Medicaid managed care lowered disparities in having a source of primary care for African-Americans and Hispanic-Americans. Managed care has been associated with a decrease in hospital utilizations (Bindman et al. 2005) and use of emergency rooms (Baker and Afendulis 2005; Garrett and Zuckerman 2005). Felland et al. (2003) found that the "health care safety net" for a community has been improving. More recently, Iglehart (2011) has concluded that Medicaid managed care does reduce program costs but is concerned about potential negative effects on access and quality of care. Burns (2009), on the other hand, found higher costs for adults with disabilities in managed care vs. fee-for-service Medicaid plans.

Veterans Affairs and Military Health Insurance Programs

Veterans Affairs Health System

The Department of Veterans Affairs (VA) operates the largest health care system in the United States (Kizer and Dudley 2009). In this section, we will explore the unique eligibility requirements and the benefit package offered to veterans who utilize this system. Veterans' health benefits date to the beginning of the country and the government's sense of responsibility to care for those who have served in the military. By the mid-1990s, veterans' health care was widely viewed as "dysfunctional...fragmented, disjointed and insensitive to individual needs" (Kizer and Dudley 2009). Today, VA health systems are recognized to be top performers in the quality and efficiency of health care delivery. Occupational therapists and physical therapists are important members of the VA health care team. Therapists provide services to the thousands of veterans who have experienced disability as a result of military service. Like Medicaid, the VA health system is an important component of the health care safety net for poor or disabled veterans (Hughes 2003).

Table 9-7 lists the eligibility categories that qualify an individual for veterans' health benefits. The basic criterion for eligibility is a minimum of two years service and an honorable discharge from the military. Except for Priority Group 8, veterans who meet the criteria for at least one of these categories are eligible for veterans' benefits. Veterans with service-related or service-aggravated disabilities are given the highest enrollment priority. Impoverished veterans also receive priority enrollment in the VA system. Non-service-connected veterans are veterans who have not incurred or aggravated a disability while in military service. Non-service-connected veterans typically have to meet income/ asset requirements or pay deductibles and co-payments to receive veterans' health benefits.

Eligible veterans are entitled to a comprehensive package of health care benefits. Table 9-8 lists the main components of this benefit package. Unlike private health insurance or Medicare/Medicaid, VA health insurance includes a rich benefit package for long-term care and support for persons with disabilities. Physical therapy and occupational therapy are mandated benefits in the VA health plan. In addition, prosthetics and orthotics are routinely covered. For veterans serving since September 11, 2001, the VA can

Table 9-7 Veterans Administration Health Program Eligibility

A. Priority Group 1
    1. Veterans with at least a 50 percent service-related disability
B. Priority Group 2
    1. Veterans with a 30 percent to 40 percent service-related disability
C. Priority Group 3
    1. Veterans who are former prisoners of war or received a Purple Heart, Medal of Honor
    2. Veterans who were discharged for disability-related reasons
    3. Veterans with a 10 percent to 20 percent service-related disability
D. Priority Group 4
    1. Veterans who are receiving homebound benefits
    2. Veterans who are classified as "catastrophically disabled"
E. Priority Group 5
    1. Veterans receiving VA pension benefits or are Medicaid eligible
F. Priority Group 6
    1. Veterans who are 0% disabled but are receiving VA compensation
G. Priority Group 7 and 8
    1. Non-service-connected veterans who do not meet the criteria for the other groups and agree to pay the required co-payment for services

Source: Department of Veterans Affairs. All Enrollment Priority Groups Accessed at http://www.va.gov /healtheligibility/eligibility/PriorityGroupsAll.asp on June 21, 2007.

provide educational and personal support, respite, and, in some cases, payment to care-givers for providing informal care to a seriously injured veteran. The inclusion of these benefits reflects the connection between disability and veterans' health benefits.

    This benefit package is not free to all eligible veterans. The VA health plan has established co-payments for prescription drugs, inpatient and outpatient hospital services, and nursing home care. Veterans with service-related disabilities do not pay these costs. Non-service-connected veterans are required to meet income and asset thresholds or

Table 9-8 Veterans Health Uniform Benefit Package

A. Inpatient and outpatient hospital care
B. Prescription drugs
C. Physician services
D. Mental health care
E. Home health and hospice
F. Rehabilitation therapies
G. Prosthetics and orthotics
H. Home improvements to improve structural access
    1. $4,100 for service-connected disability and $1,200 for non-service-connected disability
I. Vocational rehabilitation and supported employment programs
J. Services for veterans who are blind
K. Long-term care
L. Disability compensation
M. Automobile adaptations (one time up to $11,000)
N. Annual clothing allowance
O. Caregivers

Source: Department of Veterans Affairs. Federal Benefits for Veterans, Dependents and Survivors. Chapter 1 VA Health Care Benefits. Accessed at http://www.va.gov/opa/publications/benefits_book/benefits_chap01.asp on April 24, 2012.

demonstrate financial hardship to avoid making the required co-payments. The private insurance companies of insured veterans who receive care in VA health care facilities are routinely billed for the services.

TRICARE

Active military personnel receive their health care through a system of military hospitals. Certain services or services for eligible dependents, however, are provided in the civilian health care system. In addition, retired military members and their families are eligible for health care insurance. The government insurance plan for active military personnel and their families is called **TRICARE**. TRICARE covers 9.6 million Americans world-wide (Department of Defense 2012). Both physical therapists and occupational therapists provide health care to members of the military.

TRICARE consists of three insurance options for military personnel: TRICARE Prime, TRICARE Extra, and TRICARE Standard (Department of Defense 2012a). TRICARE Prime uses military hospitals and clinics as the primary provider of care. Active duty military personnel are required to enroll in TRICARE Prime. Retired military may access TRICARE Prime for an annual enrollment fee and pay other out-of-pocket costs. TRICARE Prime is a health maintenance organization model of care that utilizes primary care case management. As a result, care in network is provided at no cost to the member. TRICARE Extra and Standard are available to nonactive duty military members (e.g., retired or nonactivated National Guard members). Both of these programs utilize fee-for-service insurance models. These programs utilize a preferred provider organization model that utilizes contracted civilian providers in the community. Members must use these providers and pay plan deductibles and co-payments. Annual out-of-pocket expenses for TRICARE beneficiaries are limited to $1,000 for active military personnel and $3,000 for other eligible participants.

TRICARE covers occupational therapy and physical therapy that is "medically necessary and considered proven" (Department of Defense 2012b). Five criteria are used to determine "nationally accepted medical practice":

1. Well-controlled studies of clinically meaningful endpoints, published in refereed medical literature
2. Published formal technology assessments
3. Published reports of national professional medical associations
4. Published national medical policy organization positions
5. Published reports of national expert opinion organizations

These criteria provide an excellent example of the application of evidence-based practice to health policy.

Indian Health Service

The Indian Health Service (I.H.S.) is an agency of the federal government to provide health care to 2.1 million American Indians and Alaska Natives from one of 566 recognized tribes living in 35 states (Indian Health Service 2012a). Health care is provided to this population, which often lives in rural and isolated communities with poor access to the health care system. Health care is provided through one of two mechanisms: direct delivery by the Indian Health Service and health care developed and administered by the tribes (**tribal self-determination**). The I.H.S. operates 138 hospitals, health centers, health stations, and urban Indian health projects. The tribes operate 514 hospitals, health centers, residential treatment centers, health stations, and Alaska village clinics. Either delivery model operates primarily through a global budgeting system. Unlike funding mechanisms in the civilian system, most I.H.S. resources come from direct appropriations by the Congress. The per-person expenditure for I.H.S. beneficiaries in 2010 was $2,741 vs. $7,239 per-person spending on the entire U.S. population. Physical therapy and occupational therapy services have been provided through I.H.S. since the early 1960s. Therapists provide services either as civilians or as commissioned members of the

Public Health Service. The distribution of therapists in the I.H.S. is unequal, with most therapists working in the southwest U.S. and Alaska (Indian Health Service 2012b).

Active Learning Exercise

Learn more about physical rehabilitation services in the Indian Health Service at http://www.ihs.gov/PhysicalRehab/.

Conclusion

In this chapter, we have explored health insurance plans other than Medicare that are operated by the federal and state governments. Combined with Medicare, these governmental plans fund nearly half of the United States health care system. Eligibility for these programs reflects a public consensus that government should provide health insurance for the poor, children, persons with disabilities, active military personnel, and veterans. Because these classifications include so many people of so many different backgrounds, the eligibility criteria, types of included benefits, and provider payment methods are some of the largest and most influential health policy decisions made by government. Recent innovations in these programs highlight the importance of managed care as a defining mechanism for contemporary payment of health care in America.

Although Medicaid is an important source of health care insurance for low-income people with disabilities, the provision of physical therapy and occupational therapy services is a state option. The lack of a consistent national Medicaid policy for the disabled means that many of these individuals lack access to rehabilitation services, especially in community-based environments. For military personnel and veterans, rehabilitation services are a mandated benefit. This provision reflects a belief that government has a responsibility to care for people who have served the society in certain capacities.

Chapter Review Questions

1. Review the history and origins of the Medicaid program.

2. Describe the partnership arrangement between the federal government and states as it pertains to Medicaid.

3. Define the eligibility criteria in order to receive Medicaid benefits:
   a. Categorical eligibility
   b. Medically needy
   c. Medicare-Medicaid dual eligible

4. What is included in the Medicaid benefits package?
   a. Define the position of occupational therapy and physical therapy in the Medicaid program.

5. Describe how managed care is utilized in state Medicaid programs.

6. Recall how welfare reform and immigration reform affected the Medicaid program in the 1990s.

7. Define the purpose of the State Children's Health Insurance Program (SCHIP), and describe its effectiveness in achieving this purpose.

8. Identify the eligibility criteria and benefits package for Veterans Affairs health insurance benefits

9. What is TRICARE, and how is it organized?

Chapter Discussion Questions

1. Physical therapy and occupational therapy are included as benefits in the Medicaid and Department of Veterans Affairs health insurance programs. Both of these insurance plans serve persons with disabilities. Compare and contrast the benefit packages. What are the reasons for these differences? Do you agree with them?

2. The eligibility criteria for the Medicaid program are a good example of the policy "balancing act" between egalitarian and libertarian views of the role of government in health care. Examine closely the traditional criteria and the recent immigration criteria. Analyze and discuss these criteria from both the egalitarian and libertarian points of view.

3. Managed care is increasingly being used in public insurance programs. Managed care has been more easily implemented in the Medicaid, CHIP, and TRICARE programs than in Medicare. What are the reasons for this situation? How does this reflect our political and social realities?

References

Baker, L.C., and C. Afendulis. 2005. Medicaid managed care and health care for children. *Health Serv Res* 40(5 Pt 1): 1466–68.

Banerjee, S. 2012, February. Expenditure patterns of older Americans, 2001–2009. Issue Brief. Employee Benefit Research Institute. No. 338. Retrieved from http://www.ebri.org/pdf/briefspdf/EBRI_IB_02-2012 _No368_ExpPttns.pdf (accessed April 20, 2012).

Bindman, A.B., A. Chattopadhyay, D.H. Osmond, W. Huen, and P. Bacchetti. 2005. The impact of Medicaid managed care on hospitalizations for ambulatory care sensitive conditions. *Health Serv Res* 40(1): 19–38.

Burns, M.E. 2009. Medicaid managed care and cost containment in the adult disabled population. *Med Care* 47(10): 1069–76.

Centers for Medicare and Medicaid Services. 2011a. Data Compendium. Retrieved from http://cms.gov/Research -Statistics-Data-and-Systems/Statistics-Trends-and-Reports /DataCompendium/2011_Data_Compendium.html (accessed April 18, 2012).

_____. 2011b. Data Compendium. Medicaid managed care enrollment as of July 1, 2010. Retrieved from http://www .cms.gov/Research-Statistics-Data-and-Systems/Computer -Data-and-Systems/MedicaidDataSourcesGenInfo/ Downloads/2010July1.pdf (accessed April 24, 2012).

_____. 2011c. Data Compendium. Medicaid managed care program summary. Retrieved from http://www .cms.gov/Research-Statistics-Data-and-Systems/Computer -Data-and-Systems/MedicaidDataSourcesGenInfo /Downloads/ENROLLMENT2010.pdf (accessed April 24, 2012).

Cook, B.L. 2007. Effect of Medicaid managed care on racial disparities in health care access. *Health Serv Res* 42(1 Pt 1): 124–45.

Department of Defense. 2012a. TRICARE Plans. Retrieved from http://www.tricare.mil/Welcome/Plans.aspx (accessed April 4, 2013).

_____, TRICARE. 2012b. Covered services: Occupational therapy and physical therapy. Retrieved from http://www .tricare.mil/CoveredServices.aspx (accessed April 4, 2013).

Duderstadt K.G., D.C. Hughes, M.J. Soobader, and P.W. Newacheck. 2006. The impact of public insurance expansions on children's access and use of care. *Pediatrics* 118(4): 1676–82.

Felland, L.E., C.S. Lesser, A.B. Staiti, A. Katz, and P. Lichiello. 2003. The resilience of the health care safety net, 1996–2001. *Health Serv Res* 38(1 Pt 2): 489–502.

Garrett, B., and S. Zuckerman. 2005. National estimates of the effects of mandatory Medicaid managed care programs on health care access and use, 1997–1999. *Med Care* 43(7): 649–57.

Hu, H.T., and P.J. Cunningham. 2005. Public coverage provides vital safety net for children with special health care needs . *Issue Brief Cent Stud Health Syst Change* 98: 1–7.

Hughes, J.S. 2003. Can the Veterans Affairs health system continue to care for the poor and vulnerable? *J Amb Care Manage* 26(4): 344–48.

Iglehart, J.K. 2011. Desperately seeking savings: States shift more Medicaid enrollees to managed care. *Health Affairs* 30(9): 1627–29.

Indian Health Service. 2012a. Indian Health Service: A Quick Look. Retrieved from http://www.ihs.gov/factsheets/index .cfm?module=dsp_fact_quicklook (accessed April 4, 2013).

_____. 2012b. Physical Rehabilitation Services. Retrieved from http://www.ihs.gov/MedicalPrograms/PhysicalRehab/index .cfm (accessed April 25, 2012).

Kaiser Commission on Medicaid and the Uninsured. 2013a. Medicaid: A Primer. Retrieved from http://www.kff.org /medicaid/upload/7334-05.pdf (accessed April 4, 2013).

_____. 2012b, December. The Medicaid medically needy program: Spending and enrollment update. Issue Paper. Retrieved from http://www.kff.org/medicaid/upload/4096 .pdf (accessed April 4, 2013).

_____. 2012c, April. Medicaid's role for dual eligible beneficiaries. Issue Paper. Retrieved from http://www.kff .org/medicaid/upload/7846-03.pdf (accessed April 26, 2012).

_____. 2006, March. Medicaid's high cost enrollees: How much do they drive program spending? Retrieved from http:// www.kff.org/medicaid/7490.cfm (accessed June 20, 2007).

Kempe, A., B.L. Beaty, L.A. Crane, J. Stokstad, J. Barrow, S. Belman, and J.F. Steiner. 2005. Changes in access, utilization, and quality of care after enrollment into a state child health insurance plan. *Pediatrics* 115(2): 364–71.

Kenney, G., and J. Yee. 2007. SCHIP at a crossroads: Experiences to date and challenges ahead. *Health Affairs* 26(2): 356–69.

Kizer, K.W., and R.A. Dudley. 2009. Extreme makeover: Transformation of the Veterans Health Care System. *Ann Rev Publ Health* 30: 313–39.

Metlife Mature Market Institute. 2011. Market survey of long-term care costs. Retrieved from http://www.metlife.com /mmi/research/2011-market-survey-long-term-care-costs .html#graphic (accessed April 26, 2012).

Ng T., C. Harrington, and M. Kitchener. 2010. Medicare and Medicaid in long-term care. *Health Affairs* 29(1): 22–28.

Regenstein, M., and S.E. Anthony. 1998. Assessing the new federalism: Medicaid managed care for persons with disabilities. Retrieved from http://www.urban.org /UploadedPDF/occa11.pdf (accessed April 4, 2013).

Seid M., J.W. Varni, L. Cummings, and M. Schonlau. 2006. The impact of realized access to care on health-related quality of life: A two year prospective cohort study of children in the California State Children's Health Insurance Program. *J Pediatr* 149(3): 354–61.

Tu, H.T., and P.J. Cunningham. 2005. Public coverage provides vital safety net for children with special health care needs. *Issue Brief Cent Stud Health Syst Change* 98: 1–7.

The Acute Medical Care System

CHAPTER OBJECTIVES

At the conclusion of this chapter, the reader will be able to:

1. Explain the historical development of the hospital.
2. Describe the administrative structure of hospitals.
3. Define a hospital by size, ownership, and scope of services.
4. Compare and contrast primary, secondary, tertiary, and quaternary care.
5. Describe the development of integrated health care systems.
6. Discuss the development and results of physician-hospital integration in the acute medical care delivery system.

KEY WORDS

Accountable Care Organizations
Alternative Medicine
Complementary Medicine
Hospitals
Integrated Health Care System
Matrix System
Patient-Centered Medical Home
Patient-Focused Care
Physician-Hospital Organization
Primary Care
Product-Line Team
Quaternary Care
Safety Net
Secondary Care
Tertiary Care

CASE EXAMPLE ··

Jim M. Charge is the Director of Occupational Therapy in Anytown Hospital. Jim is responsible for the patient care and the supervision of four occupational therapists in his area. The administration of Anytown Hospital has decided to expand their rehabilitation services, which also include physical therapy and speech/language pathology. The reason for this expansion is that the hospital wants to develop a unit to treat persons with stroke and hip fractures. As a result of this change, Jim has been asked to lead the stroke team. This will require him to not only manage the occupational therapists in the hospital but also physical therapists and speech/language pathologists who are working with the patients with stroke. The reason for this change is to develop stronger "patient-focused care" in the hospital. This is an example of a matrix management system where people with similar skills are pooled together to accomplish certain tasks.

Case Example Questions:

1. What are some reasons or benefits for using a matrix management system?

2. Discuss how making this change impacts the hospital's organizational structure?

Introduction

In the preceding chapters, we have introduced and focused on health care policy and reimbursement. With this chapter, we will begin to discuss the health care system. Upcoming chapters will discuss the post-acute care system, mental health care system, public health, educational environments, and alternative medical providers.

When we think of the U.S. health care system, we commonly break it down into two broad categories—an acute medical delivery system and a post-acute care delivery system (see Figure 10-1). The acute medical delivery system includes primary, secondary, and tertiary care systems. The post-acute care system consists of a mix of subacute care, long-term care, outpatient services, home health care, and hospice. This chapter focuses mainly on the acute medical care delivery system and in particular on one of the biggest players in this system, the hospital. This is the site (along with school-based and mental health environments [see Chapter 12]) where most occupational therapists and physical therapists work. Much of our acute medical care system is centered on the bioscientific, allopathic medical care model. As we discussed in Chapter 1, the growth of the health care system in the 20th century developed in response to this framework for understanding

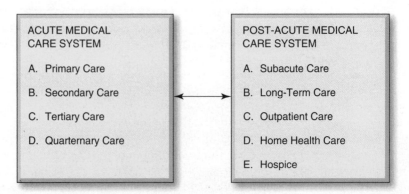

FIGURE 10-1 The United States Health Care System

and treating disease. **Alternative medicine** providers, (e.g., chiropractors or naturopaths), continue to deliver health care in the United States. Some providers, (e.g., physical therapist or occupational therapists), utilize alternative medical procedures in their practice. Conventional health care providers who do so are practicing **complementary medicine**. Given the increasing emphasis on evidence-based practice tied to payment for health care services, the future growth of alternative and complementary medicine is uncertain. It is important, however, that you understand these terms and recognize the role of complementary and alternative medicine in health care.

Active Learning Exercise

Visit the website of the National Center for Complementary and Alternative Medicine to learn more about this type of health care: http://nccam.nih.gov. How is research into complementary and alternative medicine affecting the delivery of health care services?

Hospitals are arguably one of the most recognized entities of the health care system. Hospitals are home to many activities related to health care, including patient care, medical education, and research functions. Additionally, hospitals are usually one of the major employers in a community. In this chapter, we examine hospitals and the acute care medical system more closely and explain their role in the health care system. We discuss the historical development of hospitals, their diverse functions and characteristics, their management structures, and their position within the primary, secondary, tertiary, and quaternary health care system. We will conclude with a discussion of the various forces that both constrain and promote change in the hospital industry. An understanding of the hospital's role in the health care system and the external forces that influence them is critical to therapists because it represents, in large part, the health care environment in which they must interact.

Hospitals

Historical Development

The hospitals that existed in early America were very different from the hospitals that we have today. The first hospitals were primarily charitable religious organizations whose missions were focused more on providing care to those they served than on curing their illnesses (Freymann 1974; Starr 1982). Early hospitals tended to care for and shelter the poor, elderly, orphaned, and homeless, in addition to protecting society from those who were contagious or dangerously insane (Sultz and Young 1999). Thus, these early hospitals were nothing more than infirmaries for the sick and the poor and were focused on caring for individuals and not necessarily curing them. Hospitals were commonly characterized as dirty and overcrowded environments with limited medical capabilities. While the early hospitals only served the poor, people with sufficient financial resources received care at home.

From the late 1800s to the early 1900s, hospitals began to evolve into the physician's workshop. Advances in biomedical science and technology made it more difficult and complex for physicians to have everything they needed in their "black bags" (Kovner 1995). While earlier hospitals had provided more care than cure, hospitals during this period were better able to provide a cure and a means of intervention. Because of improvements in science and technology, the hospital industry experienced a large growth in the number of hospitals, and by 1909 there were more than 4,300 hospitals in the United States, compared to just 178 in 1873 (Stevens 1971).

A second major era of growth took place between 1945 and 1980. Two major events contributed to this growth: (1) federal monies became available to build new hospitals under the Hill-Burton Act and (2) the rapid growth of hospital insurance, including Medicare and Medicaid, increased the diversity and number of services offered to a hospital's inpatients (Kovner 1995). Without clear and consistent oversight, however, these policies resulted in creating a hospital environment characterized by overbuilding and overcapacity, which resulted in a call for hospitals to become more accountable and efficient. During this era, the number of hospitals grew to more than 6,000.

In part, because of this overbuilding and overcapacity, hospitals in the 1990s experienced consolidation through the formation of networks and through closure. One of the several reasons for these changes included the cost of building and maintaining a hospital, especially in a period of cost control. In some cases, hospitals have closed because of a declining demand for their services. Mergers or consolidations were pursued to establish integrated delivery systems. **Integrated health care systems** are discussed in more detail later in this chapter. In part due to mergers and consolidation, the total number of community hospitals for the years 2000 through 2010 has been relatively stable and is approximately 4,900 hospitals per year (Kaiser State Health Facts 2010).

In the next sections, we briefly examine the managerial structure of hospitals and their unique characteristics that help to describe these organizations.

Hospital Structure

Hospitals have a complex administrative structure that is reflective of the growth of hospitals into an established organizational institution. Since physicians have the ability to control the type and amount of services patients consume, physicians have always had, and still have, an important role in the organization and management of hospitals. For years, physicians or leaders of religious organizations managed hospitals. However, the complexity of hospital management led to the creation of the field of health services management. A traditional hospital structure includes a board of directors, an administrative structure, and a medical staff structure (see Figure 10-2). Physical therapy and occupational therapy services may be positioned under the health services administrator or the medical director.

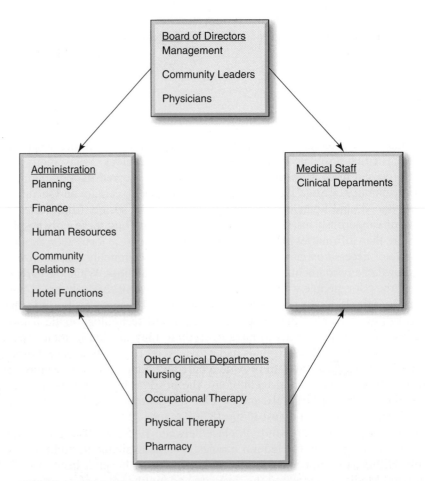

FIGURE 10-2 Traditional Structure of Hospitals

A board of directors is selected that retains fiduciary responsibility to manage and govern the hospital. This includes the hiring of a management team. Physicians are commonly represented on the hospital's board of directors. Historically, hospital administrators were primarily responsible for nonclinical matters, such as finance, personnel, community/public relations, and the hospital's "hotel" functions (laundry, housekeeping, etc.). However, in today's environment, strategic planning and negotiating ability are critical skills for the successful health care executive.

A hospital structure will also include a medical division, usually headed by a physician known as the chief of the medical staff, who is the liaison to the hospital administration and commonly serves on the board of directors. A medical division is commonly divided into departments by medical specialty (e.g., internal medicine, surgery). The medical division has important oversight over credentialing of health care professionals (i.e., determining their right to admit patients, perform surgery, etc.) and provides consultation about the quality of care in the hospital.

Other clinical professions are represented in various ways. Organizationally, these professions may be placed under the hospital administration component of the structure or under the medical division. The largest unit is usually the nursing division, which is traditionally organized into subunits by types of patient treatment/pathology (e.g., orthopedics, pediatrics). Physical therapy, occupational therapy, and the other rehabilitation disciplines are traditionally organized by discipline.

The development of **patient-focused care** has resulted in a radical reorganization of this system. Patient-focused care organizes providers around perceived patient needs rather than around professional disciplines or procedures. This avoids certain problems typical of traditional structures, such as poor communication and redundancy of services. Therapists may be organized into **product-line teams** organized around common patient types (e.g., stroke teams, joint-replacement teams). In this case, occupational therapists and physical therapists may be responsible to a team leader for their activities and performance. In some cases a dual-management structure called a **matrix system** is established whereby a physical therapist may be responsible to a team leader for clinical matters and to a physical therapy manager for nonclinical matters (e.g., personnel issues) (Boissoneau 1983) (see Figure 10-3).

Hospital Characteristics

Hospitals differ along various dimensions, including size and scope, ownership, general vs. specialty hospitals, acute care vs. long-term care hospitals, teaching vs. nonteaching hospitals, and independent hospitals vs. those in multihospital systems or networks. This section explores these issues in greater detail.

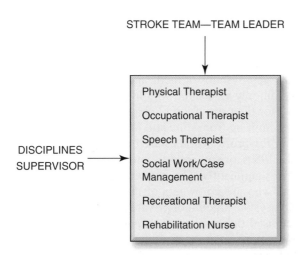

FIGURE 10-3 "Matrix" Hospital Organizational Structure

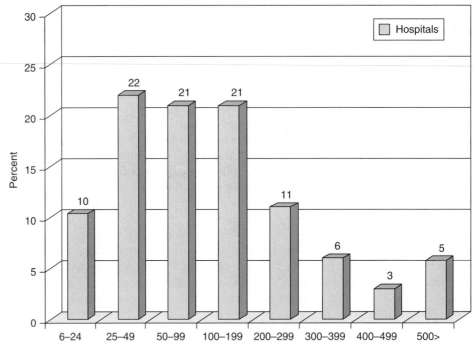

FIGURE 10-4 Percentage of U.S. Hospitals by Bed Size, 2012

Source: AHRQ (2012) Hospital Survey on Patient Safety cutlure: 2012 User Comparitive Database Report.

SIZE   The number of inpatient beds that are set up and staffed is one indicator of the size of a hospital. Figure 10-4 shows the distribution of hospitals by bed size and that most hospitals are under 200 beds. The larger hospitals most likely represent large tertiary care centers that care not only for a general population but also for a large indigent population and persons in need of advanced specialty services (e.g., trauma care).

OWNERSHIP   Hospital organizations generally have one of three types of ownership classification:

1. Hospitals operated by nonprofit organizations are referred to as not-for-profit hospitals.
2. Hospitals owned and operated by profit-making corporations are known as investor-owned or for-profit hospitals.
3. Hospitals owned and managed by either federal, state, or local government bodies are referred to as public hospitals.

Almost 60 percent of all community hospitals are not-for-profit organizations (Kaiser State Health Facts 2012) that are managed by community boards or religious organizations (see Figure 10-5). For example, religious orders within the Roman Catholic Church operate some of the largest systems of medical care facilities in the United States. These hospitals are more commonly associated with local decision making and the provision of charity care. In return for their provision of charity care, the federal government has historically granted an exemption from state and federal taxation.

Investor-owned or for-profit hospitals are dominated by national chains (e.g., Tenet Healthcare). Since the 1980s, private investment in hospitals and the development of hospital chains has grown significantly. The net revenue from for-profit hospitals is shared with outside investors who are co-owners of the hospital. Investor participation in the hospital industry increases the amount of private capital available for medical care investment. It also has increased the emphasis on financial management of all hospitals. For-profit companies own approximately 21 percent of the hospitals in the United States (Kaiser State Health Facts 2012).

One of the main distinguishing aspects between for-profit and not-for-profit facilities pertains to how net revenue is used. Whatever its profit status, every hospital must

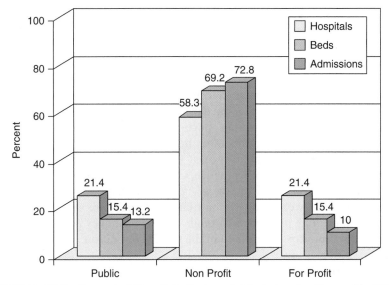

FIGURE 10-5 Percent of Hospitals, Beds, and Admissions by Ownership, 2010

generate some type of profit—the difference is how that profit is used. In a not-for-profit facility, profits are returned to the organization or community, whereas a for-profit organization distributes the profits to its shareholders.

The last type of ownership structure discussed here is the public hospital. The public hospital was the primary source of health care for the poor and indigent before the advent of Medicaid in 1965. Examples of public- and government-controlled hospitals include city and county hospitals (e.g., John H. Stroger Jr. Hospital of Cook County in Chicago), military hospitals, VA hospitals, and U.S. Public Health Service hospitals (e.g., Indian Health Service hospitals). Public hospitals provide an important safety net for the poor and for populations where private organizations have chosen not to provide services.

In addition to these three distinct categories, a number of hybrid ownership structures exist. Some hospitals have multiple owners. For example, when a not-for-profit hospital is sold to a for-profit company, the not-for-profit organization may retain some ownership short of a majority. Additionally, some local government hospitals may be leased and managed by a for-profit organization while the government retains ownership of the hospital.

GENERAL VS. SPECIALTY A general hospital provides general medical services, such as ambulatory surgery, pediatric inpatient care, rehabilitation outpatient care, emergency services, open heart surgery, angioplasty, obstetric services, and community health promotion. Alternatively, specialty hospitals provide services for either specific diseases or specifically defined populations. Examples of specialty hospitals include children's hospitals, long-term care centers, rehabilitation hospitals, mental health or psychiatric hospitals, and substance abuse centers.

ACUTE CARE VS. LONG-TERM CARE Many general hospitals are classified as acute care facilities as well. Acute care hospitals serve inpatients that have an average length of stay of no more than 30 days. Most of the patients admitted to these hospitals actually stay for less than 10 days. Patients in these hospitals have acute short-term illnesses, as compared to patients with chronic illness that may require prolonged treatment.

Long-term care hospitals include such facilities as nursing homes, psychiatric hospitals, and rehabilitation hospitals as well as home health agencies. Long-term care provides care for those experiencing diminishing functional capabilities. The level of functioning may vary across age categories and chronic conditions. Care provided to these individuals may be continuous or intermittent, but will be carried on over a long time or throughout the patient's life (Kane and Kane 1987). In some cases both the long-term facility and acute care hospital will have a common owner or be located in close proximity.

TEACHING HOSPITALS   Teaching hospitals are an important part of America's health care system. In addition to their sophisticated technology and cutting-edge research, they deliver a large percentage of health care services throughout the country (Iglehart 1993). They also deliver a disproportionate share of charity and indigent care. Although only a small percentage (approximately 6%) of all short-term nonfederal acute care hospitals are classified as members of the Council of Teaching Hospitals and Health Systems (COTH), they represent approximately 47 percent of all the discharges across the country (HCUPnet 2012).

The Council of Teaching Hospitals, part of the Association for Academic Medical Centers (AAMC), specifies (1) that member hospitals must sponsor four approved medical residency programs and (2) that at least two of the four programs must be either medicine, surgery, pediatrics, family practice, OBGYN, or psychiatry. Teaching hospitals have the additional responsibility of educating our nation's physician base and conducting medical research as well as providing quality patient care. Though other hospitals may participate in training physicians through various residency programs, they have not demonstrated the commitment outlined in the COTH definition.

Safety-Net Hospitals

Many different types of provider organizations, including hospitals, come together to make up the nation's **safety net** that provides care for vulnerable patient populations, including those without health care insurance or the ability to pay for health care services. Every year these hospitals provide uncompensated care that is worth billions of dollars (Bazzoli et al. 2005). These hospitals are typically considered to consist of both academic medical centers and public hospitals. From a policy perspective, it is important to understand the role that these hospitals play in care for the poor and uninsured. These hospitals receive funding from local, state, and federal government agencies. They will also bill for Medicare, Medicaid, and private insurers. Thus, policies or environmental changes that impact these payment sources have a relatively greater negative impact on safety-net hospitals than their "non–safety-net" hospital counterparts.

For example, from the late 1990s through early 2000s, a number of forces affected the hospital industry in general. During the late 1990s, health maintenance organizations gained power and used their leverage to negotiate deals with hospitals that lowered the hospital's reimbursement for services (Bazzoli et al. 2005). Additionally, during this time, hospitals felt the impact of the Balanced Budget Act of 1997 (BBA) (see Chapter 8) in terms of Medicare and Medicaid payments. Despite changes to the BBA in 1999 and 2000, hospitals still saw a decline in their payment growth coupled with higher expenses resulting from higher operating cost (Strunk and Ginsburg 2003). As this short review indicates, safety-net hospitals operate in a competitive, price-sensitive market where policy changes have a direct impact on their viability. Policy makers and providers must consistently be concerned and vigilant to evaluate how these hospitals are affected and if any of these hospitals fall through the cracks.

Multihospital Systems and Networks

According to the American Hospital Association, multihospital systems (MHS) are defined as two or more hospitals that are owned, leased, or contract-managed by the same organization (AHA 1998). These systems can be either for-profit or not-for-profit and may be limited to the local area or part of a national company. The AHA defines alliances as formal organizations that work for the benefits of their members to provide services and products as well as the promotion of activities and ventures. Though many hospitals participate in one or both of these activities, some hospitals remain independent and unaffiliated in any way.

Active Learning Exercise

On the World Wide Web go to the Kaiser Family Foundation at http://www.statehealthfacts .org and get the last data on number of hospitals, admissions, outpatient visits, and more. You can also examine the data by state.

Table 10-1 Characteristics of Professionals Employed in Health Care

Profession	No. Employed	No. Employed in Hospitals	Education	Avg. Salary ($)
General Medicine	202,800	17,750	Post-Doctorate	177,300
Surgeons	42,340	6,510	Post-Doctorate	231,550
Registered Nurses	2,724,570	1,556,930	Associate Degree	69,110
Respiratory Therapists	113,980	87,520	Associate Degree	56,260
Occupational Therapists	103,570	23,820	Masters Degree	74,970
Physical Therapists	185,440	48,100	Clinical Doctorate	79,830

Source: Bureau of Labor Statistics. Occupational Employment Statistics. 2011. Accessed at http://www.bls.gov/oes/ on August 1, 2012.

Professionals Working in Hospitals

Historically, hospitals have been considered to be the "physician's workshop." As was discussed earlier in this chapter, the development of hospitals in the 20th century was closely tied to the development of a bioscientific model of medicine. Today, hospitals are a center of health care technology applied to disease and injury. As a result, a number of professions have sizable workforces in hospitals (see Table 10-1).

Levels of Acute Care

Hospitals are capable of providing various levels of care. Some hospitals are known as tertiary facilities, while others are primary or secondary care hospitals. In this section, we focus on the three most common levels of care: primary, secondary, and tertiary. The main features of these levels of care are summarized in Table 10-2.

Primary Care

The first level of care in the U.S. health care system is known as **primary care** and represents the main entry point by which most people come into contact with the health care delivery system. It deals with illnesses that are general, episodic, common, and nonchronic in nature. In 1995, the Institute of Medicine offered a revised definition of primary care: "Primary care is the provision of integrated, accessible health care services

Table 10-2 Characteristics of Primary, Secondary, Tertiary, and Quaternary Care

A. Primary care	Treats common, nonchronic, episodic disorders Provides care in context of family and community Coordinator of care in managed care systems
B. Secondary care	Treats common, chronic-type disorders Long-term care required (e.g., diabetes, hypertension management)
C. Tertiary care	Treats complex, acute, and chronic disorders Utilizes specialized diagnostic and treatment procedures
D. Quaternary care	Treats uncommon acute and chronic disorders Associated with academic medical centers For example, organ transplantation

by clinicians who are accountable for addressing a large majority of personal health care needs, developing a sustained partnership with patients, and practicing in the context of family and community." Central to this definition are the concepts of access, accountability, and integrated services, all of which are discussed throughout this text.

Primary care provides most of the health care that people usually need and is the vehicle used to integrate the delivery of health care services. Primary care physicians include family medicine, internal medicine, pediatrics, and obstetrics/gynecology.

THERAPISTS WORKING IN PRIMARY CARE The development of direct access to therapy services and the growth of an outpatient model of therapy care has resulted in more therapists working in disease and injury prevention, triage in the emergency room, and in assessment of patients without physician referral. The best known model of direct access in primary care physical therapy is in the military. Moore et al. (2006) examined nearly 51,000 physical therapist direct access encounters with patients over a 40-month period and found no adverse events. In 2006, over 48,000 physical therapists and 18,000 occupational therapists worked in an outpatient office model of care (Bureau of Labor Statistics 2007).

SECONDARY CARE **Secondary care**, like primary care, may be provided in an ambulatory setting or on an inpatient basis. Secondary care is more intense than primary care, and often extends over a longer period. Unlike primary care, where illnesses or injuries are acute, secondary care focuses on injuries or illnesses that are chronic and require continuing care. Examples of conditions that require secondary care include arthritis, diabetes, and hypertension.

TERTIARY AND QUARTENARY CARE The last level of care discussed here is referred to as **tertiary care**. This care is highly specialized, complex, and costly, and delivery takes place in an inpatient setting. Teaching hospitals or academic medical centers were once the main setting for tertiary care services. However, because of the advances being made and the fierce competition among health care providers, many community hospitals can now offer these services. Examples of tertiary care include such procedures as coronary artery bypass grafting and specialized diagnostic devices (Blumenthal et al. 1997). With the continual advances being made, an even higher level of care known as **quartenary care** is available, and is predominantly provided at academic medical centers. Quartenary care services include burn units, trauma centers, transplant services, and so forth.

Hospital Integration

During the 1990s, an increase in public awareness of the problems of the uninsured and the costs of health care services coupled with the threat of government reform set in motion a number of consolidation activities and other market responses from hospital organizations and other health care providers. These responses include outright mergers, vertical integration, and the formation of hospital alliances between various health care organizations (e.g., physician-hospital alliances).

The hospital industry went through significant restructuring over the past several decades, beginning with multihospital system growth in the 1970s and 1980s (Alexander and Morrisey 1988; Ermann and Gabel 1986; Shortell 1988) and shifting to local market consolidation in the 1990s (Luke 1991). The formation of local hospital collectives helped hospitals defend themselves against increasingly powerful competitors and improve their market positions relative to such rivals as managed care organizations, consolidating physician populations, active business coalitions, large businesses, and government agencies (Zelman 1996).

Efforts to reform the delivery of health care have emphasized the importance of providing cost-effective, comprehensive patient care. One mechanism that has the capability of providing this comprehensive care is the integrated delivery system (Enthoven 2009). Integrated delivery systems often consist of a variety of delivery components and payment mechanisms. Many players are involved in the creation of integrated delivery systems, including insurers, managed care organizations, health care systems, hospitals, and medical groups (Shih et al., 2008). It is argued that the benefits of joining together in this way include the achievement of greater efficiency. Sterns (2007) reported that

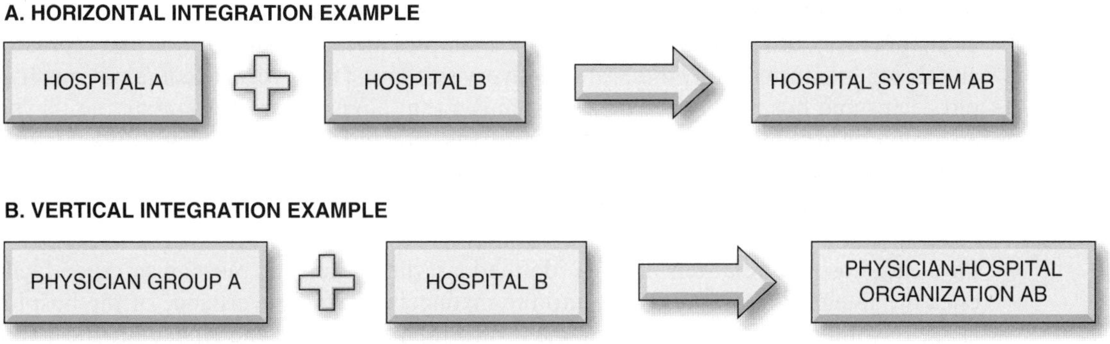

A. HORIZONTAL INTEGRATION EXAMPLE

HOSPITAL A ➕ HOSPITAL B ➡ HOSPITAL SYSTEM AB

B. VERTICAL INTEGRATION EXAMPLE

PHYSICIAN GROUP A ➕ HOSPITAL B ➡ PHYSICIAN-HOSPITAL ORGANIZATION AB

FIGURE 10-6 Horizontal and Vertical Integration

integrated delivery systems linking hospitals and physicians do appear to be better at providing efficient care and better overall outcomes. While there are many models of integrated delivery systems, Shih et al. identified four basic models. The first model is a single entity system that includes hospitals, physicians, and a health plan. Kaiser Permanente and Geisinger Health Systems are examples of this model. The second model includes a single entity delivery system but without the health plan, such as the Mayo Clinic. Model 3 consists of multiple independent providers that make up organizations that allow them to share and coordinate services. There are many types of integration formats that would fall under model 3, including physician-hospital organizations, group practices without walls, and IPAs to name a few. The last model includes government-facilitated networks of providers. These systems are usually created to help care for Medicaid beneficiaries.

There is a wide variety of integrated delivery system models. Integrated delivery systems are commonly formed through a process of horizontal or vertical integration (see Figure 10-6). Horizontal integration occurs when two or more firms producing similar services join to become a single organization. Hospitals merging or forming strategic hospital alliances (Luke, Olden, and Bramble 1998) and the consolidation of smaller solo practices into larger multispecialty group practices (see Kralewski et al. 1999) are examples of horizontal integration. Alternatively, vertical integration occurs as hospitals and physicians join with other organizations to provide a continuum of care within a single organization, including therapy services, nursing home care, health plans, and so forth.

In the early 1990s, the American Hospital Association advocated the formation of local "integrated delivery systems" (American Hospital Association 1990). These integrated systems were intended to improve the efficiency of care, increasing system accountability for both community needs and health outcomes (American Hospital Association 1992). Although some hospitals have begun to move toward a system that integrates a variety of providers, the most common activity is the horizontal combination of hospitals into local systems of networks within local markets.

There are many reasons why organizations come together to form strategic partnerships. In health care, unique and specific reasons precipitate their formation (Luke, Olden, and Bramble 1998). Foremost was the threat of managed care in the market (Olden, Roggenkamp, and Luke 2002). As hospitals combine to form local hospital systems and networks, they collectively increase their geographic presence. By thus offering greater spatial coverage, they increase their leverage in negotiations for managed care contracts. Joining together at the local level also allows organizations to develop health care products that enhance their positions in the markets.

In addition to forming horizontal relationships, hospitals are also joining vertically with physician organizations. Physician-hospital relationships are sometimes called **physician-hospital organizations** (PHOs) and represent a vertical integration strategy.

Vertical integration refers to the combination of two or more firms that were previously separate and whose products or services are inputs (or outputs) from the production of another service into a single firm. One possible advantage of these types of integration is transaction cost savings (see D'Aunno and Zuckerman 1987). Combinations of clinical group practices and acute care facilities are examples of vertical integration and represent an essential feature of fully integrated delivery systems. These vertical combinations (i.e., physicians and hospitals) provide a mechanism that aligns incentives among the players and make it possible to unify marketing efforts directed at managed care organizations (Burns and Thorpe 1993; Morrisey et al. 1999).

Physician-Hospital Relationships

Physician-hospital relationships are defined as the structural mechanism that facilitates the integration of physicians into the management and governance of the hospital as well as the integration of management into the activities of the clinical-medical staff (Alexander, Morrisey, and Shortell 1986). The purpose of these relationships is to link patient entry points to the health care delivery system, forming a continuum of services for the patient (Harris, Hicks, and Kelly 1992). Over the last five years, physician-hospital organizations have been cited with increased frequency. In the changing health care environment, physician groups are forging closer ties with hospitals as a means of lowering expenses and taking advantage of managed care contracting opportunities (Zajac, D'Aunno, and Burns 2006).

Having recognized the use of primary care physicians as gatekeepers to manage the entrance of patients into the system (Burns and Thorpe 1993), hospitals are trying to establish linkages with physician groups to ensure a constant flow of patients. Linking up with physician groups increases their leverage over managed care firms by allowing them to pool their contracting activities with other providers to achieve economies and efficiencies of scale (Burns and Thorpe 1993). Hospitals are facing growing competitive threats to their market share and profitability. Large multispecialty group practices are one source of competition. In the face of this threat, hospitals have sought to gain control over the ambulatory care of physicians in the market, thus preempting possible competitive initiatives from physicians.

Physician-system integration and clinical integration include developing mechanisms for joint hospital-physician planning and patient care services. Many new organizations attempt to integrate physicians vertically with acute care facilities, using various mechanisms to achieve this goal. Hospital-physician organizations can be arranged in a variety of ways and with different types of governance structures in which one or another of the founding entities takes a leadership role. The simplest categorization of these organizations is the four-level model developed by Shortell and his colleagues. The integrated delivery system may be hospital/health system led, physician/group practice led, insurance company led, or a hybrid model where the hospital organization and the physician groups are codominant (Shortell et al. 1994).

As a therapist, it is important to understand that the environment in which you may find yourself working consists of many different models. Early on, four overarching models were introduced, but within those models there are many different structures. These include the group practice without walls model (GPWW), the independent practice association (IPA), the management services organization (MSO), the physician-hospital organization (PHO), the salary staff models, the foundation model, and the physician equity model (Conners 1997). While newer terms for these organizations have been introduced, such as joint-operating agreements, franchise agreements, master affiliation agreements, gain-sharing models, and regional service organizations (Zajac, D'Aunno, and Burns 2006), many of the goals and purposes of these organizations remain the same. These goals and purposes include increased leverage in negotiating managed care contracts, capital and information systems sharing, quality improvement and efficiency, creating a broad continuum of care, sharing administrative expenses, and increasing physician involvement in the process of managed care contracting (Burns and Thorpe 1993; Coile and Grant 1997; Dowling 1995; Fine 1997; Shortell et al. 1996). In part to reduce uncertainty in an increasingly complex and competitive environment, hospitals and physicians continue to engage in integration activities (Zajac, D'Aunno, and Burns 2006).

Accountable Care Organizations and Patient-Centered Medical Homes

The drive to control health care costs and to improve access to services has necessitated much of the integration of the health care system, such as physician-hospital organizations. The Patient Protection and Affordable Care Act of 2010 (PPACA) encourages the development of risk-taking physician-hospital organizations called **accountable care organizations** and an integrated outpatient team: the **patient-centered medical home**. Accountable care organizations are integrated health delivery systems that manage populations of patients across all levels of care (Centers for Medicare and Medicaid Services 2012). Patient-centered medical homes are coordinated ambulatory care systems comprised of patient teams led by a physician that work together to comprehensively manage populations. Patient-centered medical homes are characterized by five primary care features: patient-centeredness, comprehensive care, coordinated care, excellent access to care, and use of information to improve quality and safety (AHRQ 2011) Both of these models of care are intended to be able to accept and manage capitated contracts to successfully deliver comprehensive health services to its population. In both cases, they are intended to address known problems with the expensive, fragmented delivery of health care in the United States and improve patient outcomes. The PPACA provides for financial incentives ("shared savings") from the government to these organizations who provide care for Medicare beneficiaries (Longworth 2011). Data, information technology, quality assessment, collaboration, and provider control will be critical to the success or failure of these forms of integrated health system (Emanuel 2012). Currently, this program is not widespread. The effect of ACOs and medical homes on therapists (e.g., therapists in private practice) has yet to unfold.

Conclusion

The 20th century saw the development of the hospital as the cornerstone of the acute medical care delivery system. Advances in biomedical science and policy decisions to fund hospital services were important catalysts in the development of the hospital. The provision of tertiary and quarternary care was the pinnacle of these 20th-century trends. However, the increasing utilization of hospital services and the high costs associated with hospital growth have factored into the move toward community-based primary care to prevent illness and injury. As a result, the acute medical care delivery system has seen the development of integrated health systems in many markets as providers align with one another both vertically and horizontally to provide services in a more cost-effective manner. With the recent changes due to the PPACA, this trend is expected to strengthen.

Chapter Review Questions

1. Describe the development of the U.S. hospital in three periods:

   a. pre-1900
   b. 1900–1945
   c. 1946–present

2. How are hospitals administratively organized?

3. Define patient-focused care, product-line teams, and matrix management in a hospital.

4. Identify common characteristic descriptors of a hospital.

5. Define primary care, secondary care, tertiary care, and quaternary care.

6. Describe the incentives for and process of development of integrated health systems in the United States.

7. Summarize the relationship of physicians and hospitals over the last century.

8. Define an accountable care organization and patient-centered medical home.

Chapter Discussion Questions

1. Discuss how the administrative structure of hospitals enhances and limits the professional autonomy of occupational therapists and physical therapists. What are the historical reasons for this situation?

2. Clinical occupational therapists and physical therapists working on product-line teams may report directly to a nontherapist supervisor on a regular basis. Discuss the pros and cons of this form of hospital organization for the role of physical therapists and occupational therapists in a hospital.

3. Integrated health delivery systems that coordinate and, in some cases, consolidate primary, secondary, and tertiary care in a community are a contemporary form of acute medical care delivery. What effect could you expect to observe on small, private-practice providers (e.g., physicians, therapists) in communities with large integrated health delivery systems? Discuss some strategies that would be necessary to compete or collaborate with such systems.

References

AHRQ. 2011. What is the PCMH? AHRQ's definition of the medical home. Retrieved from http://pcmh.ahrq.gov/portal /server.pt/community/pcmh__home/1483/what_is_pcmh_ (accessed on April 18, 2013).

_____. 2012. Hospital survey on patient safety culture: 2012 User comparitive database report. Retrieved from http://www.ahrq.gov/qual/hospsurvey12/hosp12tab3-1.htm (accessed June 2012).

Alexander, J.A., G.J. Bazzoli, L.R. Burns, and S.M. Shortell. 1999. Measures of physician-system integration. Paper presented at the annual meeting of the Association for Health Service Research, Chicago.

_____, and M.A. Morrisey. 1988. Hospital-physician integration and hospital costs. *Inquiry* 25(4): 388–401.

_____, M.A. Morrisey, and S.M. Shortell. 1986. Effects of competition, regulation, and corporatization on hospital-physician relationships. *J Health and Soc Behav* 27: 220–35.

American Hospital Association. 1990. *Renewing the U.S. health care system*. Washington DC: Section for Health Care Systems, Office of Constituency Sections.

_____.1992. *Overview: AHA's national reform strategy*. Chicago: American Hospital Association.

_____.1998. *AHA guide, 1999–2000 edition*. Chicago: American Hospital Association.

Bazzoli, G.J., R. Kang, R. Hasnain-Wynia, R.C. Lindrooth. 2005. An update on safety-net hospitals: Coping with the late 1990s and early 2000s. *Health Affairs* 24 (4): 1047–1056.

Blumenthal D., E.G. Campbell, and J.S. Weissman. 1997. The social missions of academic health centers. *N Engl J Med* 337(21): 1550–53.

Boissoneau R. 1983. Matrix management in the health care organization. *Health Care Sup* 2(1): 22–36.

Bureau of Labor Statistics. 2007. Occupational employment statistics for physical therapists and occupational therapists. Retrieved from http://www.bls.gov/oes (accessed September 17, 2007).

Burns, L.R., and D.P. Thorpe. 1993. Trends and models in physician-hospital organization. *Health Care Manag Rev* 18(4): 7–20.

_____. 1995. Managed care and integrated health care. *Health Care Manag* 2(1): 101–108.

Centers for Medicare and Medicaid Services. 2012. Accountable care organization 2013 program analysis. Retrieved from http://www.cms.gov/Medicare/Medicare-Fee-for-Service -Payment/sharedsavingsprogram/Downloads/ACO -NarrativeMeasures-Specs.pdf (accessed April 18, 2013).

Coile, R.C., and P.N. Grant. 1997. Group practice affiliation structures. In R.B. Conners, ed., *Integrating the practice of medicine* (307–31). Chicago: American Hospital Publishing.

Conners, R.B., ed. 1997. *Integrating the practice of medicine*. Chicago: American Hospital Publishing.

D'Aunno, T.A. and H.S. Zuckerman. 1987. The emergence of hospital federations: An integration of perspectives from organizational theory. *Med Care Rev* 44(2): 323–43.

Dowling, W.L. 1995. Strategic alliances as a structure for integrated delivery systems. In A.D. Kaluzny, H.S. Zuckerman, and T.C. Ricketts, eds., *Partners for the dance: Forming strategic alliances in health care* (139–76). Ann Arbor: Health Administration Press.

Emanuel, E.J. 2012. Why accountable care organizations are not 1990s managed care redux. *JAMA* 302(21): 2263–64.

Enthoven, A.C., 2009. Integrated delivery systems: The cure for fragmentation. *Am J Manag Care* 15(10 Suppl): S284–90.

Ermann, D., and J. Gabel. 1986. Investor-owned multihospital systems: A synthesis of research findings. In B.H. Gray, ed., *For-profit enterprise in health care* (474–491). Washington DC: National Academy Press.

Fine, A. 1997. Integrated delivery systems. In R.B. Conners, ed., *Integrating the practice of medicine* (273–87). Chicago: American Hospital Publishing.

Freymann, J.G. 1974. *The American health care system: Its genesis and trajectory.* New York: Medcom Press.

Harris, C., L.L. Hicks, and B.J. Kelly. 1992. Physician hospital networking: Avoiding a shotgun wedding. *Health Care Manag Rev* 17(4): 17–28.

HCUPnet. 2012. Healthcare Cost and Utilization Project National Statistics. Retrieved from http://hcupnet.ahrq.gov/ (accessed August 2012).

Iglehart, J.K. 1993. The American health care system: Teaching hospitals. *N Engl J Med* 329(14): 1052–56.

Institute of Medicine. 1995. *Primary care: America's health in a new era.* Washington DC: National Academy Press.

Kaiser State Health Facts. 2010. Total Hospitals. Retrieved from http://www.statehealthfacts.org/ (accessed January 2013).

_____. 2012. Kaiser State Health Facts. The Kaiser Family Foundation. Retrieved from at http://www.statehealthfacts.org (accessed June 2012).

Kane, R.A., and R.L. Kane. 1987. *Long-term care: Principles, programs, and policies.* New York: Springer Publishing.

Kovner, A.R. 1995. Hospitals. In A.R. Kovner, ed., *Health care delivery in the United States* (162–83). New York: Springer Publishing.

Kralewski, J.E., W. Wallace, T.D. Wingert, D.J. Knutson, and C.E. Johnson. 1999. The effects of medical group practice organzational factors on physician's use of resources. *J Healthcare Manag* 44 (3): 167–82.

Kralewski, J.E., E.C. Rich, R. Feldman, B. Dowd, T. Bernhardt, C. Johnson, and W. Gold. 2000. The effects of medical group practice and physician payment methods on costs of care. *Health Serv Res* 35(3): 591–613.

Longworth, D.L. 2011. Accountable care organizations, the patient-centered medical home, and health care reform: What does it all mean? *Cleve Clin J Med* 78(9): 571–82.

Luke. R.D. 1991. Spatial competition and cooperation in local hospital markets. *Med Care Rev* 48(2): 207–47.

_____, P.C. Olden, and J.D. Bramble. 1998. Strategic hospital alliances: Countervailing responses to restructuring health care markets. In W.J. Duncan, L.E. Swayne, and P.M. Ginter, eds., *Handbook of health care management* (81–116). Cambridge MA: Blackwell Publishers.

Moore, J.H., D.J. McMillian, M.D. Rosenthal, and M.D. Weishaar. 2006. Risk determination for patients with direct access to physical therapy in military health care facilities. *J Orthop Sports Phys Ther* 35(10): 674–78.

Morrisey, M.A., J. Alexander, L.R. Burns, and V. Johnson. 1999. The effects of managed care on physician and clinical integration in hospitals. *Medical Care* 37(4): 350–61.

Moy, E., E. Valente, R.J. Levin, K.J. Bhak, and P.F. Griner. 1996. The volume and mix of inpatient services provided by academic medical centers. *Acad Med* 71(10): 1113–22.

Olden, P.C., S.D. Roggenkamp, and R.D. Luke. 2002. A post 1900s assessment of strategic hospital alliances and their marketplace orientation: Time to refocus. *Health Care Manag Rev* 27(2): 33–49.

Shih A., K. Davis, S. Schoenbaum, A. Gauthier, R. Nuzum, D. McCarthy, et al. 2008. Organizing the U.S. Health care delivery system for high performance: The Commission on a High Performance Health System. Commonwealth Fund.

Shortell, S.M. 1988. The evolution of hospital systems: Unfulfilled promises and self-fulfilling prophesies. *Med Care Rev* 45(2):177–214.

_____, R. Gilles, and D. Anderson. 1996. *The New American Healthcare: Creating Organized Delivery Systems.* San Francisco: Jossey-Bass.

_____, R.R. Gilles, and D.A. Anderson. 1994. The new world of managed care: Creating organized delivery systems. *Health Affairs* 13(5): 46–44.

Starr, P. 1982. *The social transformation of American medicine.* New York: Basic Books.

Sterns, J.B. 2007. Quality, efficiency, and organizational structure. *Health Care Finance* 34(1): 100–07

Stevens, R. 1971. *American medicine and the public interest.* New Haven: Yale University Press.

Strunk, B.C., and P.B Ginsburg. 2003. Tracking health care costs: Trends stabilize but remain high in 2002. *Health Affairs* 24(W3): 266–74.

Sultz, H.A., and K.M. Young. 1999. *Health Care USA: Understanding Its Organization and Delivery,* 2nd ed. Gaithersburg MD: Aspen.

Zajac, E.J., T.A. D'Aunno, and L.R. Burns. 2006. Managing strategic alliances In S.M. Shortell and A.D. Kaluzney, eds., *Health care management: Organization design and behaviors,* 5th ed. (356–381). New York: Thomson Delmar Learning.

Zelman, W.A. 1996. Price, quality, and barriers to integration. *Front Health Servs Manage* 13(1): 43–45.

The Post-Acute Health Care System

CHAPTER OBJECTIVES

At the conclusion of this chapter, the reader will be able to:

1 Discuss the development of the post-acute health care system in the United States during the last quarter of the 20th century.

2 Define the main components of the post-acute health care system: informal care and formal care.

3 Discuss the size, importance, and function of the informal care system of post-acute health care.

4 Identify the components, discuss the services, define likely users, and relate the effectiveness of levels of the formal post-acute health care system:

   a. Home health care
   b. Hospice
   c. Adult day services
   d. Assisted living
   e. Skilled nursing facilities
   f. Subacute care
   g. Inpatient rehabilitation facilities

5 Identify and characterize the sites of community-based mental health practice.

6 Define the role of occupational therapy and physical therapy in the post-acute health care system.

CASE EXAMPLE ··

Mr. Johnson is a 78-year-old man living at home. Since his wife died, he has become less independent and more dependent upon his daughter and son who live nearby. His daughter checks on him regularly, takes him to physician appointments, and performs light housekeeping tasks. At his latest visit, Mr. Johnson was diagnosed with Type II diabetes and now needs to take insulin injections. His daughter did not feel comfortable giving Mr. Johnson his injections, so a home health agency was arranged to provide these injections. A nurse visited Mr. Johnson and noted that he was having increasing problems with walking and transferring from the toilet due to pain in his hip. She arranged for a physical therapist and occupational therapist to visit Mr. Johnson. The physical therapist provided Mr. Johnson with exercises and a cane to use at home. The occupational therapist arranged for a grab bar to be installed near his toilet to assist with transfers. With the assistance of home health care, Mr. Johnson is able to live in the community.

Case Example Question:

1. Consider and discuss the skills and abilities needed by therapists to work in a home setting.

Introduction

Occupational therapists and physical therapists are important providers of rehabilitation services in the post-acute care system. Patients who survive a serious medical illness or an injury often require a lengthy recuperative period. Smith and Feng (2010) have described five phases of development of long-term care in the United States (see Table 11-1). Prior to 1950, the policy response to long-term care needs was small (almost nonexistent prior to 1930) and focused on cash payments to needy persons. The delivery system was either government-sponsored institutions for the poor or private boarding houses that offered few, if any, services. With the creation of Medicare and, especially, Medicaid, new sources of funding for the growth of institutional long-term care were available. The growth and development of a post-acute health care system parallels the policy changes in health care financing and the desire to move away from the hospital to a community-based

Table 11-1 Phases of Long-Term Care Delivery System Development in the United States

1910–1930	Controlling Indigent Care Costs	Opening of Poorhouses
1930–1950	Old-Age Income Security	Closure of Poorhouses Rise of Private Boarding Homes
1950–1970	Medicare and Medicaid	Boom in Nursing Homes
1970–1990	Addressing Provider Abuses	Alternatives to Nursing Homes
1990–2010	Market Reform	Community-Based Alternatives

Source: Based on Smith D.B. and Feng Z. 2010. The accumulated challenges of long-term care. Health Affairs 29: 29–34.

care system. With the initiation of Medicare Diagnosis-Related Groups prospective payment in 1983, the incentives for extended post-acute care increased. The world of post-acute care has created multiple alternatives for patient treatment after an acute illness or injury. In 1999, the Supreme Court issued a landmark ruling (the **Olmstead decision**) that persons with disabilities have a right to integrated, community-based services (Fleming Cottrell 2005). The implications of this decision are still being played out today, but they reinforce the need for alternatives to institution-based care for persons with long-term care needs. Each **level of care** provides different services and has different costs. The complexity of the system has created a need for a case manager to assist the patient in navigating the system (see Chapter 6).

The development of the post-acute care continuum has not been even, complete, or without challenges. The problems include unequal access to care and an inability to finance care. Certain populations continue to lack access to necessary services that would permit full restoration of function. Feng et al. (2011) reported that between 2000 and 2008 the numbers of minority Americans in nursing homes grew while the number of white Americans declined, indicating fewer noninstitutional alternatives for these populations. Hispanic-Americans and African-Americans are more dependent upon informal care systems than formal long-term care services (Li and Fries 2005; Weiss et al. 2005). Racial and socioeconomic segregation of long-term care facilities and a difference in the quality of care in these facilities have been documented (Konetzka and Werner, 2009).

The preceding chapter introduced the acute health care system. For patients with chronic disease and disablement, the need for health care extends well beyond the acute health care system. In this chapter, we will explore the multiple levels of care that make up the post-acute care continuum. In the broad sense, the post-acute care continuum has two fundamental components: **informal care** and **formal care**. Informal care consists of the care provided by the family unit. Formal care is a continuum of services that begins with services to supplement informal care (e.g., home health care), extending to services that replace informal care (e.g., skilled nursing facilities, intermediate care for persons with developmental disabilities). Formal care, then, consists of a mix of nonprofessional services, professional services, and residential care. Physical therapy and occupational therapy are critical professional services on many levels of the formal care continuum. The complexity of each individual patient situation and the availability of services will dictate which level of care is most appropriate. This chapter will explain the structure and services of each level of the post-acute care continuum and what we understand as to each level's effectiveness.

Informal Care

What Is Informal Care?

Informal care is a component of the post-acute care system that provides personal care for people with chronic disease and disabilities. The foundation of long-term care in the United States is the informal care system, namely, the family (Montgomery 1999; Robinson 1997; Wolf 1999). Typical informal care activities include household chores, prevention of accidents, personal care, and dressing (McCann and Evans 2002).

Who Receives Informal Care?

About 12 percent of the U.S. population (more than 30 million persons) living in the community has a disability. The prevalence of disability increases with age (see Table 11-2). About 1 in 20 American children and 1 in 3 elderly Americans has a disability. About half of community-living persons with disability report difficulty walking and climbing stairs (see Table 11-3). Four in 10 are reported to have "serious difficulty concentrating, remembering, or making decisions." About one in three persons with disabilities has difficulty performing tasks such as attending doctor's appointments or shopping. Wolff and Kasper (2006) found that the average person in need of informal care was older than age 75, female, lives alone or with a spouse, rates their health as fair or poor, and needs help with instrumental activities of daily living (ADLs) or 1–2 basic ADLs.

Table 11-2 Total Population, Number of Persons and Percent of the Population Living in the Community with a Disability, by Age, 2010

Age (Years)	Total Population	Number of Persons Living in the Community with a Disability	Percent of the Population of Persons Living in the Community with a Disability
5–17	53,885,453	2,798,597	5.2
18–64	191,138,060	19,048,426	10.0
>65	39,132,252	14,351,651	36.7

Source: U.S. Census Bureau. 2010 American Community Survey, American FactFinder, Table B18101. Accessed at http://factfinder.census.gov on May 18, 2012.

In a study of informal vs. formal care for patients with dementia, Chiu et al. (1999) found that if family labor costs were considered, nursing home care costs would actually be lower than the cost of informal care. One study describing the major values of elderly Americans who are facing the need for long-term care found that a sense of independence and participation in life decisions were important in determining whether to access post-acute care services (Forbes and Hoffart 1998). Among other concerns considered by persons in potential need of informal or formal care were cost, stress on the family, personal preference, and premorbid attitudes about levels of care in the post-acute care continuum (Keysor, Desai, and Mutran 1999). Typically, older Americans prefer to stay at home, but this attitude changes if a significant illness will overburden the informal care system (Fried et al. 1999; Wielink and Huijsman 1999).

WHO PROVIDES INFORMAL CARE? The burden of informal caregiving typically falls on female spouses and the adult female children of aging relatives (Lee and Tussing 1998; Montgomery 1999). Boaz and Hu (1997) report that depending on marital status, networks of family and friends of elderly persons with disabilities can typically provide 10 to 40 hours per week of informal assistance. The typical informal caregiving situation is a 46-year-old female caregiver providing 21 hours of care each week to her mother (National Alliance for Caregiving 2004). The average period of caregiving is 4.3 years (see Table 11-4).

Table 11-3 Number of Americans with Disabilities, Ages 18–64, Living in the Community by Type of Disability, 2010

Type of Disability	Number of Persons with Disability, by Type	Percent of Persons with Disability, by Type
Hearing	3,924,360	20.6
Vision	3,209,067	16.8
Cognitive	7,943,002	41.7
Ambulatory	9,856,708	51.7
Self-Care	3,444,202	18.1
Independent Living	6,648,058	34.9

Source: U.S. Census Bureau. 2010 American Community Survey, American FactFinder, Table B18120. Accessed at http://factfinder.census.gov on May 18, 2012.

Table 11-4 Characteristics of Family Caregivers and Recipients in the United States

Characteristics of Informal Caregivers	61% are women
	58% are between the ages of 18 and 49
	59% work full or part time outside the home
	Provide 21 hours per week for an average of 4.3 years
	Five in six caregivers rate their health as excellent, very good, or good
Characteristics of Recipients of Informal Care	65% are female and 42% are widowed
	80% are at least 50 years of age; average age is 66
	Most common reason for informal care for older recipients is "old age," and for younger recipients it is mental illness or depression

Source: Based on data from National Alliance for Caregiving in collaboration with AARP. Caregiving in the U.S. Executive Summary. 2004. Available online at http://assets.aarp.org/rgcenter/il/us_caregiving_1.pdf on May 18, 2012.

The family is the predominant source of care for persons with developmental disabilities. The experience of providing informal care affects the lives of the caregivers. Parents caring for children with disabilities experience anxiety and increased responsibility for the care of the child (McDermott et al. 1997). Nearly 90 percent of the nation's 3 million people with developmental disabilities are cared for by family members (Fujiura 1998). About 4 in 10 adults with disabilities live in homes with primary earners age 60 or older (Fujiura 2010). Family support payments from the states to care for persons with disabilities totaled $2.6 billion in 2006 and supported 428,000 families (average of $5,376 per family) (Rizzolo, Hemp, Braddock et al. 2009). Supports vary from state to state and can include cash payments, in-home services, assistive technologies, transportation, and therapies among other services.

There are a number of challenges to the use of informal care as a method of meeting long-term care needs. First, caregivers are not always available. Stewart (2006) reported a reduced availability of informal care. Wolff and Kasper (2006) found an increase in the number of primary caregivers without support and an increase in the number of disabilities reported in their sample population. A greater proportion of chronically ill or disabled elders live in the community with no informal care support. Second, the stress of caregiving can be considerable. O'Keefe et al. (2001) found many persons with multiple disabilities who lived in the community supported by Medicare home care and informal care, but their informal care network was "overextended, stressed, and vulnerable to break down." Smith et al. (2011) found that caregiver depression and stress was associated with poorer quality of care. Long et al. (2005) found that persons living in these situations were more likely to enter a nursing home. Finally, it is important to recognize that informal care is not a static system, but rather the process of caregiving changes over time and is related to social context, caregiver ability, and the often increasing burden of care (Szinovacz and Davey 2007).

The family often obtains information and referrals for problems in caregiving through **voluntary agencies**. Voluntary agencies like the American Heart Association or the National Multiple Sclerosis Society provide education, support, and advocacy services for persons with chronic illness or disease and their families. Typically, these organizations provide health education and health maintenance activities to their constituencies, disease prevention and detection programs to the general public, and advocacy in the area of public and private policy to the government. By their nature, voluntary agencies are not-for-profit organizations that primarily have an educational purpose and provide limited direct patient-care services. It is important for occupational therapists and physical therapists to understand and be involved with these organizations in order to recognize the needs and concerns of people with disabilities and their informal care systems.

How Important Is Informal Care to the Health Care System?

Informal care is vital to meet the needs of persons with chronic illness and disability. The extent of the need for care is enormous. Donelan et al. (2002) found that each year 23 percent of Americans provide informal care to other persons, and 71 percent of the caregivers do not live with the recipient of the care. In 2007, 34 million Americans provided informal care at any one time, and 52 million Americans provided informal care at some point in time during the year at an annual economic value of $375 billion (AARP Public Policy Institute 2008). This dollar amount exceeded national spending on Medicaid in 2007. The informal care system is inexpensive to the larger society and is a desirable alternative to formal care for many persons with chronic disease and disability (Chappell et al. 2004; Charles and Sevak 2005). The presence of a caregiver reduces formal long-term care costs by thousands of dollars per year (Yoo et al. 2004).

For society, the economic and social value of the informal care system is enormous. The development of formal long-term care services (e.g., home health care, skilled nursing facilities) can be traced to the need to bolster the family as primary caregiver for patients with chronic disease and disability. For occupational therapists and physical therapists, this has applications to the design and implementation of intervention plans for patients with chronic disease and disability (e.g., the incorporation of family goals into treatment plans, the development of patient/family education programs).

Formal Care

Formal care consists of a mix of residential and professional sites and types of care (see Figure 11-1). Residential services range from facilities that provide supervision and minimal assistance (e.g., assisted living facilities) to facilities that provide multiple medical and rehabilitation treatments (e.g., skilled nursing facilities, subacute care units). As we will discover, the deterioration of a person's ability to perceive the environment, think, communicate, and perform basic activities of daily living is critical to determining the appropriate level of formal post-acute care.

There are two types of formal care: nonresidential and residential (see Tables 11-5, 11-6). Nonresidential types of formal care include home health agencies, hospice, and adult day services. In these situations, the informal care system is supported and supplemented with targeted interventions based on the needs of the client and the caregiver. Much of the day-to-day care is provided by the person's family. Residential care provides a place for a person to live along with other services. Residential types of formal care replace the informal care system. Both of the types of formal care provide skilled and nonskilled services. Various professionals provide services in these settings (see Table 11-7). Settings within residential and nonresidential formal care systems provide a continuum of varying levels of care. This continuum provides several options and intensities of services for the care of persons with needs that exceed the capabilities of the informal care system.

The type of formal care and the exact mix of services provided depend on the needs of the patient and the ability of the acute care providers. Kane et al. (2006) found that professionals favored the locations where they worked or were more familiar. For example, registered nurses were likely to recommend home health care, assisted living, and adult day services. Primary care physicians favored rehabilitation and skilled nursing care. Bowles et al. (2008) found that hospital clinicians were able to properly refer patients

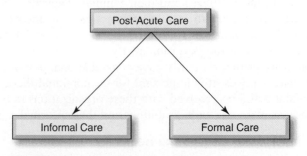

FIGURE 11-1 The Post-Acute Health Care System

Table 11-5 Common Services in Nonresidential Sites of the Post-Acute Health Care System

	Skilled	Nonskilled
Home Health	Physical therapy Occupational therapy Nursing Speech/language pathology Dietetics Pharmacy Social work	Homemaking Personal services
Hospice	Medicine Nursing Pastoral care Social work Counseling Rehabilitation therapy Dietetics Pharmacy	Homemaking Personal hygiene Volunteer companions
Adult Day Services	Nursing Social work Physical therapy Occupational therapy Recreational therapy	Transportation Meals Personal care

Table 11-6 Common Services in Residential Sites of the Post-Acute Health Care System

	Skilled	Nonskilled
Assisted Living		Meals Transportation Social activities ADL assistance Security
Skilled Nursing Facility	Nursing Physical therapy Occupational therapy Social work Dietetics	Personal hygiene Restorative care
Subacute Care	Medicine Nursing Occupational therapy Physical therapy Speech/language pathology	Personal hygiene

Table 11-7 Professionals Found in U.S. Skilled Nursing Facilities and Home Health Agencies (2011)

Profession	No. Employed	Education	Avg. Salary($)
Occupational Therapist	19,540	Master	82,250
Physical Therapist	34,870	Doctorate	85,000
Recreational Therapist	19,650	Bachelor	42,940
Registered Nurse	294,810	Associate	63,000
Social Worker	30,470	Bachelor	50,000
Speech/Language Pathologist	9,880	Master	84,500

Source: Bureau of Labor Statistics. Occupational Employment Statistics. 2011. Accessed at http://www.bls.gov/oes/ on May 21, 2012.

for post-acute services who were older, had complex medical conditions, and lacked an informal care system. However, other patients identified by a panel of experts as needing post-acute care but who were not referred for services were five times more likely to be rehospitalized than patients identified by the experts as not needing post-acute care services. Your understanding of the type and extent of services offered in these settings is important as you may be consulted to provide recommendations for the appropriate level of care for your future patients. In the remainder of the chapter, we will explore the different types of nonresidential and residential formal care.

Nonresidential Formal Care

HOME HEALTH CARE

What Is Home Health Care? Home health care is "a formal, regulated program of care, providing a range of medical, therapeutic, and nonmedical services; delivered by a variety of health care professionals in the patient's home" (Jones et al. 2012, p. 1). Home health care agencies provide services to patients who are medically stable but cannot access other community-based resources. Home health care has also developed in the gap created by the increasing orientation of medical physicians to high-technology practice environments.

Who Receives Home Health Care? About 1.4 million Americans are receiving home health care services, and there are 7.2 million discharges from home health agencies annually (National Center for Health Statistics 2007). The average length of stay is 70 days. A typical home health patient is an elderly, white female with multiple medical diagnoses and functional limitations (see Table 11-8). The most common medical diagnoses of persons utilizing home health care services are circulatory system disease, injuries and poisoning, and musculoskeletal/connective tissue system disorders. Post-acute care for orthopedic conditions accounts for about 5 percent of all reasons for home health care. Collins, Beissner, and Krout (1998) reported that patients with musculoskeletal conditions were treated most frequently by physical therapists, followed by neurological and cardiopulmonary problems. Falls are a major concern with home health patients (Lewis et al. 2004; Carroll et al. 2005, Shumway-Cook et al. 2009). Patients who have neurological or cardiopulmonary impairments, a history of falling, and who take medications intended to prevent falling are at higher fall risk at home (Lewis et al. 2004). About 4 in 10 patients receive physical therapy, and 1 in 10 receives occupational therapy. Slightly more than half of home health patients use a mobility aid (most commonly a walker), and about one-third are utilizing a self-care aid (most commonly a bedside commode or shower chair/bath bench). Home health care is most beneficial for individuals who need comprehensive care to recover from an illness or injury, desire to live in their home, and have some social

Table 11-8 **Characteristics of Patient Receiving Home Health Care (2007)**

Percent of Patients over Age 65	69%
Percent of Female Patients	60%
Percent of Patients Who Are Caucasian	80%
Average Number of Diagnoses per Patient	4.2
Percent of Patients with ADL Limitations	
4 or 5 limitations	51%
3 limitations	22%
2 limitations	17%
1 limitations	11%

Source: National Center for Health Statistics. National Home Health Care Patients and Hospice Care Discharges. 2007 National Home and Hospice Survey. Accessed at http://www.cdc.gov/nchs/data/nhhcs /2007hospicecaredischarges.pdf on May 21, 2012.

support. Individuals receiving home health care services are homebound, meaning that they are unable to leave their homes except for medical appointments or religious services.

Who Provides Home Health Care? Home health care is provided by nonprofit, for-profit, and governmental agencies that are either freestanding organizations or components of an integrated health care system. Ten percent of home health agencies also offer hospice care. In 2007, there were 10,500 home health agencies in the United States (Centers for Disease Control and Prevention 2009). Three in four home health agencies are for-profit businesses and are located in metropolitan areas. Occupational therapy is provided in 90 percent, and physical therapy is provided in 79 percent of home health agencies.

What Services Are Provided in Home Health Care? Home health care is a set of health care services organized and delivered by nurses and rehabilitation professionals under medical supervision. Home health agencies provide a package of skilled services as well as nonskilled services intended for short-term, intermittent needs after an acute illness (see Table 11-5). Skilled services include physical therapy, occupational therapy, nursing, speech/language pathology, dietetics, and pharmacy. Nonskilled services (e.g., homemaking and personal hygiene care) are provided when related to the care and recovery from a medical illness. Patients entering home health care services receive a comprehensive evaluation and care plan developed to meet their needs. A program of skilled and nonskilled services can ensure a smooth transition to the community after illness.

Overall, the most commonly utilized service in home health care is provided by a nurse (National Center for Health Statistics 2007). Eighty-five percent of home health patients receive care by a nurse. Home health aides provide assistance with activities of daily living, light housekeeping, and basic medical procedures (e.g., wound-dressing changes). About one in four home health patients will receive personal care or companion services from a home health worker (National Center for Health Statistics 2007). Skilled nursing and physical therapy are the professional services most commonly utilized in home health care. Skilled nursing services are closely related to the need for a home health aide and the presence of significant disease (Diwan, Berger, and Manns 1997). Case management, patient education, intravenous therapy, wound care, and pain control are frequently employed nursing procedures (Montauk 1998). Nursing care is limited to no more than 8 hours per day, and less than 28 hours per week. Hispanics are less likely to receive physical therapy than white Americans (Yeboah, Kleppinger, and Fortinsky 2011).

Physical therapy and occupational therapy services are important components of a home health care plan (Coke et al. 2005; O'Sullivan and Siebert 2004). Gitlin et al. (2009)

found that physical therapy and occupational therapy intervention in the home extended survivorship by 3.5 years, and this effect was sustained for 2 years. Payne, Thomas, Fitzpatrick, et al. (1998) studied patterns of home health visit length and found that case management, functional limitations, and clinical instability affected the need for professional intervention. In a study of goal achievement in home health care, O'Sullivan and Volicer (1997) reported that persons discharged to home after total hip replacement who received physical therapy home care were more likely to be discharged with their goals achieved. For total joint replacement patients who are healthy and have good social support, home health therapy services have been shown to be an effective delivery mechanism (Mallinson, Bateman, Tseng, et al. 2011). Patients with more disability are most responsive to a therapy intervention (Gitlin et al. 2008). Continuity in providing home health physical therapy is associated with improved patient outcomes (Russell, Rosati, and Andreopoulos 2012).

HOSPICE   Hospice services provide care for individuals with terminal illness and their support systems during and after the dying process. The early development of hospice services can be traced to the efforts of volunteers interested in providing services to persons with terminal illness (Petrisek and Mor 1999). The first hospice organization was St. Christopher's Hospice, which opened in London in 1967 (Leland and Schonwelter 1997; Pickett, Cooley, and Gordon 1998). The first hospice in the United States opened in New Haven, Connecticut, in 1974. Today there are approximately 3,407 hospice organizations in the United States (Hospice Association of America 2010). In 2007, 1.05 million persons received services through a hospice program (Centers for Disease Control and Prevention 2007).

Hospice is founded on a philosophy of palliative care, not curative medicine. Palliative care focuses on pain management, emotional counseling, and social support (Petrisek and Mor 1999). Byock (1996) has summarized the philosophy of hospice care: "Beyond symptom management, hospice and palliative care intervention can be directed at helping the person to attain a sense of completion within the social and interpersonal dimensions, to develop or deepen a sense of worthiness, and to find their own unique sense of meaning in life" (p. 251). As Leland and Schonwelter (1997) succinctly state, hospice is about "dying well" (p. 381). To qualify for hospice benefits, patients with terminal illness are usually expected to die within six months (Gabel, Hurst, and Hunt 1998; Petrisek and Mor 1999). Patient populations are usually older and are equally divided between males and females. The most common physical complaints of patients receiving hospice services include pain, fatigue, anorexia, dyspnea, nausea, confusion, and depression (Cleary and Carbone 1997; Ng and von Gunten 1998).

Hospice services are characterized by a patient-focused, interdisciplinary, coordinated plan of care. Besides the family, physicians, nurses, clergy, social workers, home health aides, counselors, and volunteers make up the core of the hospice team. Occupational therapists, physical therapists, speech/language pathologists, dietitians, and pharmacists are other important contributing professions to hospice care. Hospice care benefits are typically inclusive of necessary prescription drug and durable medical equipment needs. A unique Medicare benefit for hospice services is follow-up bereavement care for family members after the patient's death.

In the last 10 years, the important role of rehabilitation in hospice has been increasingly recognized. Pizzi and Briggs (2004) report that therapists can work to improve patient function and comfort, create a safe environment, engage people in meaningful occupation, and provide emotional and spiritual support. Improvements in function, mobility, endurance, pain, dyspnea, depression, and cognitive function have been reported as a result of rehabilitation intervention (Javier and Montagnini 2011). Occupational therapists have an important role in creating a safe home environment, reducing stress, and improving self care (Frost 2001). Saarik and Hartley (2010) reported improvement in cancer-related fatigue and improved functional performance with occupational therapy and physical therapy intervention. Utilization of therapy services in the hospice setting may still be quite small. Drouin et al. (2009) reported that only 3 percent of hospice patients received physical therapy. The patients who received physical therapy improved in mobility, quality of life, and safety with improved caregiver confidence.

ADULT DAY SERVICES   For the caregivers of adults with chronic disease and disability, the ongoing provision of informal care can be exhausting. A respite from providing care can alleviate this stress and allow for the continuation of informal care. For working caregivers, the ability of an agency to provide services during workday hours allows informal care to continue in the evening or during the weekend. One option in the post-acute care continuum designed to meet these needs is adult day services.

In the United States, there are over 4,600 adult day service providers, and 260,000 family members and caregivers are supported by adult day services providers (Met Life Mature Market Institute 2010). Adult day services provide transportation, meals, social services, personal care, occasional nursing services, rehabilitation services, and activities, usually during normal business hours, five days per week. About half of adult day service providers offer physical or occupational therapy. Adult day services allow for the supervision and care of an adult while the primary caregiver works or is given a respite from daily care.

A typical user of adult day services is an elderly white female who lives with a spouse, family, or friends. One-half of the recipients of adult day services have a cognitive impairment, 50 percent of persons need help with toileting, and one in three need assistance with bathing. The average daily fee for adult day care is $62, much less than the daily cost of skilled nursing facility care (MetLife Mature Market Institute 2010). Two in three participants attend adult day services at least three days per week.

A variation of adult day services is the Program of All-Inclusive Care (PACE). PACE is unusual in adult day services in that it serves populations at risk for nursing home placement (National PACE Association 2012). Persons eligible for PACE must be at least 55 years old, live in a PACE service area, and be able to live safely in the community. It originated in San Francisco's Chinatown in the early 1970s. There are 82 PACE sites in 29 states (National PACE Association 2012).

Several studies have addressed the effectiveness of PACE. Persons using PACE services have fewer hospital admissions and emergency room visits (Kane et al. 2006). Specifically, older adults who had their unmet ADL limitations addressed by PACE are less likely to be admitted to a hospital (Sands et al. 2006). PACE enrollees are also less likely to be admitted to a nursing home (Friedman et al. 2005) and have higher five year survival rates (Wieland et al. 2010).

Residential Formal Care

ASSISTED LIVING   Assisted living is a form of residential care facility (RCF) that "provides housing and supportive services to persons who cannot live independently but generally do not require the skilled level of care provided by nursing homes" (Park-Lee et al. 2011). Unlike home health care, adult day care, and many hospices, assisted living facilities provide residential care. Assisted living facilities are ideal for persons who need supervision or nonskilled services but not skilled care on a regular basis. About 733,400 Americans live in one of 31,300 assisted living facilities in the United States (Park-Lee et al. 2011). Average length of stay is three years (Golant 2004).

The typical resident is "an 80-year-old female who is ambulatory but needs assistance with about two ADLs, most likely bathing and possibly dressing or using the toilet. She also probably needs or accepts some assistance with transportation, shopping, preparing meals, housework, taking medication, and managing money" (National Center for Assisted Living 2001). This level of care is commonly called **intermediate care**. Assisted living facilities usually provide three meals per day, transportation, social activities, assistance with activities of daily living, medication monitoring, and security services (see Table 11-4). Assisted living facilities may be freestanding buildings or, in some cases, are part of a skilled nursing facility. The average, national monthly cost for assisted living is $3,477 (MetLife Mature Market Institute 2011). This is more than adult day services but less than skilled nursing facility care. Payment is primarily by private funding; although, state Medicaid programs provide 19 percent of funding of assisted living as an alternative to more expensive skilled nursing facility care (Park-Lee et al. 2011). A study of the needs of the Veterans Health Administration found that 19 percent of veterans in nursing homes were functioning at a status consistent with assisted living (Kinosian, Stallard, and Wieland 2007).

Bishop (1999) reported that assisted living facilities were replacing skilled nursing facilities as the residential choice for persons with minimal disability or post-acute care needs. The goal of many assisted living admissions is to allow the person to "age in place" (Ball et al. 2004). Providing the appropriate service mix to permit this to occur can be difficult. Cognitive decline and an increased number and severity of medical conditions is common and is associated with transfer to more medically intensive facilities (Burdick, et al. 2005; Fonda et al. 2002; Sloane et al. 2005). Exercise and walking programs have been found to be beneficial in this population (Baum et al. 2003; Taylor et al. 2003). Hatch and Lusardi (2010) reported that participation twice weekly for 9 to 12 months improved function and decreased risk of falls for residents of assisted living facilities. Bell et al. (2011) reported that use of gaming technology in assisted living facilities by occupational therapy may benefit residents. Physical therapy and occupational therapy are offered by nearly all assisted living facilities, usually through a contract relationship with therapists (National Center for Assisted Living 2001).

SKILLED NURSING FACILITIES   Skilled nursing facilities (SNFs) or nursing homes (NH) are the oldest type of long-term care facility. They have been present in the United States in one form or another for over a century. Originally designed to provide long-term **custodial care**, skilled nursing facilities have been transformed in the last two decades into facilities that are a key part of a continuum of care for patients with complex illnesses. An indication of this change is the development of specialized units in SNFs for Alzheimer's disease, AIDS, ventilator-dependent patients, and subacute care. Reschovsky (1998) classifies persons served by skilled nursing facilities into two types: post-acute and chronic. Post-acute patients receive subacute care or skilled services with the anticipation of a community discharge (e.g., short-term Medicare stay). Chronic patients receive skilled nursing and occasional skilled rehabilitation services to prevent the deterioration of function and health status, with the expectation of long-term residence in the skilled nursing facility (Table 11-9).

About 1.4 million Americans reside in 15,673 skilled nursing facilities in the United States (American Health Care Association 2012). Nationally, occupancy is about 86 percent of capacity (American Health Care Association 2012). Most skilled nursing facilities (53%) are part of a multifacility chain, and two-thirds are for-profit enterprises

Table 11-9 Characteristics of U.S. Skilled Nursing Facilities (2012)

Type of Ownership:	Multifacility/Chain	55%
	Independent	45%
	Hospital	6%
Sponsorship:	For Profit	68%
	Not For Profit	25%
	Government	7%
Medicare and Medicaid Certified:		91%
Average Number of Beds:		106
Special Beds Designated:	Alzheimers	5%
	Rehabilitation	1%
	Ventilator	0.5%
Average Number of Direct Care Staff per Facility:		66

Source: OSCAR Data Reports. 2012. Nursing Facility Operational Characteristics Report. March 2012 Update. American Health Care Association. Retrieved from http://www.ahcancal.org/research_data/oscar_data /Nursing%20Facility%20Operational%20Characteristics/OperationalCharacteristicsReport_Mar2012.pdf (accessed May 23, 2012).

(see Table 11-9). The average facility numbers 90 beds and consists of resident rooms, dining and activity areas, and therapy space. Skilled nursing facility care is the most expensive site of care in the post-acute care continuum. The average daily cost for a private room in a skilled nursing facility is $239 (MetLife Mature Market Institute 2011). The federal Medicaid program funds almost 7 in 10 persons residing in skilled nursing facilities (see Table 11-7).

Skilled nursing facility care is for patients who have complex nursing or rehabilitation needs that cannot be provided in another environment (e.g., home health, assisted living). Persons in skilled nursing facilities typically need help with at least three activities of daily living, and three in four have cognitive problems (see Table 11-10). Typically, individuals have complex care needs but are medically stable with regular nursing observation/treatment. Examples of care needs that would qualify an individual for skilled nursing care include daily injections, wound care, tube feedings, needing assistance of more than one person for mobility tasks, help for all personal hygiene tasks, and significant confusion.

Four basic services are provided in skilled nursing facilities: nursing and rehabilitation, personal care, residential services, and medical care. Each resident receives an individualized plan of care developed by a multidisciplinary team to meet their needs.

Table 11-10 Characteristics of Residents in U.S. Nursing Homes (2012)

Average Number of ADL limitations: 4.12
Percentage Requiring Assistance with Bathing: 95.9
Percentage Requiring Assistance with Dressing: 90.5
Percentage Requiring Assistance with Transferring: 92.8
Percentage Requiring Assistance with Toileting: 85.8
Percentage Requiring Assistance with Eating: 54.7
Percentage Bedbound: 3.5
Percentage Restricted to a Chair: 52.7
Percentage Ambulatory: 43.2
Percentage Physically Restrained/With Orders to be Restrained: 2.9/1.3
Percentage with Contractures: 24.6
Percentage with Dementia: 47.9
Percentage with Behavior Problems: 24.6
Percentage Experiencing Depression: 48.3
Percentage with Pressure Sores: 7.1

Payer Source:		
	Medicaid	63.5%
	Medicare	14.4%
	Other	21.9%

Source: LTC Stats: Nursing Facility Patient Characteristics Report March 2012 American Health Care Association. Accessed at http://www.ahcancal.org/research_data/oscar_data/NursingFacilityPatientCharacteristics/LTC%20 STATS_HSNF_PATIENT_2012Q1_FINAL.pdf on May 23, 2012.

All facilities have 24-hour nursing services staffed by nurses' aides for personal care, with supervision by licensed practical nurses and registered nurses. Nurses' aides assist with feeding, bathing, dressing, walking, and transfers. Professional nurses provide examination, evaluation, and technical nursing interventions.

Occupational therapists and physical therapists provide evaluation and intervention to improve function and prevent secondary conditions in this population. One in five nursing home residents are admitted for short-term, Medicare-related stays. For these patients, nursing homes are important sites to receive occupational and physical therapy (Murray et al.1999). Rehabilitation in a nursing home typically takes longer, and the post-acute care patients served have more severe deficits. An early study of nursing home rehabilitation reports that nearly two in three patients ultimately return to the community (Kosasih et al. 1998). Young age, fewer limitations in ADL performance, and rehabilitation therapy are associated with a greater likelihood of community discharge (Mehr, Williams, and Fries 1997). Kauh et al. (2005) found that persons treated in a geriatric rehabilitation unit within a skilled nursing facility had shorter length of stay, a greater likelihood of community discharge, and greater improvement in ADLs and mobility. Lee and Higgins (2008) reported that persons with lower initial function, confusion, skin ulcers, and less physical therapy had worse physical function after discharge from a short-term skilled nursing facility stay. Jette et al. (2005) found that higher physical therapy and occupational therapy intensities were associated with shorter lengths of stay and greater functional gains for patients receiving care in a skilled nursing facility.

Restorative care is an important component of rehabilitation services for persons with long-term, chronic disease in nursing homes. Porell et al. (1998) describe how the slow rate of decline in functional task performance among nursing home residents with chronic conditions is exacerbated by serious medical illness (e.g., congestive heart failure, chronic obstructive pulmonary disease, cancer). Restorative care is commonly implemented by a specially trained nursing aide. Training usually encompasses, at a minimum, basic range of motion exercise and ambulation training. Restorative care services are usually overseen by the nursing supervisor. Restorative aides can be a most useful adjunct person for the completion of rehabilitation protocols established by physical therapists and occupational therapists and for providing maintenance therapy, which is not reimbursable as a professional service. An initial evaluation by an occupational therapist or physical therapist to establish a maintenance program in a skilled nursing facility is a Medicare-reimbursable service (see Chapter 8). Improvement in mobility and balance has been reported with well-structured restorative care services (Resnick et al. 2009).

Concerns regarding the quality of care in nursing homes have been addressed on several occasions. Among the issues addressed by nursing homes are use of physical restraints and employee turnover and absenteeism. Nursing homes are criticized for excessive use of physical restraints (Castle and Engberg 2009). Currently, physical restraints are used in 9 percent and antipsychotic restraints are used in 25 percent of the U.S. nursing home population (Feng et al. 2009). In Chapter 8, we discussed the use of the Minimum Data Set of the Resident Assessment Instrument (RAI) to determine payment for skilled nursing facility care. The RAI is also used to improve the quality of care in nursing homes. Information from the MDS may "trigger" the identification of a problem area that will require a more formal assessment. The outcome of a "trigger" is to investigate, identify, document, and address the problem. A care plan is then developed to address the problem. The care plan includes an intervention and a method to evaluate the outcome of the care.

Subacute Care

Subacute care is defined as "comprehensive inpatient care designed for someone who has an acute illness, injury, or exacerbation of a disease process. It is goal-oriented treatment rendered immediately after, or instead of, acute hospitalization to treat one or more specific active complex medical conditions or to administer one or more technically complex treatments, in the context of a person's underlying long-term conditions and overall situation" (American Health Care Association 1996; American Health Care Association 2012). Subacute care occupies a unique niche in the health care delivery system. It is a "step down" from acute hospitalization intended for the short-term recuperation of a person after a significant illness or injury. Subacute care units have developed both in nursing homes and hospitals. Subacute units in hospitals are sometimes termed **swing bed units**. Other locations for subacute care units include rehabilitation hospitals and freestanding subacute care units. Subacute care facilities are licensed as skilled nursing facilities. Subacute care facilities provide an intensity of care between a hospital and skilled nursing facility.

Subacute care units tend to be organized around patient types (e.g., medically complex, respiratory/ventilator care, postsurgical, stroke or orthopedic rehabilitation, oncology). In contrast to acute hospital care, subacute care patients receive a lower intensity of physician and nursing care. Physicians typically do not visit on a daily basis; occasionally they visit only weekly. Nursing time is closely monitored and is typically four to seven contact hours per day. In general, physical therapy and occupational therapy services are provided on a daily basis. In contrast to inpatient rehabilitation facilities, subacute rehabilitation total therapy time is less than three hours per day. The goal is to move the patient to a less intense level of care (perhaps home or long-term care) as soon as possible.

INPATIENT REHABILITATION FACILITIES   Inpatient rehabilitation facilities are either independent, stand-alone institutions or dedicated units within hospitals or nursing homes that provide intensive inpatient rehabilitation. Inpatient rehabilitation facilities provide care for patients recovering from serious illness and injury in preparation for reentry into the community. Typically, these programs provide rehabilitation care for the most complex patients (e.g., traumatic brain injury and spinal cord injury survivors) (at least 60% of admissions must come from patients with complex illnesses and injuries [see Chapter 7]). Consistent with Medicare rules, patients in these facilities need to be able to tolerate at least three hours of therapy per day. Occupational therapy, physical therapy, speech/language pathology, therapeutic recreation, rehabilitation nursing, psychological and counseling services, and rehabilitation medicine (physiatry) services are common services in these centers.

Conclusion

In this chapter, we have explored the range of care options for persons in need of rehabilitation and recuperation after serious illness or injury (see Figure 11-2). Given these options, the informal care system remains the largest and most important component of the post-acute care system. The experience of disablement increases the risk of the need for formal post-acute care services. For physical therapists and occupational therapists, the implications of this fact are important. Therapists make important contributions to reducing the risk of disablement. Rehabilitation services exist to promote and restore the ability to live in the community for patients with

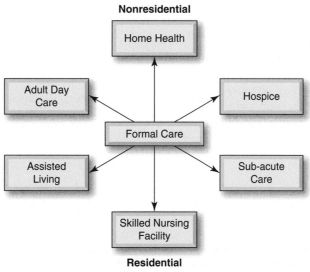

FIGURE 11-2 The Formal Care System

chronic disease and disability. For most of them, community living will depend on the strength of the informal care system. The strength of this system is the care provided by parents, female spouses, and adult female children.

The formal care system consists of professional services, nonprofessional services, and residential care to either support or replace the informal care system. The majority of the residents in formal post-acute care sites are older women, which reflects the longer life span of women and the disproportionate share of informal care provided to males in our society by women. Home health care and adult day services provide professional and nonprofessional services to support the informal care system. Assisted living facilities, skilled nursing facilities, subacute care facilities, and inpatient rehabilitation facilities provide a continuum of residential, professional, and nonprofessional services for the short-term or long-term care of persons with chronic disease and disability. Finally, the majority of mental health practice is provided in community environments and, increasingly, in nontraditional settings (e.g., schools, the justice system, and the workplace).

Chapter Review Questions

1. Consider how the post-acute care continuum evolved over the last 20 years. What are the reasons for these changes?

2. Identify the two components of the post-acute care continuum. Consider how they are related to one another.

3. What are the characteristics of the informal care system? Describe its strengths and weaknesses.

4. Identify the levels of the formal care system. Identify the professional services and residential features, if any, of each level of care.

5. Define home health care. Describe the services common to home health care, the types of patients served, and the effectiveness of home health care.

6. Define hospice. Describe the services common to hospice, the types of patients served, and the effectiveness of hospice care.

7. Define adult day services and the PACE program. Describe the services common to adult day care, the types of patients served, and the effectiveness of adult day care.

8. Define assisted living. Describe the services common to assisted living, the type of patients served, and the effectiveness of assisted living services.

9. Define skilled nursing facilities. Compare and contrast post-acute care services and chronic care services in skilled nursing facilities. Describe the services common to skilled nursing facilities, the types of patients served, and the effectiveness of skilled nursing facility care.

10. Define subacute care. Describe the services common to subacute care, the types of patients served, and the effectiveness of subacute care services.

11. Define inpatient rehabilitation. Describe the services common to inpatient rehabilitation facilities and the types of patients served.

Chapter Discussion Questions

1. Consider and discuss how societal gender roles have influenced the development of the post-acute care system.

2. Consider the development of the post-acute care continuum in light of the medical and social disability models of disablement. Which model has been most influential in the development of the system to date? Why?

3. A primary purpose of occupational therapy and physical therapy is to promote independence in the living environment. Compare and contrast the settings in the post-acute continuum as they affect the ability of physical therapists and occupational therapists to complete these roles.

References

American Association of Retired Persons. 2008. Valuing the Invaluable: The economic value of family caregiving, 2008 update. Retrieved from http://assets.aarp.org/rgcenter/il /i13_caregiving.pdf (accessed May 18, 2012).

American Health Care Association. 1996. Nursing facility subacute care: The quality and cost-effective alternative to hospital care. Business Journal Serving Southern Tier, CNY, Mohawk Valley, Finger Lakes, North 10(23): p1B. 11/ 96.

_____. 2012. OSCAR Data Reports. Nursing Facility Operational Characteristics Report. March 2012 Update. Retrieved from http://www.ahcancal.org/research_data /oscar_data/Nursing%20Facility%20Operational%20 Characteristics/OperationalCharacteristicsReport _Mar2012.pdf (accesssed May 23, 2012).

_____. 2012. LTC Stats: Nursing Facility Patient Characteristics Report. Retrieved from http://www.ahcancal.org/research _data/oscar_data/NursingFacilityPatientCharacteristics /LTC%20STATS_HSNF_PATIENT_2012Q1_FINAL.pdf (accessed May 23, 2012).

Ball, M.M., M.M. Perkins, F.J. Whittington, B.R. Connell, C. Hollingsworth, S.V. King, C.L. Elrod, and B.L. Combs. 2004. Managing decline in assisted living: The key to aging in place. *J Gerontol B Psychol Sci Soc Sci* 59(4): S202–12.

Baum, E.E., D. Jarjoura, A.E. Polen, D. Faur, and G. Rutecki. 2003. Effectiveness of a group exercise program in a long-term care facility: A randomized pilot trial. *J Am Med Dir Assoc* 4(2): 74–80.

Bell, C.S., E. Fain, J. Daub, S.H. Warren, S.H. Howell, K.S. Southard, C. Sellers, and H. Shadoin. 2011. Effects of Nintendo Wii on quality of life, social relationships, and confidence to prevent falls. *Phys Ther Occup Ther Ger* 29: 213–21.

Bishop, C.E. 1999. Where are the missing elders? The decline in nursing home use. 1995. *Health Affairs* 18(4): 146–55.

Boaz, R.F., and J. Hu. 1997. Determining the amount of help used by disabled elderly persons at home: The role of coping resources. *J Gerontol B Psychol Sci Soc Sci* 52(6): S317–24.

Bowles, K.H., S.J. Ratcliffe, J.H. Holmes, M. Liberatore, R. Nydick, and M.D. Naylor. 2008. Post-acute referral decisions made by multidisciplinary experts compared to hospital clinicians and the patients' 12 week outcomes. *Med Care* 46: 158–166.

Burdick, C.J., A. Rosenblatt, Q.M. Samus, C. Steele, A. Baker, M. Harper, L. Mayer, J. Brandt, P. Rabins, and C.G. Lyketsos. 2005. Predictors of functional impairment in residents of assisted–living facilities: The Maryland Assisted Living study. *J Gerontol A Biol Sci Med Sci* 60(2): 258–64.

Byock, I.R. 1996. The nature of suffering and the nature of opportunity at the end of life. *Clin Geriatr Med* 12(2): 237–52.

Carroll, N.V., P.W. Slattum, and F.M. Cox. 2005. The cost of falls among the community-dwelling elderly. *J Manag Care Pharm* 11(4): 307–16.

Castle, N.G., and Engberg J. 2009. The health consequences of using physical restraints in nursing homes. *Med Care* 47: 1164–73.

Centers for Disease Control and Prevention. 2009a. 2007 National Home and Hospice Care Survey. Retrieved from http://www.cdc.gov/nchs/data/nhhcs/2007hospicecaresurvey .pdf (accessed May 22, 2012).

_____. 2009b. Home health care patients and hospice care discharges. 2007 National Home and Hospice Care Survey. Retrieved from http://www.cdc.gov/nchs/data/nhhcs /2007hospicecaredischarges.pdf (accessed May 22, 2012).

Chappell, N.L., B.H. Dlitt, M.J. Hollander, J.A. Miller, and C. McWilliam. 2004. Comparative costs of home care and residential care. *Gerontologist* 44(3): 389–400.

Charles, K.K,. and P. Sevak. 2005. Can family caregiving substitute for nursing home care? *J Health Econ* 24(6): 1174–90

Chiu, L., K.Y. Tang, Y.H. Liu, W.C. Shyu, and T.P. Chang. 1999. Cost comparisons between family-based care and nursing home care for dementia. *J Adv Nurs* 29(4): 1005–12.

Cleary, J., and J. Carbone. 1997. Palliative medicine in the elderly. *Cancer* 80(7): 1335–47.

Coke, T., R. Alday, K. Biala, S. Luna, and P. Martines. 2005. The new role of physical therapy in home health care. *Home Healthc Nurse* 23(9): 594–99.

Collins, J., K.L. Beissner, and J.A. Krout. 1998. Home health physical therapy: Practice patterns in western New York. *Phys Ther* 78(2): 170–79.

Diwan, S., C. Berger, and E.K. Manns. 1997. Composition of the home care service package: Predictors of type, volume, and mix of services provided to poor and frail older people. *Gerontologist* 37(2): 169–81.

Donelan, K., C.A. Hill, C. Hoffman, K. Scoles, P.H. Feldman, C. Levine, and D. Gould. 2002. Challenged to care: Informal caregivers in a changing health care system. *Health Affairs* 21(4): 222–31.

Drouin, J.S., K. Martin, N. Onowu, A. Berg, and L. Zuellig. 2009. Physical therapy utilization in hospice and palliative care settings in Michigan: A descriptive study. *Rehab Oncol* 27: 3–8.

Feng, Z, M.L. Fennell, D.A. Tyler, M. Clark, and V. Mor. 2011. Growth of racial and ethnic minorities in US nursing homes driven by demographics and possible disparities in options. *Health Affairs* 30: 1358–1366.

_____, J.P. Hirdes, T.F. Smith, H. Finne-Soveri, I. Chi, J. Du Pasquier, R. Gilgen, N. Ikegami, and V. Mor. 2009. Use of physical restraints and antipsychotic medications in nursing homes: A cross-national study. *Int J Ger Psychiatr* 24: 1110–18.

Fleming Cottrell, R.P. 2005. The Olmstead decision: Landmark opportunity or platform for rhetoric? Our collective responsibility for full community participation. *Am J Occup Ther* 59: 561–68.

Fonda, S.J., E.C. Clipp, and G.L. Maddox. 2002. Patterns of functioning among residents of an affordable assisted living housing facility. *Gerontologist* 42(2): 178–187.

Forbes, S., and N. Hoffart. 1998. Elders' decision making regarding the use of long-term care services: A precarious balance. *Qual Health Res* 8(6): 736–50.

Fried, T.R., C. van Doorn, J.R. O'Leary, M.E. Tinetti, and M.A. Drickamer. 1999. Older persons' preferences for site of terminal care. *Ann Intern Med* 131(2): 109–12.

Friedman, S.M., D.M. Steinwachs, P.J. Rathouz, L.C. Burton, and D.B. Mukamel. 2005. Characteristics predicting nursing home admission in the Program of All-Inclusive Care for elderly people. *Gerontologist* 45(2): 157–66.

Frost, M. 2001. The role of physical, occupational, and speech therapy in hospice: Patient empowerment. *Am J Hosp Palliat Care* 18: 397–402.

Fujiura, G.T. 1998. Demography of family households. *Am J Ment Ret* 103(3): 225–35.

———. 2010. Aging families and the demographics of family financial support of adults with disabilities. *J Dis Pol Stud* 20: 241–50.

Gabel, J.R., K.M. Hurst, and K.A. Hunt. 1998. Health benefits for the terminally ill: Reality and perception. *Health Affairs* 17(6): 120–27.

Gitlin, L.N., L. Winter, M.P. Dennis, and W.W. Hauck. 2008. Variation in response to support daily function by age, race, sex, and education. *J Gerontol A Biol Sci Med Sci* 63(A): 745–50.

———, W.W. Hauck, M.P. Dennis, L. Winter, N. Hodgson, and S. Schinfeld. 2009. Long-term effect on mortality of a home intervention that reduces functional difficulties in older adults: Results from a randomized trial. *J Am Geriatr Soc* 57: 476–81.

Golant, S.M. 2004. Do impaired older persons with health care needs occupy U.S. assisted living facilities? An analysis of six national studies. *J Gerontol B Psychol Sci Soc Sci* 59(2): S68–79.

Hatch, J., and M.M. Lusardi. 2010. Impact of participation in a wellness program on functional status and falls among aging adults in an assisted living facility. *J Ger Phys Ther* 33: 71–77.

Hospice Association of America. 2010. Hospice facts and statistics. Retrieved from http://www.nahc.org/assets/1/7 /HospiceStats10.pdf (accessed April 18, 2013).

Javier, N.S.C., and M.L. Montagnini. 2011. Rehabilitation of the hospice and palliative care patient. *J Palliative Med* 14: 638–674.

Jette, D.U., R.L. Warren, and C. Wirtalla. 2005. The relation between therapy intensity and outcomes of rehabilitation in skilled nursing facilities. *Arch Phys Med Rehabil* 86(3): 373–79.

Jones, A.L., L. Harris-Kojetin, and R. Valverde. 2012. Characteristics and use of home health care by men and women aged 65 and over. National Health Statistics Reports. No. 52. Retrieved from http://www.cdc.gov/nchs /data/nhsr/nhsr052.pdf (accessed May 23, 2012).

Kane, R.L., P. Homyak, B. Bershadsky, and S. Flood. 2006. Variations on a theme called PACE. *J Gerontol A Biol Sci Med Sci* 61(7): 689–693.

———, B. Bershadsky, and J. Bershadsky. 2006. Who recommends long-term care matters? *Gerontologist* 46(4): 474–482.

Kauh, B., T. Polak, S. Hazelett, K. Hua, and K. Allen. 2005. A pilot study: post-acute geriatric rehabilitation versus usual care in skilled nursing facilities. *J Am Med Dir Assoc* 6(5): 321–326.

Keysor, J.J., T. Desai, and E.J. Mutran. 1999. Elders' preferences for care setting in short-and long-term disability scenarios. *Gerontologist* 39(3): 334–44.

Kinosian, B., E. Stallard, and D. Wieland. 2007. Projected use of long-term care services by enrolled veterans. *Gerontologist* 47(3): 356–64.

Konetzka, R.T., and R.M. Werner. 2009. Review: Disparities in long-term care: Building equity into market-based reforms. *Med Care Res Rev* 66: 491–521.

Kosasih, J.B., H.H. Borca, W.J. Wenninger, and E. Duthie. 1998. Nursing home rehabilitation after acute rehabilitation: Predictors and outcomes. *Arch Phys Med Rehabil* 79(6): 670–73.

Lee, J., and P.A. Higgins. 2008. Predicting posthospital recovery of physical function among older adults after lower extremity surgery in a short-stay skilled nursing facility. *Rehabil Nurs* 33: 170–177.

Lee, M., and A.D. Tussing. 1998. Influences on nursing home admissions: The role of informal caregivers. *Abstr Book Assoc Health* 15: 55–56.

Leland, J.Y., and R.S. Schonwelter. 1997. Advances in hospice care. *Clin Geriatr Med* 13(2): 381–401.

Lewis, C.L., M. Moutoux, M. Slaughter, and S.P. Bailey. 2004. Characteristics of individuals who fell while receiving home health services. *Phys Ther* 84(1): 23–32

Li, L.W., and B.E. Fries. 2005. Elder disability as an explanation for racial differences in informal home care. *Gerontologist* 45(2): 206–15.

Long, S.K., K. Liu, K. Black, J. O'Keefe, and S. Molony. 2005. Getting by in the community: Lessons from frail elders. *J Aging Soc Policy* 17(1): 19–44.

Mallinson, T.R., J. Bateman, H.Y. Tseng, L. Manheim, O. Almagor, A. Deutsch, and A.W. Heinemann. 2011. A comparison of discharge functional status after rehabilitation in skilled nursing, home health, and medical rehabilitation settings for patients after lower-extremity joint replacement surgery. *Arch Phys Med Rehabil* 92: 712–20.

McCann, S., and D.S. Evans. 2002. Informal care: The views of people receiving care. *Health Soc Care Community* 10(4): 221–28.

McDermott, S., D. Valentine, D. Anderson, D. Gallup, and S. Thompson. 1997. Parents of adults with mental retardation living in home and out of home: Caregiving burdens and gratifications. *Am J Orthopsychiatry* 67(2): 323–29.

Mehr, D.R., B.C. Williams, and B.E. Fries. 1997. Predicting discharge outcomes of VA nursing home residents. *J Aging Health* 9(2): 244–65.

MetLife Mature Market Institute. 2010. The MetLife national study of adult day services: Providing support to individuals and their family caregivers. Retrieved from http://www .metlife.com/assets/cao/mmi/publications/studies/2010/mmi -adult-day-services.pdf (accessed May 22, 2012).

———. 2011. The 2011 MetLife survey of long-term care: The 2011 MetLife market survey of nursing home, assisted living, adult day services, and home care costs. Retrieved from http://www.metlife.com/mmi/research/2011-market -survey-long-term-care-costs.html#findings (accessed May 22, 2012).

Montauk, S.L. 1998. Home health care. *Am Fam Physician* 58(7): 1608–14.

Montgomery, R.J. 1999. The family role in the context of long-term care. *J Aging Health* 11(3): 383–416.

Murray, P.K., M.E. Singer, R. Fortinsky, L. Russo, and R.D. Cebul. 1999. Rapid growth of rehabilitation services in traditional community-based nursing homes. *Arch Phys Med Rehabil* 80(4): 372–78.

National Alliance for Caregiving. 2004. Caregiving in the U.S. Executive Summary. Retrieved from http://assets.aarp.org /rgcenter/il/us_caregiving_1.pdf (accessed May 18, 2012).

National Center for Assisted Living. 2001. Facts and trends: The assisted living sourcebook. Retrieved from http://www .ahcancal.org/ncal/resources/Documents/alsourcebook2001 .pdf (accessed May 22, 2012).

National Center for Health Statistics. 2007. Home Health Care Patients and Hospice Care Discharges. 2007 National Home and Hospice Care Survey. Retrieved from http://www .cdc.gov/nchs/data/nhhcs/2007hospicecaredischarges.pdf (accessed May 21, 2012).

National PACE Association. 2012. What is PACE? Retrieved from http://www.npaonline.org/website/article.asp?id=12 (accessed May 22, 2012).

Ng, K., and C.F. von Gunten. 1998. Symptoms and attitudes of 100 consecutive patients admitted to an acute hospice/ palliative care unit. *J Pain Symptom Manage* 16(5): 307–16.

O'Keefe, J., S.K. Long, K. Liu, and M. Kerr. 2001. How do they manage? Disabled elderly persons in the community who are not receiving Medicaid long-term care services. *Home Health Care Serv Q* 20(4): 73–90.

O'Sullivan, A., and C. Siebert. 2004. Occupational therapy and home health: A perfect fit. *Caring* 23(5): 10–16.

O'Sullivan, M.J., and B. Volicer. 1997. Factors associated with achievement of goals for home health care. *Home Health Care Serv Q* 16(3): 21–34.

Park-Lee, E., C. Caffrey, M. Sengupta, A.J. Moss, E. Rosenoff, and L.D. Harris-Kojetin. 2011. Residential care facilities: A key sector in the spectrum of long-term care providers in the United States. NCHS Data Brief, No. 78. Hyattsville MD: National Center for Health Statistics.

Payne, S.M., C.P. Thomas, T. Fitzpatrick, M. Abdel-Rahman, and H.L. Kayne. 1998. Determinants of home health visit length: Results of a multisite prospective study. *Med Care* 36: 1500–14.

Petrisek, A.C., and V. Mor. 1999. Hospice in nursing homes: A facility level analysis of the distribution of hospice beneficiaries. *Gerontologist* 39(3): 279–90.

Pickett, M., M.E. Cooley, and G.B. Gordon. 1998. Palliative care: Past, present, and future perspectives. *Semin Oncol Nurs* 14(2): 86–94.

Pizzi, M.A., and R. Briggs. 2004. Occupational and physical therapy in hospice: The facilitation of meaning, quality of life, and well-being. *Topics Ger Rehabil* 20: 120–30.

Porell, F., F.G. Caro, A. Silva, and M. Monane. 1998. A longitudinal analysis of nursing home outcomes. *Health Serv Res* 33(4 Pt. 1): 835–65.

Reschovsky, J.D. 1998. The demand for post-acute and chronic care in nursing homes. *Medical Care* 36(4): 475–90.

Resnick, B., A.L. Gruber-Baldini, S. Zimmerman, E. Galik, I. Pretzer-Aboff, K. Russ, and J.R. Heber. 2009. Nursing home resident outcomes from the Res-Care intervention. *J Am Geriatr Soc* 57: 1156–1165.

Rizzolo, M.C., R. Hemp, D. Braddock, and A. Schindler. 2009. Family support services for persons with intellectual and developmental disabilities: Recent national trends. *Intel Develop Dis* 47: 152–155.

Robinson, K.M. 1997. The family's role in long-term care. *J Geront Nurs* 23(9): 7–11.

Russell, D., R.J. Rosati, and E. Andreopoulos. 2012. Continuity in the provider of home-based physical therapy services and its implications for outcomes of patients. *Phys Ther* 92: 227–35.

Saarik, J., and J. Hartley. 2010. Living with cancer-related fatigue: Developing an effective management programme. *Int J Palliative Nurs* 16: 6, 8–12.

Sands, L.P., Y. Wang, G.P. McCabe, K. Jennings, C. Eng, and K.E. Covinsky. 2006. Rates of acute care admissions for frail older people living with met versus unmet activity of daily living needs. *J Am Ger Soc* 54(2): 339–344.

Shumway-Cook, A., M.A. Ciol, J. Hoffman, B.J. Dudgeon, K. Yorkston, and L. Chan. 2009. Falls in the Medicare population: Incidence, associated factors, and impact on health care. *Phys Ther* 89: 324–332.

Sloane, P.D., S. Zimmerman, A.L. Gruber-Baldini, J.R. Hebel, J. Magaziner, and T.R. Konrad. 2005. Health and functional outcomes and health care utilization of persons with dementia in residential care and assisted living facilities: Comparison with nursing homes. *Gerontologist* 45 Spec No 1(1): 124–32.

Smith, D.B., and Z. Feng. 2010. The accumulated challenges of long-term care. *Health Affairs* 29: 29–34.

Smith, G.R., G.M. Williamson, L.S. Miller, and R. Schulz. 2011. Depression and quality of informal care: A longitudinal investigation of caregiving stressors. *Psych Aging* 26: 584–91.

Stewart, K. 2006. Perspectives on the recent decline in disability at older ages. *Policy Brief (Cent Home Care Policy Res)* 27: 1–6.

Szinovacz, M.E., and A. Davey. 2007. Changes in adult child caregiver networks. *Gerontologist* 47(3): 280–95.

Taylor, L., F. Whittington, C. Hollingsworth, M. Ball, S. King, V. Patterson, S. Diwan, C. Rosenbloom, and A. Neel Jr. 2003. Assessing the effectiveness of a walking program on physical function of residents living in an assisted living facility. *J Community Health Nurs* 20(1): 15–26.

U.S. Census Bureau. 2010 American Community Survey, American FactFinder, Table B18101. Retrieved from http://factfinder.census.gov (accessed May 18, 2012).

Weiss, C.O., H.M. Gonzalez, M.U. Kabeto, and K.M. Langa. 2005. Differences in amount of informal care received by non-Hispanic whites and Latinos in a nationally representative sample of older Americans. *J Am Geriatr Soc* 53(1): 146–51.

Wieland, D., R. Boland, J. Baskins, and B. Kinosian. 2010. Five-year survival in a Program of All-Inclusive Care for elderly compared with alternative institutional and home and community-based care. *J Gerontol A Biol Sci Med Sci* 65: 721–726.

Wielink, G., and R. Huijsman. 1999. Elderly community residents' evaluative criteria and preferences for formal and informal in-home services. *Int J Aging Hum Dev* 48(1): 17–33.

Wolf, D.A. 1999. The family as provider of long-term care: Efficiency, equity, and externalities. *J Aging Health* 11(3): 360–82.

Wolff, J.L., and J.D. Kasper, 2006. Caregivers of frail elders: Updating a national profile. *Gerontologist* 46(3): 344–356.

Yeboah, A., A. Kleppinger, and R.H. Fortinsky. 2011. Racial and ethnic variations in service use in a national sample of Medicare home health care patients with type 2 diabetes mellitus. *J Am Geriatr Soc* 59: 1123–29.

Yoo, B.K., J. Bhattacharya, K.M. McDonald, and A.M. Garber. 2004. Impacts of informal caregiver availability on long-term care expenditures in OECD countries. *Health Serv Res* 39(6 Pt. 2): 1971–92.

12

Special Education and Mental Health Systems

CHAPTER OBJECTIVES

At the conclusion of this chapter, the reader will be able to:

1 Define special education and the educational system for children with special needs.

2 Describe the educational system and structure for children with special needs in relation to occupational and physical therapists' roles and responsibilities.

3 Identify the members of and the role of the Individualized Education Program team.

4 Relate the needs of children with special education needs and the role of occupational therapists and physical therapists in meeting those needs.

5 Describe the history of mental health policy in the United States.

6 Discuss key perspectives of public policy and mental health legislation.

7 Describe mental health practice settings.

8 Explain the role of occupational therapy and physical therapy in meeting the needs of children with special education needs and persons diagnosed with mental disorders.

KEY WORDS

Early Intervention
Mental Health Policy
Mental Health Settings
Related Services
School-Based Practice
Special Education
Services

Stephanie is an occupational therapist working in an area agency that serves several rural school districts. Each day she provides services to infants with physical disabilities in their parents' home. She consults with teachers in the schools she serves to assist children in the classroom. Later this afternoon, she is participating in a conference with special education teachers, a child, and their parents to determine the plan for care over the next year.

Case Example Question:

1. How is Stephanie's workday similar or different from a therapist's workday in a hospital or long-term care setting?

Introduction

In previous chapters, traditional medical systems, including acute medical and post-acute medical care, were covered. In this chapter, two additional specialized systems will be addressed placing an emphasis on their unique perspectives. For therapy services delivered in a special education setting, the structure is different from other medical settings. This model of practice is unique in its delivery, focus, and roles. Pediatric therapists working in the special education setting should be aware of these unique perspectives in order to maximize effectiveness of services to children with special needs. Similarly, the provision of services for persons with mental disorders is distinctive in settings, focus, and roles of practitioners. Health care practitioners should have knowledge and understanding of mental disorders in order to provide effective services in all areas including mental, physical, spiritual, and environmental health.

Special Education

There is a great need for **special education services** within the United States, as can be seen through the number of children receiving these services at any given time. The U.S. Department of Education reported in the fall of 2010 that 6,552,766 children from the ages of 3 to 21 were receiving services under Part B of the Individuals with Disabilities Education Improvement Act (IDEA) within the United States including Washington, DC, and Puerto Rico (U.S. Department of Education 2010). Special education services are specifically designed services that are put in place to meet the unique needs of a child with a disability. This specialized instruction ensures the child is able to access the educational environment and that they can best meet the standards set forth for them (Jackson 2007; McEwen 2009). Special education is provided at no cost to the child or family and can be implemented in settings including the school, home, hospital, institution, or other settings (Pape and Ryba 2004). Special education services are to be provided as part of Free Appropriate Public Education (FAPE) and should take place in the least restrictive environment (LRE) for the child as outlined by IDEA (Bazyk and Case-Smith 2010).

Legislation and public policy is essential for a therapist to be aware of as it drives practice and funding in the special education setting (Davies 2012; Pope 2011). As was previously outlined in Chapter 4, Part B of IDEA is the Assistance for Education of all Children with Disabilities. Occupational therapy and physical therapy are considered **related services** for children with special needs in the educational system (see Chapter 4). The term *related services* as stated by the IDEA 2004 Title I "means transportation and such developmental, corrective, and other supportive services as may be required to assist a child with a disability to benefit from special education, and includes the early identification and assessment of disabling conditions in children." It is important to recognize that in this related service role, therapy services are only a portion of what is often required for students to benefit from their educational environment. Therapy services in **school-based practice** are intended to minimize obstacles in this setting but not necessarily maximize all skills or function as you may be more accustomed to in a medical model. (Hanft and Place 1996; Hinder and Ashburner 2010). Services are provided when they are viewed as educationally appropriate and will help the child benefit from their educational programming.

As of the 2009–2010 school year, the total number of occupational therapists and physical therapists serving children 3 to 21 years of age as related service providers totaled 27,240 (U.S. Department of Education 2010). With a large number of therapists working within the school system, therapists should have an understanding of employment factors that are present. In a rural area, related service professionals may often be responsible for services in multiple schools and multiple districts through an educational service agency. Special education services may be organized through cooperative districts or at a statewide level. In contrast, school districts in larger metropolitan areas will likely address special education services through the local school district. Physical therapists as well as occupational therapists can be involved as related service providers in these various systems through direct employment in a school district, working with an intermediate provider, or contracting with a clinic or other outside agency (APTA 2009). The type of employment and environment will impact how services are funded and what roles these types of professionals will play in each setting.

Individualized Education Program (IEP)

In order for an occupational therapist or physical therapist to provide services to a child in the educational setting, an Individualized Education Program (IEP) must be in place. This document is created to identify a student's educational needs and how these will be addressed (Pape and Ryba 2004). This document also outlines who the team members are that are directly involved with the implementation of the plan, along with when, where, and how the needs will be addressed and ultimately met. The members of this team are the individuals that an occupational or physical therapist will regularly be consulting with in the educational setting. Members of the team will change as needed, and the level of involvement for each member may not remain the same throughout the duration of the IEP (Hanft and Shepherd 2008). Ideally, though, all team members will contribute on some level to the success of the student in his or her educational environment. The required members of an IEP team are listed in Table 12-1.

Team member collaboration and communication are an essential part of school-based practice for therapists (Asher 2010; Effgen, Chiarello, and Milbourne 2007). This process to provide program support and information that will benefit the child is considered to be a part of indirect service, while interactions with the child directly, therapy sessions, modifications of the school environment, and other direct student interactions are considered direct service (Bazyk and Case-Smith 2010; McEwen 2009). While the IEP team members listed in Table 12-1 make up many of the individuals a therapist would interact

---

Table 12-1 Required Members of an Individualized Education Program

- The parent(s) of a child with a disability
- Not less than one regular education teacher of the child (if the child is participating in the regular education environment)
- Not less than one special education teacher or provider of the child
- A representative of the local educational agency (may be referred to as LEA)
- An individual who can interpret the instructional implications of the evaluation results
- At the discretion of the parent or the agency, other individuals who have knowledge or special expertise regarding the child, including related services personnel as appropriate
- Whenever appropriate, the child with a disability

Source: Individuals with Disabilities Education Improvement Act of 2004, Pub. L. No. 108-446. Retrieved June 14, 2012, from: http://frwebgate.access.gpo.gov/cgi-bin/getdoc.cgi?dbname=108_cong_public_laws&docid=f:publ446.108.pdf

Table 12-2 Required Components of an IEP

- A statement of the child's present level of educational performance and how disability affects participation in the curriculum.
- Measurable annual goals.
- A statement of special education and related services, and supplementary aids and services to be provided for the child.
- A statement of the extent, if any, to which the child will not participate with children without disabilities in the regular classroom.
- A statement of any modifications in the administration of state- or district-wide assessments of student achievement or an explanation of why the assessment is not appropriate for the child and an alternative assessment measure.
- Projected date for initiating services.
- Statement on how student progress towards measurable goals will be assessed, how the parent(s) will be informed of progress on a regular basis, and the extent to which progress is sufficient to allow the child to achieve goals by the end of the school year.

Source: Adapted from L. Pape, and K. Ryba. 2004. *Practical considerations for schoolbased occupational therapists.* Bethesda, MD: AOTA, Inc.

with regularly while providing services, there are other individuals to consider within a school-based setting. Members of the student's team could also consist of paraprofessionals and paraeducators, speech/language pathologists, school psychologists, school principals, school district administrators, custodial staff, physical education teachers, music teachers, art teachers, and other individuals that are integral to the everyday functioning of a child in the school setting (AOTA 2010).

The IEP is required to address several items and has an emphasis on student-driven and family-centered practices to increase participation and ensure understanding (Dole, Arvidson, Byrne, Robbins, and Schasberger 2003). The required components of an IEP are listed in Table 12-2. The occupational and/or physical therapist should be involved in the creation of the IEP including the creation of student-centered, meaningful, and functional goals and objectives (Dole et al. 2003).

Team Communication Case Example

Janie is a seven-year-old first-grade student who has qualified for special education along with related services of occupational and physical therapy at her public elementary school. Janie has difficulty participating in writing, cutting, and coloring activities in the classroom environment. She also has difficulty accessing her school environment independently. An IEP has been established, and her therapists have been working with numerous individuals within her school to increase her ability to successfully participate in her academic setting. Collaborations have been successful as all team members are assuming responsibility in implementing solutions and working together to meet the same goals that were established on the IEP. In the table below are several examples of positive team communication and collaboration as well as the potential outcomes related to Janie and other students in her school.

Collaboration	Outcome
The occupational therapist and physical therapist communicate with Janie's teacher during a prescheduled meeting time to discuss Janie's daily schedule and adjustments that can be made to increase transition time and/or reduce number of transitions.	1. Janie's teacher is able to revise Janie's schedule to allow her a few extra minutes to transition to classes outside of the classroom with a peer buddy (PE, art, music, lunch, and special events).
	2. Janie is provided with an organizer by her desk to allow her to switch materials without having to carry items back and forth from her cubby at the back of the room.

Continued

Collaboration	Outcome
The physical therapist collaborates with the physical education teacher to assist with Janie's participation in required activities including basketball, which is the current unit in PE class.	1. The PE teacher is able to provide Janie with a modified PE environment (i.e., lower basketball hoop, lighter ball) that allows her to participate in class instead of sitting on the sideline as she had been doing. 2. The PE teacher is able to apply the suggestions provided by the physical therapist in other classes as well and increases participation for Janie and other students who previously were struggling.
The occupational and physical therapist consult with the custodial staff at the school to see what modifications can be made to Janie's school-issued chair and desk as it does not provide her the optimal support and positioning she needs in the classroom.	1. The custodial staff is able to adjust her chair to the correct height and seat depth and find a different desk that can be adjusted to the new chair height. This desk has increased storage options which also help with Janie's need to store additional items by her desk to decrease transition time.
The occupational therapist communicates with the principal about a need for more education for Kindergarten and first-grade teachers regarding modified cutting and coloring activities for children with decreased bilateral coordination and visual motor deficits. After talking to many teachers, the occupational therapist finds they are avoiding these skills with students who struggle similarly to Janie and realizes a need to advocate at the administrative level.	1. Janie's teacher, along with others, is provided with an in-service time when Janie's occupational therapist presents strategies and techniques for the classroom that could better address the needs of children struggling at this school. 2. Janie's teacher applies some of these techniques in her classroom with Janie and other children and is able to see improvement. 3. The school principal expresses interest in providing additional in-services by related service providers on other topics of teacher interest.

Related Services in the School Setting

After an IEP has been established, how therapy is provided can vary greatly by school district. Services may be provided directly to students in a one-to-one environment similar to what you may see in a therapy clinic (Bazyk and Case-Smith 2010). However, the trends in school-based therapy have been moving away from this model in order to best support the child's learning needs in the least restrictive environment (Effgen, Chiarello, and Milbourne 2007). This means that therapists may be providing services within the classroom context directly with the student, but also consultatively with the educators, paraeducators, and other school staff to increase a child's ability to benefit from the educational environment (Bazyk and Case-Smith 2010). The model of service provided is directed by the IEP but also through national, state, and local policies as well as the individual school setting (Jackson 2007; McEwen 2009). This service model may change as the child progresses in skill and ability if the setting allows.

Children with disabilities may enter the special education system through various pathways. Many children are identified with a disability during the ages of two to five years of age (NICHY 2010). When in this age range, a child may qualify for services in a preschool setting that is provided through IDEA. These children can be identified and referred for an evaluation through a pediatrician during well-baby check-ups but some are also identified through Child Find services provided by the state. According to IDEA 2004, "each State must have comprehensive systems of Child Find in order to identify, locate, and evaluate children with disabilities residing in the State who are in need of special education and related services" (NICHCY 2010). Children that have already been identified prior to age three may have been receiving early intervention services through Part C of IDEA, which was described in greater detail in Chapter 4. These children will often transition into school-based services at the preschool age and will move from the Individualized Family Service Plan (IFSP) to an IEP.

Some students are not identified until later in their educational careers. This can occur through teacher referral or parent request, but therapists have also found themselves to

Table 12-3 Disability Categories

Autism	Orthopedic Impairments
Deaf-Blindness	Other Health Impairments
Deafness	Specific Learning Disability
Emotional Disturbance	Speech or Language Impairments
Hearing Impairments	Traumatic Brain Injury
Mental Retardation	Visual Impairments (including blindness)
Multiple Disabilities	Developmental Delay (applies to children ages 3–9)

Source: U.S. Department of Education, Office of Special Education Programs, Data Analysis System (DANS),OMB #1820-0043: "Children with Disabilities Receiving Special Education Under Part B of the Individuals with Disabilities Education Act," 2010. Data updated as of July 15, 2011.

have increased involvement in identifying these students and providing input for such processes as early intervening services, Response to Intervention (RtI), and plans addressing Section 504 of the Rehabilitation Act (Jackson 2007). Refer back to the discussion in Chapter 4 regarding the Rehabilitation Act. Section 504 affects school service provision, as education is included in this legislation, but no additional funding is available under ADA for schools to address these needs (Jackson 2007). On the other hand, early intervening services and RtI are supported through provisions in IDEA 2004. These services are intended to increase aid to students that struggle in the regular education environment and prevent discrimination against individuals living with disabilities (Jackson 2007; Pope 2011). Occupational therapists and physical therapists have seen increased involvement in these processes and this should be considered a part of a therapist's role in the educational institution.

Once children have been referred in a school-based setting, they can qualify for services under a variety of disabilities. Disability categories provided services under IDEA are detailed in Table 12-3. Numerous children receive special education services under these categories each year. In 2010, the greatest number of four-year-old children receiving special education services were classified under the disability categories of developmental delay and speech or language impairments (U.S. Department of Education 2010). Since the category of developmental delay can only apply to children from ages three to nine, as children grow older, there seems to be a significant increase in children receiving services in the categories of specific learning disabilities and other health impairments. The percentages of children being served in 2010 in each disability category for specified ages under IDEA can be found in Table 12-4. The changes in disability category can result in children being identified for related services at varying times in their educational careers. A better understanding of the disability categories and how children are categorized within a specific school district will assist a therapist in advocating for children and their needs.

Early Intervention Services
Early intervention services are also provided under IDEA 2004 in Part C. These services are provided to children between birth and three years of age. Part C provides support to states to maintain and implement these required early intervention services but does not establish mandatory programs as is done through Part B for school-aged services (Myers, Stephens and Tauber 2010). If infants or toddlers are identified as having a disability, they and their family are then eligible for early intervention services. Once a child has been assessed and necessary services determined, an Individualized Family Service Plan (IFSP) is put in place to address the family's needs. Regulations specify that the IFSP

Table 12-4 Percentage of Children Served by Disability Category under IDEA, Part B

Disability Category	4 Years	13 Years	18 Years
Specific Learning Disabilities	0.81	52	52
Speech or Language Impairments	43	7.6	2.2
Mental Retardation	1.2	7.5	14
Emotional Disturbance	0.25	7.7	9.1
Multiple Disabilities	0.83	2	3.3
Hearing Impairments	1.1	1.2	1.3
Orthopedic Impairments	0.94	0.94	1
Other Health Impairments	2	15	11
Visual Impairments	0.43	0.43	0.46
Autism	5.9	5.7	5.3
Deaf-Blindness	0.03	0.01	0.03
Traumatic Brain Injury	0.13	0.44	0.63
Developmental Delay	43	NA	NA

Source: U.S. Department of Education, Office of Special Education Programs, Data Analysis System (DANS),OMB #1820-0043: "Children with Disabilities Receiving Special Education Under Part B of the Individuals with Disabilities Education Act," 2010. Data updated as of July 15, 2011.

along with outcomes must be established with the participation of the family and assistance from the service providers as needed to create an effective plan (McEwen 2009).

Occupational and physical therapists working in early intervention can be the sole providers of service for a child or may work in conjunction with other early intervention providers (Myers, Stephens, and Tauber 2010). This is in contrast to school-based practice where therapists are considered to be only a related service. Children are often identified as requiring early intervention services due to multiple factors; one common factor is delay in developmental milestones. Interventions in this setting may focus on developmental skills, minimizing or preventing future impairments, addressing functional skills and/or motor skills, and assistive technology (APTA 2010; Myers, Stephens, and Tauber 2010)

Occupational and physical therapists may provide services to children receiving early intervention through a variety of models. A common model for these services is to work in a transdisciplinary team, where members collaborate to provide the most effective services to the child and family. This model can also support a primary service provider where a therapist or other team member is the primary contact and provider for the child and family. The primary provider is coached by the other discipline members of the team to ensure they are addressing all the goals previously set for the child (Myers, Stephens, and Tauber 2010). The model of service in this setting will vary by state, and all have their benefits and drawbacks. One of the most important elements for a therapist working in early intervention is to have a good understanding of policies influencing practice and an ability to communicate effectively with a variety of stakeholders, including team professionals, physicians, community resources, extended family, day care providers, parents, and the child (APTA 2010; Myers, Stephens, and Tauber 2010).

Special Considerations in School-Based and Early Intervention Practice

There are other factors that should be taken into consideration in the special education environment. One of those factors is the changing school-based environment. Depending on the school district, a therapist may find that many roles and practices are changing (Davies 2012). While traditional school-based practice often took place by pulling children out of the classroom for services, there has been an increasing push to follow an inclusionary and collaborative model in education (AOTA 2006). This results in a therapist's role expanding to not only include working with children in the natural environment but also providing support and education to staff and teachers in the classroom and throughout the school district (Asher 2010). Therapists may also see an increase in time spent observing groups of students for early intervening services and providing instruction to large groups of parents and educators in the facilities. This is a beneficial role to assume in these settings and allows therapists to showcase their value as a vital team member.

Therapists should also be aware of the impact that mental health can have on children and their ability to participate in their educational environments. Learning is affected by cognitive skill development, but increasing evidence is showing that social-emotional health of children also has a large impact on this (Bazyk and Case-Smith 2010). There has been a push to increase all personnel's understanding of mental health concerns for children in the school systems, resulting in occupational therapists and physical therapists also becoming involved in services for these children (Bazyk and Case-Smith 2010). While this may still be considered an emerging area of practice, it is important to be prepared to work with these children as well and to know the policies and legislation that support these services in the special education system.

Mental Health

It is estimated that 450 million people worldwide are treated for some type of mental disorder (World Health Organization [WHO] 2010), and in the United States about 26.2 percent of adults will be diagnosed with a mental disorder (Kessler, Chiu, Demler, and Walters 2005). Of those adults, approximately 6 percent, or 1 in 17 (Kessler et al., 2005), experience a severe and persistent mental illness. Additionally, Kessler et al. (2005) estimate 13 percent of children are identified with a mental disorder; of those children, 5 to 9 percent experience severe emotional disturbances (Center for Mental Health Services [CMHS] 2006). The purpose of this section is to provide an overview of **mental health policy**, mental health practice settings, and the roles of occupational therapists and physical therapists in current and future mental health practice.

In the DSM-V, set for release in 2013, a proposed definition of a mental disorder is "a health condition characterized by significant dysfunction in an individual's cognitions, emotions, or behaviors that reflects a disturbance in the psychological, biological, or developmental processes underlying mental functioning" (American Psychological Association [APA] 2012). As noted in the DSM IV-TR, mental disorders vary according to individual, culture, environment, and severity (APA 2000). Throughout this section, the term *mental illness* will be utilized and will refer specifically to persons diagnosed with severe and persistent clinical diagnoses identified in Axis I of the DSM IV-TR.

Mental Health Policy

In 1775, persons diagnosed with mental disorders were admitted to the first psychiatric hospital in Philadelphia under the care of Dr. Benjamin Rush (National Institutes of Health [NIH] 1998) as a safe, calm retreat (Peters 2011). Over the next two centuries, institutions were the primary treatment facilities for mental illnesses (Fisher, Geller, and Pandiani 2009; Peters 2011). In the mid-18th century, concerns grew in regard to care and treatment provided in these locked hospitals. From that time, the moral treatment movement and the mental hygiene movements influenced both mental health policy and practice (Dixon and Goldman 2004) serving as a basis for future movements (Cutler, Bevilacqua, and McFarland 2003).

In the 1940s, there was growing concern about the mental health of soldiers returning from World War II as soldiers experienced anxiety and stress referred to as shell shock

(Cutler, Bevilacqua, and McFarland 2003). These concerns prompted the government to provide mental health services. The National Mental Health Act (P.L. 79–487) was passed in 1946 establishing the National Institute for Mental Health (NIMH) to address the need for improved services and better understanding of mental disorders (Cutler, Bevilacqua, and McFarland 2003; NIH 1998). From the 1940s, until the 1960s the majority of persons with mental illnesses received treatment in psychiatric hospitals (Bruce and Borg 2002; Cutler, Bevilacqua, and McFarland 2003). In 1948, the first community mental health center was established (Dixon and Goldman 2004) and more practitioners began working in community-based settings (Cutler, Bevilacqua, and McFarland 2003).

During the 1960s, tensions rose between advocates for persons with severe and persistent mental illnesses and supporters of persons with mental disorders (Goldman and Grob 2006) in regard to policies and services. Paradoxical to this growing tension, there was a growth in the knowledge and understanding of mental disorders, specifically the impact of psychotropic medications on symptoms (Cutler et al. 2003; Drake, Green, Mueser, and Goldman 2003). Services available at this time focused on managing symptoms, remaining stable, and remaining out of the hospital (Drake et al. 2003). In 1961 the Joint Commission on Mental Health and Mental Illness recommended a community-based mental health system supporting the release of persons from long-term psychiatric facilities (Cutler et al. 2003; Dixon and Goldman 2004; Goldman and Grob 2006). President Kennedy signed the Community Mental Health Centers Act in 1963 in order to create noninstitutionalized services based in communities. The passage of this act marked the first time that the federal government assumed a direct role in the provision of **mental health services** (Cutler et al. 2003).

Community mental health centers (CMHCs) were established by this act with the intent to "provide inpatient and outpatient services as well as consultation and education, day treatment, and crisis services" (Cutler et al. 2003, p. 386). The implementation of community mental health centers resulted in the decrease of numbers of persons in long-term psychiatric hospitals (Dixon and Goldman 2004). The shift toward community-based services also caused negative outcomes, such as higher rates of homelessness and incarceration for persons with mental illnesses (Bruce and Borg 2002; Dixon and Goldman 2004; Peters 2011). Additionally, older adults were shifted from inpatient psychiatric facilities to long-term nursing facilities (Dixon and Goldman 2004; Scott and Mahaffey 2010), creating new institutions for adults with mental illnesses.

During the late 1970s, the needs of persons with chronic mental illnesses were not being supported by the national mental health system (Manderscheid et al. 2010) as community mental health centers provided limited services to persons with severe mental illnesses (Cutler et al. 2003; Dixon and Goldman 2004; Goldman and Grob 2006). In 1977, President Carter created the President's Commission on Mental Health, and again differences arose between "those who favored a broad definition of mental health and those who favored a narrower focus on mental illness" (Goldman and Grob 2006, p. 741). One outcome of the commission's findings was creation of the Mental Health Systems Act of 1980. The purpose of this act was to improve mental health services by (a) prioritizing mental health services for the most vulnerable, (b) restructuring guidelines to give states more control, (c) requiring planning for implementing programs, (d) improving links between mental and general health care, and (e) improving advocacy (Cutler et al. 2003; Goldman and Grob 2006). However, President Reagan's administration did not fund this policy (Goldman and Grob 2006). Instead, the 1980s ushered in an era of emphasis on rehabilitation where the goal of mental health "became to help people function in adult societal roles, such as worker, student, parent, or spouse" (Drake et al. 2003).

By the start of the 1990s, two new movements were influencing shifts in mental health policy and practice. The evidence-based movement began to influence policy as questions arose about quality of care and the effectiveness of care (Dixon and Goldman 2004; Drake and Latimer 2012). Concerns about fraud and efficacy in community mental health systems drove a need for evidence-based practices (Cutler et al. 2003). Evidence-based practice is composed of researched interventions with consistent positive outcomes (Drake et al. 2003). In 1992, the federal government created the Substance Abuse and Mental Health Services Administration (SAMHSA) to support, fund, and disseminate information on evidence-based practices (SAMHSA 2012). Since then, SAMHSA has identified numerous evidence-based practices including but not limited to Illness Management and Recovery, Supported Employment, and Family Psychoeducation.

The second movement was the recovery movement, which has been influential in changing mental health services (Drake and Latimer 2012). Recovery is "a journey of healing and transformation enabling a person with a mental health problem to live a meaningful life in a community of his or her choice while striving to achieve his or her full potential" (CMHS 2005, p. 5). Recovery is a lifelong process in which the role of mental health systems "is to help people pursue independence, self-management, personally meaningful activities, and better quality of life" (Drake et al. 2003). The influence of the recovery movement can be seen in the improvement of services across the United States, specifically in the increase of rehabilitative services and the decreased use of restraints and seclusion (Drake and Latimer 2012).

In addition to these two movements, the Supreme Court issued a decision in 1999 that further supported the establishment of community-based services (Merryman 2010). The Court ruled in *Olmstead v. L.C.* that "under the Americans with Disabilities Act (ADA) unjustifiable institutionalization of a person with a disability who, with proper support, can live in the community is discrimination" (Department of Health and Human Services [DHHS] 2000).

In 2003, the president's New Freedom Commission on Mental Health (NFCMH) Committee released a final report, *Achieving the Promise: Transforming Mental Health Care in America.* The report detailed the status of, made recommendations for changes in, and highlighted the fragmented nature of both federal and state mental health systems. The committee set forth goals of a transformed mental health system (see Table 12-5) in order for persons with severe and persistent mental illnesses to "live, work, learn, and participate fully in their communities" (NFCMH 2003, p. 5).

One aspect of change supported by the committee addressed the inequality of "insurance plans that place greater restrictions on treating mental illnesses than on other illnesses" (NFCMH 2003, p. 21) and called for parity between mental health and general health care. Parity is "the drive to integrate and equalize mental health coverage in the mainstream of private health insurance" (Goldman and Grob 2006, p. 744). Connecticut was the first state to pass parity legislation, and by 2001, at least 37 states had followed (Goldman and Grob 2006). Not until 1992 was parity addressed on a national level by Senators Domenici and Wellstone who proposed separate federal parity legislation (Goldman and Grob 2006).

By 1996, the senators, in conjunction with advocacy efforts of national organizations such as NAMI and APA, had succeeded in passing the first Federal Mental Health Parity Act (P.L. 104–204) (Cutler et al. 2003; Swarbrick 2010). However, the bill was a compromise and narrowly focused on annual and lifetime limits (Goldman and Grob 2006; Merryman 2010). As such, both senators continued to champion passage of a broader federal parity act. Then in 2008, as part of the Emergency Economic Stabilization Act of 2008 (H.R. 1424) the Paul Wellstone–Pete Domenici Mental Health Parity and Addiction Equity Act of 2008 (P.L. 110–343) passed. The law went into place for most mental health providers in January 2010 and "ensures fair and equal coverage of mental health and substance abuse disorders for those in large self-insured plans, as well as for 31 million

---

Table 12-5 Goals of a Transformed Mental Health System in the United States

- Americans understand that mental health is essential to overall health.
- Mental health care is consumer- and family-driven.
- Disparities in mental health services are eliminated.
- Early mental health screening, assessment, and referral to services are common practices.
- Excellent mental health care is delivered and research is accelerated.
- Technology is used to access mental health care and information.

Source: Achieving the Promise: Transforming Mental Health Care in America (NFCMH, 2003, p. 5).

more people in fully insured large group plans" (NAMI 2009, p. 1). It is important to note that the law does not require health insurance plans that did not previously cover mental health services to provide coverage.

In the mid-2000s, the health and wellness movement began to influence mental health policy and practice as concerns were raised about morbidity and mortality of persons with mental illnesses (Insel 2009; Lawrence and Kisely 2010). Current research indicates that persons with severe mental illnesses die on average 25 years sooner than their peers who are not diagnosed with a mental illness (Druss and Bornemann 2010; Swarbrick 2010a; Swarbrick 2010b). The campaign of this new movement is that it is imperative to address the whole health of the person (Manderscheid et al. 2010; Swarbrick 2010b). Traditionally, mental health and physical health are treated separately by different health care professionals (Lawrence and Kisely 2010; Manderscheid et al., 2010). Building on the recovery movement, the health and wellness movement seeks to address the health disparities of persons with mental illnesses, to design and implement effective health and wellness services, and to promote well-being (Manderscheid et al., 2010).

Mental Health Practice Settings

TRADITIONAL   *Acute and Subacute Hospitalization.* An acute hospitalization setting is utilized for persons in crisis, experiencing acute symptoms, and who are either a danger to themselves or a danger to someone in the community. The goal of an inpatient unit is to "provide a safe and structured environment in which to manage issues of inability to care for oneself, clear and present danger to self or others, and/or deterioration in condition that cannot be managed at a lesser level of care" (Hopkins, Loeb, and Fick 2009, p. 928). Inpatient units provide "a protective environment that includes medical stabilization, support, treatment for psychiatric and/or addictive disorders, and supervision" (Commission on Accreditation of Rehabilitation Facilities [CARF] 2012, p. 10). Once an acute exacerbation of psychiatric symptoms subsides, a person may require further inpatient treatment in a subacute unit. Depending on state regulations for length of stay in acute and subacute inpatient units, an individual who is still experiencing symptoms such that he or she is unable to return to the community may be transferred to another more appropriate treatment setting such as long-term hospitalization (Lutterman, Berhane, Phelan, Shaw, and Rana 2009, p. 46).

Long-Term hospitalization. Originally intended "for persons in need of the most intensive level of mental health services" (Lutterman et al. 2009, p. 19) long-term psychiatric hospitals were built to protect and treat individuals with mental illnesses (Peters 2011). Yet, the unique experience of symptoms of a mental illness may result in a person needing long-term hospitalization: for example, a person who is unable to live and function in the community because of safety concerns or committed by court order (Exley, Thompson, Hays 2011; Fisher et al. 2009). The goal of long-term care is to provide stabilization, support, and supervision with an expected outcome of reintegration into the community.

Partial Hospitalization. Partial hospitalization provides a structured program for persons who are either (a) ready for discharge from inpatient hospitalization but who still require a higher level of support than community-based programming may provide or (b) are at a high risk of rehospitalization without partial hospitalization (DHHS 2012). In partial hospitalization, a person attends a program tailored to his or her needs and "treatment may be arranged for day, evening, night, or weekends, within the framework of the recommended minimum number of hours per week" (Association for Ambulatory Behavioral Healthcare [AABH] 2010). The flexibility of partial hospitalization programs supports persons with mental illnesses in being able to remain in community, return to work, and/or interact with family and friends while receiving the best of inpatient and outpatient care (AABH 2010).

Crisis Stabilization. Crisis Stabilization Programs provide services for persons struggling in the early stages of crisis. A person with a mental illness may voluntarily check in and receive immediate, short-term, individualized crisis-oriented treatment in order to minimize the impact of the crisis and possibly deter hospitalization. These programs "are organized and staffed to provide the availability of overnight residential services 24 hours a day, 7 days a week for a limited duration" (CARF 2012, p. 8).

COMMUNITY-BASED The next section will review community-based settings; however, the types of settings, including name, vary by state, requiring health care practitioners to review individual state regulations.

Community Mental Health Centers. In 1963, President Kennedy envisioned community mental health centers (CMHC) that "were to be comprehensive, providing services not only to the severely mentally ill, but also to children, families, and adults suffering from the effects of stress" (Cutler et al. 2003, p. 384). Today, these centers are "the main source of public outpatient mental health services" (SAMHSA 2009b, p. 342) and, depending on the state in which an individual resides, may or may not be available in all areas. A CMHC must provide core services including outpatient services, 24-hour emergency care, day treatment or partial hospitalization, and screening for admission to long-term psychiatric facilities (Centers for Medicare and Medicaid Services [CMS] 2012). Furthermore, in order to be eligible to receive Medicare payment for services, a CMHC must also "provide at least 40 percent of its services to individuals who are not eligible for benefits under Medicare" (CMS 2011).

Day Rehabilitation Programs. Day Rehabilitation Programs are an option for adults with mental illnesses to receive "comprehensive, intensive, individually planned, coordinated, and structured services" (CARF 2012, p. 8). The goal of a day program is to address social, educational, and leisure needs of participants by "promoting daily routine, a sense of belonging to the program community, as well as the community at large" (Griswold, Evenson, and Roberts 2011, p. 1085). These programs are typically open at least five days a week and offer some evening and weekend outings (CARF 2012, p. 8). Unlike partial hospitalization programs, day rehabilitation programs do not provide services similar to inpatient care.

Adult Day Service Programs. Older adults with a mental illness may require different services as they age, including more support for social, leisure, and medical needs. Adult Day Service programs are located within communities and provide services during the day. Similar to day rehabilitation programs, these programs focus on providing support and structure "to increase the quality of life and health status of day care participants" (Griswold et al. 2009, p. 1084) who are 65 years of age and older.

Clubhouse Model Programs. Clubhouse model programs are similar to day rehabilitation programs; however, a clubhouse also provides support and structure to meet the vocational needs of participants. The term "clubhouse" was originally utilized "to communicate the work and vision of Fountain House, the very first clubhouse, which was started in New York in 1948" (International Center for Clubhouse Development [ICCD] 2009). Additionally, the term conveys a sense of membership, participation, and ownership. In the clubhouse model, participants are referred to as *members*, as membership in a club or organization indicates belonging (ICCD 2009). A clubhouse model program creates, implements, and emphasizes a work focus to all programming. Members of the clubhouse participate equally, alongside staff, in the operation and maintenance of the program providing services in all units (Stoffel 2011, p. 561). A typical clubhouse is open eight hours a day, five days a week, and includes evening and weekend outings.

One of the most important aspects of a clubhouse model is the inclusion of transitional and supported employment opportunities for members. Transitional employment consists of part-time employment (ICCD 2009) where members work at a job for a set amount of time in a specific work setting to build their work experience and skills (Bennett and Logsdon 2010). After the allotted time, members can either change to a different transitional job, or members can move on to supported employment or independent employment. Supported employment is long-term competitive employment in the open labor market (SAMHSA 2009a) and may continue for as long as the member wants the position, as the expected outcome is competitive employment. In both transitional and supported employment, job coaches provide on- and off-site support to workers, and workers are paid at or above minimum wage. Additionally, both may be part of other programs and are not solely part of clubhouse model programs. Supported employment is designated by SAMHSA (2009a) as an evidence-based practice.

Programs of Assertive Community Treatment. Occurring in the community in which the participant resides, PACT is a service-delivery model that consists of comprehensive, flexible, community-based treatment support and services 24 hours a day, 7 days a week, 365 days a year (SAMHSA 2008). P/ACT programs incorporate a multidisciplinary team including psychiatrists, nurses, mental health workers, therapists, peer specialists, and more. Participants in a P/ACT program are diagnosed with severe and persistent mental illnesses, have a history of difficulty keeping themselves safe, and experience difficulty in completing daily activities of living and maintaining housing (Dallas 2011, p. 576). The purpose of a P/ACT program is to provide services at one location in order to support participants living in the community and includes "case management, initial and ongoing assessments, psychiatric services, employment and housing assistance, family support and education" (Assertive Community Treatment Association [ACTA] 2007) and more.

P/ACT is effective for persons who have a history of multiple hospital admissions in a year, a history of long hospitalizations, and who are diagnosed with a co-occurring substance abuse disorder. P/ACT is recognized as an evidence-based practice (SAMHSA 2008) and is the most implemented evidence-based adult service in the United States (Lutterman et al. 2009).

Consumer-Operated Service Programs. Also known as consumer-run services and peer support programs, these programs provide a "different worldview, structure, and approach to 'helping' than traditional treatment services" (SAMHSA 2011, p.3). Built on the foundation of consumers providing support and structure for other consumers, these programs offer a variety of services in multiple settings. One example of these programs is a drop-in center. The goal of a drop-in center is to meet the social and leisure needs of the participants resulting in centers being open in the evening, on weekends, and on holidays (Swarbrick 2011, p. 509). Activities provided at a drop-in center may include support groups, social events, and information for support services (SAMHSA 2011). For consumers in early crisis stages, some consumer-run programs may provide crisis response support and respite information and education (SAMHSA 2011). These services are limited up to a 24-hour stay but may be further limited to only open program hours. If a participant requires beginning of the profession occupational more intensive support, consumer-operated service programs are able to refer out to community resources such as Crisis Stabilization Programs.

CHILDREN'S MENTAL HEALTH   Services for children differ from those for adults. The unique experience for both the child and the family dealing with an emotional disturbance resulted in the development and implementation of systems of care. The system consists of "coordinated networks of community-based services and supports" (CMHS 2006, p. 1) and includes both public and private service organizations. The goal of the system is to provide support to both the child and the family in a client-centered, family-centered, culturally appropriate manner so that the children may "reach their full potential at home, at school, and in their communities" (CMHS 2006, p. 1). Within the systems of care, services are delivered in community-based settings either at home, in school, or at local outpatient clinics. The outcomes of these systems of care result in "an increase in behavioral and emotional strengths and a reduction in mental health problems" (NFCMH 2003, p. 29). If a child is unable to remain in the home or a foster home, there are other residential treatment options available such as children's residential treatment, institutions, and jail/correctional facilities (Lutterman et al. 2009). Within these residential facilities, children and adolescents receive services in-house.

Role of Occupational Therapy

Occupational therapy has a rich and detailed history in the mental health field. Practitioners agree that the profession of occupational therapy began in 1917 as part of the mental hygiene movement (Bonder 2010; Bruce and Borg 2002; Kavanaugh Scheinholtz 2010; Peters 2011). At the beginning of the profession, occupational therapists were working with persons with mental illnesses to engage in interests and "normal activities" (Bruce and Borg 2002, p. 3) as a way to reduce symptoms (Kavanaugh Scheinholtz 2010). As

Table 12-6 Practice Settings in Mental Health for Occupational Therapists

• Adult Day Service Programs	• Psychiatric Hospitals/Units
• Day Rehabilitation Programs	• Community Mental Health Centers
• Clubhouse Programs	• Outpatient Psychiatric Clinics
• P/ACT Programs	• Group Homes
• Employment Programs	• Home Health Agencies

Source: Based on American Occupational Therapy Association. [AOTA] (2007). *OT and Community Mental Health.*

the profession grew, occupational therapists also engaged in adapting activities of interest in order to address a multitude of issues stemming from a mental illness (Bruce and Borg 2002). By the 1950s occupational therapists were working in psychiatric facilities as well as community programs, especially vocational rehabilitation settings such as sheltered workshops (Bruce and Borg 2002). Today occupational therapists work in a variety of mental health practice settings (see Table 12-6) and "may work in traditional clinical roles or, with increasing frequency, in new roles" (Bruce and Borg 2002, p. 6) focusing on prevention and rehabilitation.

Within these settings, an occupational therapist provides services in order to "help people develop the skills and obtain the supports necessary for independent, interdependent, productive living" (AOTA 2007, para. 1). The therapist, in collaboration with the client, will obtain an occupational profile to gain information about the client's needs, wants, strengths, and challenges (Bonder 2010). Similar to other practice settings, an occupational therapist working in mental health will conduct interviews, complete assessments, and communicate with other providers to create a detailed narrative of a client's lived experience (Brown 2011; Roberts and Evenson 2009). Additionally, occupational therapists engage in partnerships with consumers and collaborate on the creation of goals and intervention plans using client-centered, occupation-based interventions in order to promote recovery, health, and wellness (Brown 2011; Champagne and Gray 2011).

The role of an occupational therapist may include direct care, consultation, case management, advocacy, education, or administration (Bruce and Borg 2002; Champagne and Gray 2011). As part of these roles, occupational therapists may provide a wide assortment of clinical services. Occupational therapists collaborate with consumers and other providers on the creation of discharge plans as well as support and reinforce behavioral or therapy plans of other service providers (Roberts and Evenson 2009). Other clinical services provided by an occupational therapist may include creating, implementing, and/or modifying programming as well as providing education and/or training for other clinical staff and family members (Griswold et al. 2009). Furthermore, an occupational therapist may implement individual or group psychosocial interventions on coping skills, emotion regulation, stress management, and relapse prevention (Stoffel 2011). Mental health services provided by occupational therapists should also promote and facilitate recovery (see Table 12-7).

Table 12-7 Occupational Therapy Service as Part of Mental Health Recovery

- Teach and support active use of coping skills to manage impact of symptoms in life
- Help identify and implement health habits, rituals, and routines to support wellness
- Support the creation and use of a wellness recovery action plan (WRAP)
- Provide information to increase knowledge and use of community-based resources
- Provide information on monitoring physical health concerns and strategize to control, recognize, and respond to acute changes

Source: From "Occupational Therapy Service as Part of Mental Health Recovery" by T. Champagne and K. Gray, 2011, Bethesda, MD American Occupational Therapy Association. Reprinted with permission.

Future Implications for Health Care Professionals

Health care professionals working in mental health settings will be aware of psychiatric diagnoses, symptoms, and treatments. In addition, health care professionals such as occupational therapists or physical therapists in other practice settings should be aware of mental disorders, as symptoms of these disorders may impact implementation of interventions (Bonder 2010). Health care professionals need to be able to communicate with mental health providers as well as understand and support mental health services being implemented for a person with mental illness.

As health issues such as cardiovascular events, metabolic syndrome, COPD, and diabetes continue to impact persons with mental illnesses at a disproportionate rate (Lawrence and Kisely 2010; Swarbrick 2010), there is a need to address both mental and physical health (Manderscheid et al. 2010). Occupational therapists and physical therapists within their scope of practice are in positions to design and implement health and wellness programs and interventions (Swarbrick 2010a). Occupational therapists may develop, implement, and oversee wellness programs (AOTA 2007; Swarbrick 2010b), whereas physical therapists may design and implement interventions such as "aerobic and strength exercises, relaxation training, and basic body awareness" (Vancampfort et al. 2012). Utilizing a multidisciplinary approach to well-being may "improve overall health, delay onset of chronic diseases, and enable personal success in family, community, and work" (Manderscheid et al. 2010, p. 4)

Health care professionals may advocate for implementation of health and wellness programs already established and available such as NAMI Hearts and Minds or the 10×10 Campaign. In addition, health care professionals, including national organizations, may partner and support federal and state legislation to improve mental health services.

Conclusion

Occupational therapists and physical therapists desiring to work in either the special education field or mental health field should be knowledgeable about both the unique policies and settings in each of these areas. As discussed in the section on special education, therapy services are provided to assist students in benefitting from their educational environment. In both of these systems, emphasis is placed on client-centered and family-centered practice as evidenced by the creation and implementation of goals and interventions. In contrast, policies and practice related to the special education field are driven by funding and regulations; however, in the mental health field, policies and practice are primarily influenced by consumers, family members, and health care practitioners. Therapists working in these fields will need to stay current on policies and practices in an ever-changing health care environment in order to provide the most effective services to clients and their families.

Acknowledgement: Special thanks to Yolanda Griffiths, OTD, OTR/L, FAOTA for assistance and editorial advice throughout the mental health section of this chapter.

Chapter Review Questions

1. Define the terms "special education," "early intervention," "related services," "IEP," and "IFSP."

2. What is the difference between early intervention and early intervening services? What IDEA supported programs exist to assist students struggling in the educational environment when they do not receive special education services?

3. What are the required elements and team members of an IEP that is based on IDEA 2004?

4. Describe some of the most common conditions addressed by occupational therapists and physical therapists in the school setting. How does age impact the classification of students in disability categories?

5. Describe the impact of one of the movements influencing mental health policy and practice.

6. Explain the different between a traditional and a community-based practice setting.

7. Compare the roles of occupational therapists and physical therapists in mental health practice.

8. Select and evaluate a SAMHSA identified evidence-based practice.

Discussion Questions

1. Reflecting on both of the systems presented in this chapter, what do you see to be commonalities, and what are some of the primary differences? How might this affect service delivery as a therapist working in either of these specialized systems?

2. What are your thoughts on providing only educationally related services in the school system when, as a therapist, you may see other skills that could be improved but are not impacting educational performance? What do you think you could you do in this situation to address the concerns?

3. Explain the importance of mental health parity in improving services for all persons affected by mental illnesses including the consumer, family members, and health care professionals. What roles have professional organizations taken in advocating for parity?

References

American Occupational Therapy Association (AOTA). 2006. Transforming caseload to workload in school-based and early intervention occupational therapy. Retrieved from http://www.aota.org/Consumers/Professionals/WhatIsOT /CY/Fact-Sheets/38519.aspx?FT=.pdf (accessed June 26, 2012).

_____. 2007. OT and Community Mental Health. Author. Retrieved from http://www.aota.org/Consumers/consumers /MentalHealth/Community/35166.aspx.

_____. 2010. Occupational therapy in school settings. Retrieved from http://www.aota.org/Consumers /Professionals/WhatIsOT/CY/Fact-Sheets/School.aspx (accessed June 14, 2012).

American Physical Therapy Association (APTA). 2009. Providing physical therapy in schools under IDEA 2004. Retrieved from http://www.pediatricapta.org/consumer -patient-information/pdfs/09%20IDEA%20Schools.pdf (accessed June 14, 2012).

_____. 2010. Early intervention physical therapy: IDEA Part C. Retrieved from http://www.pediatricapta.org/consumer -patient-information/pdfs/IDEA%20EI.pdf (accessed June 22, 2012).

American Psychological Association (APA). 2000. *Diagnostic and statistical manual of mental disorders*, 4th ed. Arlington VA: Author.

_____. 2012. Definition of a mental disorder: Proposed revision. Retrieved from http://www.dsm5.org/proposedrevision /Pages/proposedrevision.aspx?rid=465.

Asher, A. 2010. Collaboration in schools: Service providers pulling together as a team. *OT Practice* 15(14): 8–13.

Assertive Community Treatment Association (ACTA). 2007. ACT Model. Retrieved from http://www.actassociation.org /actModel/.

Association for Ambulatory Behavioral Healthcare (AABH). 2010, March. Fast facts on PHP. Retrieved from http://www .aabh.org/content/fast-facts-php.

Bazyk, S., and J. Case-Smith. 2010. School-based occupational therapy. In J. Case-Smith, and J.C. O'Brien, eds. *Occupational therapy for children*, 6th ed. (713–43). Maryland Heights MO: Mosby Elsevier.

Bennett, O., and D. Logsdon. 2010. Occupational engagement of adults with mental illness. In M. Kavanaugh Scheinholtz, M. ed., *Occupational therapy in mental health: Considerations for advanced practice* (81–95). Bethesda MD: AOTA Press.

Bonder, B. 2010. *Psychopathology and function*, 4th ed. Thorofare NJ: Slack Incorporated.

Brown, C. 2011. Introduction to the person. In C. Brown and V.C. Stoffel, eds., *Occupational therapy in mental health: A vision for participation* (73–82). Philadelphia: F.A. Davis Company.

Bruce, M.A., and B. Borg. 2002. *Psychosocial frames of reference: Core for occupation-based practice,* 3rd ed. Thorofare NJ: Slack Incorporated.

Center for Mental Health Services (CMHS). 2005. *National consensus statement on mental health recovery* (Publication No. SMA 05-4129). Washington DC: Government Printing Office.

_____. 2006. *Childrens' mental health facts: Helping children and youth with serious mental health needs: Systems of care* (Publication No. SMA-4125). Washington DC: Government Printing Office.

Centers for Medicare and Medicaid Services (CMS). 2011, June. Medicare Program: Conditions of Participation (CoPs) for community mental health centers. Retrieved from https://www.federalregister.gov /articles/2011/06/17/2011-14673/medicare-program -conditions-of-participation-cops-for-community-mental -health-centers#p-32.

_____. 2012, March. Community mental health centers. Retrieved from http://www.cms.gov/Medicare/Provider -Enrollment-and-Certification/CertificationandComplianc /CommunityHealthCenters.html.

Champagne, T., and K. Gray. 2011, May. Occupational therapy's role in mental health recovery. *Recovery to Practice Weekly Highlights.* Retrieved from http://www.dsonline.com/rtp /weekly.2011.05.19/WH.2011.05.19.html.

Commission on Accreditation of Rehabilitation Facilities (CARF) International. 2012. 2012 Behavioral health program descriptions. Retrieved from http://www.carf.org/ programdescriptions/bh/.

Cutler, D., J. Bevilacqua, and B. McFarland. 2003. Four decades of community mental health: A symphony in four movements. *Community Mental Health Journal* 39(5): 381–98.

Dallas, J. 2011. Community-based case management. In C. Brown, and V.C. Stoffel, eds., *Occupational therapy in mental health: A vision for participation* (571–81). Philadelphia: F.A. Davis Company.

Davies, P.L. 2012. Pediatric occupational therapy in the United States: Understanding laws, policies, and regulations for practice. In S.L. Lane and A.C. Bundy, eds., *Kids can be kids: A childhood occupations approach* (203–19). Philadelphia: F.A. Davis Company.

Dixon, L., and H. Goldman. 2004. Forty years of progress in community mental health practices: The role of evidence-based practices. *Adm Policy Ment Health* 31(5): 381–92.

Dole, R.L., K. Arvidson, E. Byrne, J. Robbins, and B. Schasberger. 2003. Consensus among experts in pediatric occupational and physical therapy on elements of Individualized Education Programs. *Pediatr Phys Ther* 15(3): 159–66.

Drake, R., A. Green, K. Mueser, and H. Goldman. 2003. The history of community mental health treatment and rehabilitation for persons with severe mental illness. *Community Mental Health Journal* 39(5): 427–40.

_____, and E. Latimer. 2012. Lessons learned in developing community mental health care in North America. *World Psychiatry* 11: 47–51.

Druss, B., and T. Bornemann. 2010. Improving health and health care for persons with serious mental illness: The window for US federal policy change. *JAMA* 303(19): 1972–73.

Effgen, S.K., L. Chiarello, and S. Milbourne. 2007. Updated competencies for physical therapists working in schools. *Pediatr Phys Ther* 19(4): 266–74.

Exley, S.M., C.A. Thompson, and C. Hays. 2011. State hospitals. In C. Brown and V.C. Stoffel, eds., *Occupational therapy in mental health: A Vision for participation* (546–58). Philadelphia: F.A. Davis Company.

Fisher, W., J. Geller, and J. Pandiani. 2009. The changing role of the state psychiatric hospital. *Health Affairs* 28(3): 676–84. doi:10.1377/hlthaff.28.3.676.

Goldman, H., and G. Grob. 2006. Defining mental illness in mental health policy. *Health Affairs,* 25(3): 737–49. doi:10.1377/hlthaff.25.3.737.

Griswold, L., M. Evenson, and P. Roberts. 2011. Appendix C: Community-based settings for adults. In E. Crepeau, E. Cohn, and B. Boyt Schell, eds., *Willard and Spackman's occupational therapy,* 11th ed. (1084–87). Philadelphia: Wolters Kluwer-Lippincott Williams & Wilkins.

Hanft, B.E., and P.A. Place. 1996. *The consulting therapist: A guide for OT's and PT's in schools.* San Antonio, TX: Therapy Skill Builders.

_____, and J. Shepherd. 2008. *Collaborating for student success: A guide for school-based occupational therapy.* Bethesda, MD: AOTA Inc.

Hinder, E.A., and J. Ashburner. 2010. Occupation-centered intervention in the school setting. In S. Roger, ed., *Occupation-centered practice with children: A practical guide for occupational therapists.* Malden MA: Wiley-Blackwell.

Hopkins, J., S. Loeb, and D. Fick. 2009. Beyond satisfaction, what service users expect of inpatient mental health care: A literature review. *Journal of Psychiatr Ment Health Nurs* 16: 927–37. doi:10.1111/j.1365-2850.2009.01501.x.

Individuals with Disabilities Education Improvement Act of 2004. P.L. No. 108–446. Retrieved from: http://frwebgate .access.gpo.gov/cgi-bin/getdoc.cgi?dbname=108_cong_public _laws&docid=f:publ446.108.pdf (accessed June 14, 2012).

Insel, T. 2009. Translating scientific opportunity into public health impact: A strategic plan for research on mental illness. *Arch Gen Psychiatry* 66(2): 128–33.

International Center for Clubhouse Development (ICCD). 2009. What is a clubhouse? Retrieved from http://www.iccd.org /whatis.html.

Jackson, L. 2007. *Occupational therapy services for children and youth under IDEA,* 3rd ed. Bethesda MD: AOTA Inc.

Kavanaugh Scheinholtz, M. 2010. Foundation for advanced occupational therapy practice in mental health. In M. Kavanaugh Scheinholtz, ed., *Occupational therapy in mental health: Considerations for advanced practice* (3–13). Bethesda MD: AOTA Press.

Kessler, R., W. Chiu, O. Demler, and E. Walters. 2005. Prevalence, severity, and comorbidity of 12-month DSM-IV disorders in the national comorbidity survey replication. *Arch Gen Psychiatry* 62(6): 617–27.

Lawrence, D., and S. Kisely. 2010. Inequalities in healthcare provision for people with severe mental illness. *Psychopharmacol* 24(11): 61–68.

Lutterman, T., A. Berhane, B. Phelan, R. Shaw, and V. Rana. 2009. Funding and characteristics of state mental health agencies, 2007. (HHS Publication. No. SMA 09-4424). Rockville MD: Center for Mental Health Services, Substance Abuse, and Mental Health Services Administration.

Manderscheid, R., C. Ryff, E. Freeman, L. McKnight-Eily, S. Dhringra, and T. Strine. 2010. Evolving definitions of mental illness and wellness [Special topic]. *Prev Chronic Dis* 7(1): 1–6.

McEwen, I.R. 2009. *Providing physical therapy services: Under Parts B & C of the Individuals with Disabilities Education Act (IDEA).* Alexandria VA: Section on Pediatrics, American Physical Therapy Association.

Merryman, M. 2010. Mental health policy and regulation. In M. Kavanaugh Scheinholtz, ed., *Occupational therapy in mental health: Considerations for advanced practice* (267–92). Bethesda MD: AOTA Press.

Myers, C.T., L. Stephens, and S. Tauber. 2010. Early intervention. In J. Case-Smith and J.C. O'Brien, eds., *Occupational therapy for children,* 6th ed. (681–711). Maryland Heights MO: Mosby Elsevier.

National Alliance on Mental Illness (NAMI). 2009, June. NAMI fact sheet: Federal parity for mental illness and addictions. Retrieved from http://www.nami.org

/Template.cfm?Section=Issue_Spotlights&template=
/ContentManagement/ContentDisplay.
cfm&ContentID=94885.

National Dissemination Center for Children with Disabilities
(NICHY). 2010. Special education services for preschoolers
with disabilities. Retrieved from http://nichcy.org/schoolage
/preschoolers (accessed June 22, 2012).

National Institute of Health. 1998. NIH Almanac 1998.
National Institutes of Health Office of the Director. (NIH
Publication No. 98-5).

New Freedom Commission on Mental Health (NFCMH). 2003.
*Achieving the promise: Transforming mental health care
in America final report* (DHHS Publication No. SMA-03-
3832). Rockville, MD.

Pape, L., and K. Ryba. 2004. *Practical considerations for school-
based occupational therapists.* Bethesda, MD: AOTA Inc.

Peters, C. 2011. History of mental health: Perspectives of
consumers and practitioners. In C. Brown, and V.C.
Stoffel, eds., *Occupational therapy in mental health:
A vision for participation* (17–30). Philadelphia: F.A.
Davis Company.

Pope, E. 2011. Impact of federal policy on services for children
and families in early intervention programs and public
schools. In W. Dunn, ed., *Best practice occupational therapy:
For children and families in community settings,* 2nd ed.
(15–23). Thorofare, NJ: Slack Incorporated.

Rapport, M.J., and S.K. Effgen. 2004. Personnel issues in school-
based physical therapy: A look at supply and demand,
professional preparation, licensure, and certification.
Journal of Special Education Leadership 17(1): 7–15.

Roberts, P., and M. Evenson. 2009. Appendix A: Settings
providing medical and psychiatric services. In E. Crepeau,
E. Cohn, and B. Boyt Schell, eds., *Willard and Spackman's
occupational therapy,* 11th ed. (1074–79). Philadelphia:
Wolters Kluwer-Lippincott Williams & Wilkins.

Scott, J., and L. Mahaffey. 2010. Occupational engagement
of older adults with mental illnesses. In M. Kavanaugh
Scheinholtz, ed., *Occupational therapy in mental health:
Considerations for advanced practice* (97–113). Bethesda,
MD: AOTA Press.

Stoffel, V. 2011. Psychosocial clubhouses. In C. Brown and
V.C. Stoffel, eds., *Occupational therapy in mental health:
A vision for participation* (559–70). Philadelphia:
F.A. Davis Company.

Substance Abuse and Mental Health Services Administration
(SAMHSA). 2012, April. About the Agency (SAMHSA).
Retrieved from http://www.samhsa.gov/about/.

Swarbrick, M. 2010a. Lived experiences: Recovery and wellness
concepts for systems transformation. In M. Kavanaugh
Scheinholtz, ed., *Occupational therapy in mental health:
considerations for advanced practice* (233–48). Bethesda,
MD: AOTA Press.

_____. 2010b. Occupation-focused community health and
wellness programs. In M. Kavanaugh Scheinholtz, ed.,
*Occupational therapy in mental health: Considerations for
advanced practice* (27–43). Bethesda, MD: AOTA Press.

_____. 2011. Consumer-operated services. In C. Brown and
V.C. Stoffel, eds., *Occupational therapy in mental health:
A vision for participation* (503–15). Philadelphia:
F.A. Davis Company.

U.S. Department of Education. 2010. Office of Special
Education Programs, Data Analysis System (DANS),OMB
#1820-0043: "Children with disabilities receiving special
education under Part B of the Individuals with Disabilities
Education Act." Data updated as of July 15, 2011. Retrieved
from www.ideadata.org (accessed June 14, 2012).

U.S. Department of Health and Human Services. 2000.
Administration for Children & Families. Administration on
Intellectual and Developmental Disabilities. *The Olmstead
decision: Fact sheet.* Retrieved from http://archive.acf.hhs
.gov/programs/add/otherpublications/olmstead.html

_____. 2006. Substance Abuse and Mental Health Services
Administration, Center for Mental Health Services
(CMHS). *Children's mental health facts: Helping children
and youth with serious mental health needs: Systems of care*
(SAMHSA Publication No. SMA-4125/2006).

_____. 2008. Substance Abuse and Mental Health Services
Administration (SAMHSA). *Evidence-based practices KIT:
Assertive Community Treatment (ACT)* (HHS Publication
NO. SMA08-4345).

_____. 2009a. Substance Abuse and Mental Health Services
Administration, Center for Mental Health Services (CMS).
Evidence-based practices KIT: Supported Employment
(DHHS Publication No. SMA-08-4365).

_____. 2009b. Substance Abuse and Mental Health Services
Administration, Center for Mental Health Services (CMS).
*Illness management and recovery: Practitioner guides and
handouts* (HHS Publication No. SMA-09-4462).

_____. 2011. Substance Abuse and Mental Health Services
Administration (SAMHSA). *Evidence-based practices
KIT: Consumer operated services* (HHS Publication No.
SMA-11-4633).

_____. 2012. Centers for Medicare & Medicaid Services
(CMS) *Mental health services* (CMMS Publication No.
ICN 903195).

Vancampfort, D., M. Probst, L. Skjaerven, D. Catalan-
Matamoros, A. Gyllensten, A. Gomez-Conesa,…, and M.
De Hert. 2012. Systematic review of the benefits of physical
therapy within a multidisciplinary care approach for people
with schizophrenia. *Phys Ther* 92(1), 11–23. doi:10.2522/
ptj.20110218.

World Health Organization (WHO). 2010. *Mental health:
Strengthening our response.* Fact Sheet No. 220.
Retrieved from http://www.who.int/mediacentre/factsheets
/fs220/en/.

Web-Based Resources—Special Education

Updated statistics on the state of special education services and children being served through IDEA can be found by utilizing the IDEA Data Accountability Center, www.ideadata.org.

AOTA Children and Youth Section, http://www.aota.org /Consumers/consumers/Youth.aspx

Useful link for PT references, http://www.pediatricapta.org/pdfs /References%20for%20SB%20SIG1_23.pdf.

National Center on Educational Outcomes, http://www.cehd .umn.edu/nceo.

National Dissemination Center for Children with Disabilities, http://nichcy.org/.

Web-Based Resources—Mental Health

Center for Mental Health Services (CMHS), www.samhsa.gov/about/cmhs.aspx.

National Institute of Mental Health (NIMH), www.nimh.nih.gov.

Substance Abuse and Mental Health Services Administration (SAMHSA), www.samhsa.gov.

Program-Related Resources

Assertive Community Treatment Association (ACTA), www.actassociation.org.

Commission on Accreditation of Rehabilitation Facilities (CARF), www.carf.org.

Depression and Bipolar Support Alliance (DBSA), www.dbsalliance.org.

International Center for Clubhouse Development (ICCD), www.iccd.org.

Mental Health America (MHA), www.mentalhealthamerica.net.

National Alliance on Mental Illness (NAMI), www.nami.org.

National Federation of Families for Children's Mental Health (NFFCMH), www.ffcmh.org.

Schizophrenia and Related Disorders Alliance of America (SARDAA), www.sardaa.org

Recovery-Related Resources

Copeland Center for Wellness and Recovery, www.copelandcenter.com.

National Empowerment Center, www.power2u.org.

Parity-Related Resources

Wellstone Action, www.wellstone.org.

National Organizations

American Psychiatric Association (APA), www.psychiatry.org.

United States Psychiatric Rehabilitation Association (USPRA), www.uspra.org.

13

Global and Population Health

CHAPTER OBJECTIVES

At the conclusion of this chapter, the reader will be able to:

1. Identify the common problems across diverse health systems.
2. Discuss the key features of health care systems in other countries.
3. Examine the U.S. health care system from a comparative perspective.
4. Define and discuss the importance of population health.
5. Discuss the role of public health.

KEY WORDS

Core Functions
Determinants
Epidemiologist
Population Health
Public Health

CASE EXAMPLE ··

Rory and Jim are therapist-owners of a private therapy practice with a large patient base originating in workers' compensation claims from a local manufacturing facility. Over time, they have noted a significant number of patient cases related to rotator cuff injuries from this facility in their practice. They have learned that most of these injuries occur with overhead activities in one section of the plant. Rory and Jim decided to take their data about the number, type, and probable cause of the claims to the facility manager to discuss possible methods to reduce workplace injury. After their presentation, the manager agrees to contract with Rory and Jim for a worksite analysis of the ergonomics of the workplace where a majority of the injuries are occurring and to provide education about proper ergonomics to the employees. As a result, Rory and Jim are moving the walls of their practice into the community.

Case Example Question:

1. Discuss how the focus of Rory and Jim's practice changes when they consider the needs of their patient population.

Introduction

In this book, we have introduced and discussed the U.S. health care system as it affects the practice of occupational and physical therapists. In this final chapter, we compare the U.S. system to those of other industrialized nations. Many of the challenges faced by the United States also exist in other countries. However, the way in which other countries approach those challenges are much different than in the United States. Every country has some form of health care system that consists of organizations, individuals, and other resources whose primary mission is to attend to and improve the health of those living within their country. Strengthening and improving one's health care system is a perennial topic for most countries. This chapter explores the health care system in various other countries. Exploring other health care systems helps us to inform policy here in the United States. Since many of the health care issues across nations are common, studying and learning from other health care systems is not just an academic exercise, but may be very fruitful. This chapter will focus on the health systems of various countries and specifically examine the structures and processes they use to manage and deliver health care services to their populations.

A second purpose of this chapter is to introduce and explore **population health**. Increasingly, more information is available about the health status of groups of people or whole nations. This information can be used to develop and evaluate health policy. Many improvements in the health status of populations can be explained by **public health** interventions. Therapists need to be aware of the role of public health in improving the health of their communities. Some of the largest threats to population health are best addressed by public health. The case example at the start of this chapter presents an application of public health principles by therapists. Therapists need to consider their role in advocating for healthy lifestyles and behaviors that are a part of public health. Let's begin by examining how health care is delivered in five other large industrialized democracies. Table 13-1 provides an overview of how health care is financed in these countries.

An Overview of Five Countries' Health Care Systems

Canada

Canada has a publicly funded single-payer system that was legislated by the Canadian government in 1966 and became fully operational in 1971 (Taylor 1990). Through this system, Canada provides universal access to health care services for its citizens. To achieve

Table 13-1 **An Overview of Public and Private Health Care Financing in Five Industrialized Nations**

	Government Role	Public Financing	Private Insurance
Canada	Regionally administered universal insurance.	Provincial/federal income tax.	Approximately 67% buy coverage for extra benefits.
France	Statutory health insurance system.	Employer/employee payroll tax and general tax revenue.	90% buy coverage to pay for cost sharing and some extra benefits.
Germany	Statutory health insurance system. High income can opt out for private insurance.	Employer/employee payroll tax and general tax revenue.	Approximately 20% buy private insurance to cover cost sharing and amenities; 10% opt out of the SHI system for private insurance only.
United Kingdom	National health insurance.	General tax revenue.	About 10% buy private insurance for private facilities.
United States	Medicare, Medicaid.	Medicare is funded by federal tax, payroll tax, and premiums. Medicaid is funded by federal and state tax revenue.	Private insurance through employers or individuals covers more than half of the population.

Source: International Profile of Health Systems, 2011, Commonwealth Fund pub. no. 1562

universal health care and pay for the services provided by physicians and hospitals, the federal and provincial governments set physician fees and hospital budgets (O'Neill and O'Neill 2007). Under the Canadian health care system, citizens receive preventive care services and medical treatments from primary care physicians as well as access to hospitals (http://www.canadian-healthcare.org/).

The Canadian Health Act sets the policy by which Canadian provinces may receive funding for health care services. The act states that five principles must be followed: 1) the administration of the provincial insurance must be carried out by an accountable public authority; 2) all necessary services, including physician and hospital services, must be insured; 3) all insured residents must be able to receive the same level of care; 4) the residents who move to different provinces must retain their home province insurance for a minimum grace period; and 5) there must be reasonable access to health care services (Allin, Watson, and The Commonwealth Fund 2011). The funding for this universal coverage comes from both the federal and provincial level via taxing both personal and corporate income. Additional funds are secured through sales and lottery proceeds as well. As seen in Table 13-3, Canadians spend just over $4,000 per capita on health expenditures, accounting for approximately 10.9 percent of the GDP; in comparison, the United Sates spends over 16 percent of its GDP on health care, or $7,410 per capita.

As in the United States, health care in Canada is a major part of politics. One of the issues is the federal involvement in health care when it is the provinces that are responsible for the actual administration and delivery of health care services. Similar debates occur in the United States in terms of what the federal government can mandate. Additionally, there are some who feel that health care providers are not adequately compensated, thus leading to a shortage of medical workers. Again, there are similarities to the United States. While compensation is relatively high, there are often strong debates about compensation levels being set too low for some services (Allin, Watson, and The Commonwealth Fund 2011).

United Kingdom

In 1948, the National Health Service (NHS) in the United Kingdom (UK) was established (Sidel and Sidel 1983). The NHS is a centralized, single-payer system that is funded by general revenues from national taxation and provides health care services to all residents of the UK. Services that are typically covered include preventive services, physician services, hospital care, prescription medication, and some long-term rehabilitation. Most of the funding comes from general taxation (75%) or a payroll tax on all employees (20%) (Harrison, Gregory, Mundle, and Boyle 2011). Insurance coverage is not tied to employment as in the United States, and the United Kingdom makes no distinction between social insurance and public assistance (Bodenheimer and Grumbach 2002). Patients in the NHS can purchase private insurance that allows them to "hop" over the lines to receive services faster and have a wider choice of specialists (Foubister et al. 2006).

The NHS employs general practitioners, nurses, ambulance staff, and other health care workers to provide covered services. Patients must see a general practitioner first and receive a referral before seeing a specialist. In addition to providers, the NHS unifies all of the hospitals (Bodenheimer and Grumbach 2002). This allows the NHS to control patient flow in the system. For example, patients see their general practitioner for common illness and only move to a regional hospital for illnesses that are more severe. Finally, for very complex cases, patients can be moved to a tertiary care center or national teaching hospital. The management of this patient flow and control of the governmental single-payer system are two of the factors that help the United Kingdom to control health care costs.

Germany

Germany became the first nation to enact compulsory health insurance with a groundbreaking law passed in 1883 that required employers and employees to pay into existing sickness funds designed to pay for the medical care of covered employees (Bodenheimer and Grumbach 2002). While initially the eligible population for this coverage was limited, the Statutory Health Insurance (SHI) now covers about 85 percent of the population, while around another 10 percent are covered through private health insurance. For those that earn less than approximately $6,000, coverage is through the SHI. People who earn more than the minimum can choose to either remain covered through the SHI or purchase private insurance. Those receiving SHI are covered for a wide range of services including preventive services, hospital care, mental health services, physician service, prescription drugs, rehabilitation, hospice care, and sick leave compensation (Busse and Blümel 2011).

The SHI has set up over 150 sickness funds that are autonomous, not-for-profit, nongovernmental entities regulated by law (Busse and Blümel 2011). Funds collect money from their members and their members' employers and may not exclude people due to illness or raise contribution amounts due to medical condition (Bodenheimer and Grumbach 2002). Funds are collected through compulsory contributions that are taxed as a percentage of gross wages. When fund members retire or lose their job, they retain membership in the fund. Sickness funds are required to continue to cover their members whether they change jobs or stop working, regardless of the reason (Bodenheimer and Grumbach 2002).

As mentioned earlier, those that can afford to may purchase private health insurance. Private health insurance is still regulated by the government to ensure that those opting out of SHI do not experience large premium increases as they age or have overwhelming premiums if their income decreases (Busse and Blümel 2011). It has been reported in the past that private insurance pays physicians at a higher rate, thus allowing their policy holders to receive special treatment (Iglehart 1991).

Physicians are generally paid on a fee-for-service fee schedule from regional associations. Ambulatory care physicians are required to join a regional association, which then in turn negotiates with the sickness fund. The regional association receives a lump sum payment from the sick funds and pays physicians based on a structured fee schedule. Hospitals in Germany are paid by the sickness fund on a similar basis as DRG payments in the United States and include salary payment for physicians (Bodenheimer and Grumbach 2002).

France

The French employ a universal coverage system that covers all residents and is publically financed through Statutory Health Insurance (SHI). However, SHI does not cover 100 percent of expenditures, and most of the population has access to voluntary health insurance through their employers or vouchers (Durand-Zaleski and Chevreul 2011). Compared to Germany, the French system covers limited services, which include ambulatory care, hospital care, and prescription drugs. Some of SHI expenditure provides cash benefits for daily allowances for maternity, sickness, or occupational accident leave and disability.

The French system employs three forms of cost sharing that include co-insurance, co-payments, and extra billing (Durand-Zaleski and Chevreul 2011). Co-insurance can be fully reimbursed by the voluntary health insurance; however, that is not the case with co-payments. The amount of co-insurance and co-payment vary by type of service. Extra billing is the difference between the reference price set by the SHI and the physician charges for services. This extra billing has to be paid by the patient and may or may not be reimbursed by voluntary health insurance.

The majority of SHI is financed through employer and employee payroll taxes as well as a national income tax. These funds are managed by a board that has representatives from employers and employees. In recent years there have been strong financial incentives to encourage adults to have coordinated care through a voluntary gatekeeping system, and more than 85 percent of the population has registered with a primary care physician (Durand-Zaleski and Chevreul 2011).

United States

The United States has a fragmented health care system funded by a mix of private and public sources. The system is characterized by large numbers of uninsured and many that are underinsured. The Affordable Care Act is expected to decrease the number of uninsured over the years. Covered benefits vary by the type of insurance and typically will include physician and hospital services, preventive services, physiotherapy, mental health care, and prescription drug coverage.

The private insurance market is financed by individuals or tax-free premium contributions shared by employers. Medicare, which is a federal government-run insurance program for the elderly and disabled who are under 65, is financed by payroll taxes, premiums, and general revenues. Medicaid, which covers the poor, is administered by states that operate within federal guidelines and is financed through tax revenue.

Comparing Performance of Health Care Systems

A compelling rationale for comparing health systems is to evaluate the value and performance of the system for the amount of time, resources, and money spent on health care. Important issues to consider when evaluating health care systems include access to care, level of health care expenditures, the satisfaction of patients with health care services, and the overall quality of care that is provided. Evaluating and comparing across systems can offer opportunities to learn from others.

Using patient and provider self-reported experiences, the Commonwealth Fund was able to examine performance on various dimensions (Davis, Schoen, and Stremikis 2010). The report found that the United States, despite having one of the most expensive system (see Table 13-2), is not at the top of most dimensions of performance. In fact, the report concludes that the U.S. health care system is last or next to last in five dimensions of health care performance, including access, quality, efficiency, equity, and healthy lives. A couple of highlights from the report are discussed below.

Access and Level of Expenditures

As discussed in Chapter 2, access to care encompasses many dimensions. However, the lack of universal health coverage in the United States directly impacts access to health care services and results in people going without needed care. The United States, for the most part, is fundamentally funded by private insurance through a market approach. Countries such as Canada and the United Kingdom have national health insurance systems. This is one of the major differences between the United States and other countries and may be one of the major reasons that the United States continues to realize problems related to the cost and access of health care services. In the Commonwealth Fund report, 54 percent of

Table 13-2 Selected Safety and Access Performance Indicators

		Canada	France	Germany	United Kingdom	United States
Access	Able to Get Same/Next Day Appointment When Sick	45%	62%	66%	70%	57%
	Waited Two Months or More for Specialist Appointment	41%	28%	7%	19%	9%
	Experienced Access Barrier Due to Cost in Past	15%	13%	25%	5%	33%
Safety	Experienced Medical, Medication, or Lab Test Error in Past 2 Years	17%	14%	10%	8%	18%
	Experienced Coordination Problems with Medical Tests/ Records in Past 2 Years	25%	22%	26%	20%	34%
	Specialist Did Not Have Information about Medical History During Appointment	16%	28%	32%	14%	22%
	Physicians' Use of EMRs (% of Primary Care Physicians)	37%	68%	72%	96%	45%
Satisfaction	Works Well, Minor Changes Needed	38%	42%	38%	62%	29%
	Fundamental Changes Needed	51%	47%	48%	34%	41%
	Needs to Be Completely Rebuilt	20%	11%	14%	3%	27%

Source: International Profile of Health Systems, 2011, Commonwealth Fund pub. no. 1562

U.S. citizens say they experience access problems (Davis, Schoen, and Stremikis 2010). Of those in the United States who experience health problems, 41 percent have out-of-pocket costs that are greater than $1,000 as compared to only 4 percent in United Kingdom.

Though patients in the United States have significant financial barriers that may keep them from care, if they are insured, they have relatively timely access to specialized health care services (see Table 13-2). This is in contrast to patients in United Kingdom, who may have short waiting periods for basic health care, but face much longer wait times for specialist care and elective surgery. Canada also ranks low in terms of wait times. Universal insurance is often associated with longer waits; however, that is not always true. For example, patients in Germany experience a comparable wait time to patients in the United States with regard to getting an appointment with a specialist.

Quality

The quality dimension consists of four categories: 1) effective care, 2) safe care, 3) coordinated care, and 4) patient-centered care. The United States had positive findings relating to providing preventive and patient-centered care. For example, U.S. respondents indicated they were more likely than their counterparts in other countries to receive preventive care services such as reminders and advice on diet and exercise from their physicians. However, the converse was true for the areas of safe and coordinated care (see Table 13-2) where the United States received low scores (Davis, Schoen, and Stremikis 2010).

Efficiency

The Commission on a High Performance Health System in their first National Scorecard report, defined efficiency as a health care system that maximizes the quality of care and outcomes given the committed resources as well as ensuring that additional investments yield a net value (The Commonwealth Fund 2006). The Commonwealth Report found that the United States was last overall on indicators of efficiency, including measures of timely access to records and test results, duplicative tests, rehospitalization, and physicians' use of health information technologies (see Table 13-2) (Davis, Schoen, and Stremikis 2010).

Satisfaction

There are many dimensions of satisfaction to consider when comparing health systems across countries. Complicating this measure are cultural norms. That is, what might be satisfactory to one person may not be so satisfactory for another. For example, waiting for services in one culture may be acceptable while in another culture it may be a sign of a poor system. Nonetheless, the data in Table 13-2 above show the relative satisfaction levels of people with their country's health care system. Respondents in the United States were less likely to respond that the health system works well. Only 29 percent agreed with this statement while the next-lowest countries were Canada and Germany (38%). Additionally, 27 percent of the U.S. participants in the survey thought the health care system needed to be completely rebuilt as compared to 14 percent of those in Germany, the country with the next-highest response. The data indicate satisfaction in the United States with the health care system is much lower than in other countries.

Examining responses across countries indicates that there is need for improvement across the board. However, many countries are spending a lot less on health care per capita as compared to the United States. Thus, for the huge investment that is made in health care, the United States should do much better at bringing value to the health system (see Table 13-3). There continues to be ongoing debate on health care legislation and policy in this country. Most recently, President Obama singed the Patient Protection and Affordable Care Act, which was then subsequently upheld by the Supreme Court. This act is intended to help expand the use of health information technology and encourage more efficient use of resources as well as increase access to health care services for many of the currently uninsured. While this legislation and policy will certainly not be the last and final word, and may or may not accomplish its goal, it is clear that the United States needs to continually seek ways that will allow the country to maximize its health care investment for the betterment of its population.

Table 13-3 Selected Health System Indicators

	Canada	France	Germany	United Kingdom	United States
Population*	33,573,000	62,343,000	82,167,000	61,565,000	314,659,000
Male life expectancy*	79	74	78	78	76
Female life expectancy*	83	85	83	82	81
Under 5 mortality per 1,000 live births*	6	4	4	5	8
Total health expenditure per capita[†]	$4,363	$3,978	$4,218	$3,487	$7,960
Total expenditure on health as a % of GDP[+]	11.4%	11.8%	11.6%	9.8%	17.4

Source: Data based on World Health Organizations: http://www.who.int/countries/en/

Table 13-4 Twentieth-Century Achievements in Public Health

1. Vaccination
2. Motor vehicle safety
3. Safer workplaces
4. Control of infectious diseases
5. Decline in deaths from coronary heart disease and stroke
6. Safer and healthier foods
7. Healthier mothers and babies
8. Family planning
9. Fluoridation of drinking water
10. Recognition of tobacco as a health hazard

Source: Centers for Disease Control. 1999. Ten great public health achievements. United States, 1990-1999. http://www.cdc.gov/oc/media/tengpha.htm (accessed July 2, 2007)

A Public Health and Population Health Perspective

In addition to stepping back and looking at health care from a global perspective, it is also beneficial to take a public health view of health. Just as examining health care from a global perspective broadens our view of health care so does the public health perspective. The public health perspective moves us from just viewing individuals to examining populations. While public health focuses on populations, its impact on individuals is significant, and many of the major achievements that have improved individual health can be traced to public health practices (see Table13-4). Moreover, researchers have calculated that of the 30-year increase in age longevity during the 20th century, 25 of those years were attributed to improved public health practices (Bunker, Frazier, and Mosteller 1994).

By moving beyond just focusing on individuals, public health is able to identify illnesses, injuries, and diseases in the population and begin to develop ways to reduce the resulting mortality, morbidity, and disability that result from these conditions. This is accomplished by establishing a system of surveillance across the population. Table 13-5 outlines some of the key goals of this population surveillance, which is a key component of public health.

Public health shifts our thinking and redefines health such that we begin to recognize health as a product of the contribution of many different factors that include social, economic, and environmental factors. These factors that influence health status are often referred to as the **determinants** of health. Broadly speaking, these determinants can fall into many categories including policy making, health services, and individual behaviors. As this text has addressed throughout, policies either at the local, state, or federal level impact both the health of individuals and of populations. We have also discussed how access to health services and the quality of those services affect health. Individual behavior also plays a role, and many of the public health strategies are attempts to change individual behaviors with the goal of improving the population's health. Approaching health

Table 13-5 The Goals of Public Health

1. Prevent and mitigate epidemics and the spread of disease
2. Protect against environmental hazards
3. Prevent injuries
4. Promote and encourage healthy behaviors
5. Respond to disasters and help communities recover
6. Assure individuals of their quality of life and of the accessibility of health

Source: Public Health in America. 1994. www.health.gov/phfunctions/public.htm (accessed June 12, 2000)

Table 13-6 Core Functions of the World Health Organization (2006–2015)

1. Provide leadership on matters critical to health and engage in partnerships where joint action is needed
2. Shape the research agenda and stimulate the generation, translation, and dissemination of valuable knowledge
3. Set norms and standards as well as promote and monitor their implementation
4. Articulate ethical and evidence-based policy options
5. Provide technical support, catalyze change, and build sustainable institutional capacity
6. Monitor the health situation and assess health trends

Source: World health Organization.

from this perspective has the potential to save significant money as well as years of life. For example, Mokdad and colleagues reported in 2004 that 40 percent of the mortality in the United States was a result of preventable causes such as poor diet, lack of activity, misuse of alcohol, and tobacco smoking (Mokdad, Marks, Stroup, and Gerberding 2004). Additionally, taking preventive measures such as smoking cessation counseling, colorectal cancer screening, and influenza vaccination can reduce mortality (Maciosek, Coffield, Edwards et al. 2006). Population health often focuses on prevention, which is a key source of cost savings.

One example of an organization focusing on population health is the World Health Organization (WHO). The WHO was created in 1948 as what is essentially the public health branch of the United Nations (WHO 2007). Table 13-6 lists the **core functions** of WHO, which include the surveillance of disease, development of policy, and implementation of basic health procedures for people around the world. Major accomplishments of the WHO include the eradication of smallpox and the near-eradication of poliomyelitis and leprosy through extensive immunization programs.

WHO and other public health organizations interested in population health use the science of epidemiology as the foundation to identify the multiple factors and determinants of health. The purpose of epidemiology is to identify the threats to a population and devise a control strategy to reduce them with the goal of improving the population's health. This is accomplished through routine surveillance that allows the **epidemiologist** to collect vital data, analyze the environment, investigate disease outbreaks, and determine the incidence of disablement. The purpose of this routine surveillance is to identify the cause of the problem. For example, this surveillance has been used to identify the cause of communicable diseases and subsequent strategies to treat or prevent the disease.

The analysis and interpretation of the data collected through routine surveillance is also used in the development of policies that are intended to impact the health of populations. Identifying public health problems and subsequent strategies to control them leads to setting public health policies and objectives. In the United States, the Healthy People Initiative is one example of using and analyzing data of different health care trends and then developing goals and objectives to improve population health. The Leading Health Indicators are listed in Table 13-7 with the overall goal to increase quality and eliminate health disparities.

The Importance of Population Health in Improving Health

Population health examines the distribution of health outcomes in a population along with the determinants, such as the impact of relevant policies and interventions that influence that distribution (Kindig 2007; Kindig and Stoddart 2003). The goal of population health is to preserve health and minimize the impact of morbidity both from a physical and financial perspective. To accomplish this goal, the focus is on improving health through prevention and lifestyle changes, reducing errors and waste, closing disparity gaps, and improving accountability and coordination of care (Nash 2012). It is the interrelatedness

Table 13-7 Healthy People 2020 Leading Health Indicators by Topic

Access to Health Services
- Persons with medical insurance
- Persons with a usual primary care provider

Clinical Preventive Services
- Adults who receive a colorectal cancer screening based on the most recent guidelines
- Adults with hypertension whose blood pressure is under control
- Adult diabetic population with an A1c value greater than 9%
- Children aged 19 to 35 months who receive the recommended doses of DTaP, polio, MMR, Hib, hepatitis B, varicella, and PCV vaccines

Environmental Quality
- Air Quality Index (AQI) exceeding 100
- Children aged 3 to 11 years exposed to secondhand smoke

Injury and Violence
- Fatal injuries
- Homicides

Maternal, Infant, and Child Health
- Infant deaths
- Preterm births

Mental Health
- Suicides
- Adolescents who experience major depressive episodes (MDEs)

Nutrition, Physical Activity, and Obesity
- Adults who meet current federal physical activity guidelines for aerobic physical activity and muscle-strengthening activity
- Adults who are obese
- Children and adolescents who are considered obese
- Total vegetable intake for persons aged 2 years and older

Oral Health
- Persons aged 2 years and older who used the oral health care system in past 12 months

Reproductive and Sexual Health
- Sexually active females aged 15 to 44 years who received reproductive health services in the past 12 months
- Persons living with HIV who know their serostatus

Social Determinants
- Students who graduate with a regular diploma 4 years after starting 9th grade

Substance Abuse
- Adolescents using alcohol or any illicit drugs during the past 30 days
- Adults engaging in binge drinking during the past 30 days

Tobacco
- Adults who are current cigarette smokers
- Adolescents who smoked cigarettes in the past 30 days

Source: HealthlyPeople.gov http://healthypeople.gov/2020/LHI/2020indicators.aspx (accessed Aug 2012).

of these concepts that influences the health of a population. Thus, population health is, or least should be, central to the success of any health care reform aimed at improving the American health care system.

Accountable Health Care Organizations (ACOs) represent one health care reform model that brings population health concepts to the forefront (see Chapter 9). Using measurable outcomes as criteria, ACOs bring providers together to be accountable for a defined population (McClellan et al. 2010). To be successful, these organizations should result in better communication and coordination across providers and care settings. Additionally, ACOs should employ standardized processes, measurements, and information to achieve their goals, all of which address the goal and focus of population health discussed above.

In addition to providing better personal care through ACOs or other health care delivery models, population health seeks to understand and address the reasons behind the incidences of morbidity in a population. Identifying and addressing these underlying reasons, helps care givers improve the population's health. Bringing together community stakeholders with a common goal can also have a significant impact on health, especially in terms of preventions associated with lifestyle changes such as tobacco cessation or other wellness programs (Zell 2012). As population approaches are employed, communities can be transformed to create the favorable cultural, social, economic, and environmental conditions that will better enable Americans to live healthier lives. The role of physical therapists and occupational therapists working with patients or clients in ACOs, hospitals, or private clinics is an excellent opportunity to improve the public health by addressing one or more Healthy People 2020 Leading Indicators.

Conclusion

This chapter has challenged us to take a global perspective on health in the United States. This includes moving beyond individuals and examining population health. As noted in the Healthy People 2020 Leading Health Indicators, movement, fitness, and physical activity–related public health issue is a top concern. This is an example of an area where therapists can influence population health by addressing and advocating health promotion topics aimed at achieving the goals set in Healthy People 2020.

Chapter Review Questions

1. Define population health and public health.

2. Summarize the role of government, public financing, and private financing in the health systems of the five countries discussed in this chapter.

3. Identify the key indicators of health system performance discussed in this chapter.

4. Relate the goals and core functions of public health organizations.

5. Identify the Healthy People 2020 leading indicators that can be addressed by physical and occupational therapists.

Chapter Discussion Questions

1. What are the strengths and weaknesses of the U.S. health care system when compared to those of other industrialized nations? What effect do you think the Patient Protection and Affordable Care Act of 2010 will have on the key indicators of health system performance discussed in this chapter?

2. The majority of occupational and physical therapists work in the personal health care system with individuals or small groups of patients. How does working in this system impede or promote the goals or core functions of public health?

References

Allin, S., D. Watson, and The Commonwealth Fund. 2011. The Canadian health care system, 2011. In S. Thomson, R. Osborn, D. Squires, and S.J. Reed, eds., *International profiles of health care systems, 2011* (21–31). The Commonwealth Fund. Pub. No. 1562.

Bodenheimer, T.S., and K. Grumbach. 2002. *Understanding health policy: A clinical approach*, 3rd ed. New York: McGraw-Hill.

Bunker, J.P., H.S. Frazier, and F. Mosteller. 1994. Improving health: Measuring the effects of medical care. *Milbank Q* 72: 225–58.

Busse, R., and M. Blümel. 2011. The German health care system, 2011. In S. Thomson, R. Osborn, D. Squires, and S.J. Reed, eds., *International profiles of health care systems, 2011* (57–64). The Commonwealth Fund. Pub. No. 1562.

Centers for Disease Control. 1999. Ten great public health achievements. United States, 1990–1999. *MMWR* 48(12): 241–43.

The Commonwealth Fund. 2011. The U.S. health care system, 2011. In S. Thomson, R. Osborn, D. Squires, and S.J. Reed, eds., *International profiles of health care systems, 2011*. New York: The Commonwealth Fund. Pub. No. 1562.

The Commonwealth Fund Commission. 2006, September. On a high performance health system, why not the best? Results from a national scorecard on U.S. health system performance. New York: The Commonwealth Fund.

Davis, K., C. Schoen, and K. Stremikis. 2010. Mirror, mirror on the wall: How the performance of the U.S. health care system compares internationally, 2010 update. The Commonwealth Fund. Pub. No. 1400.

Davis, K., C. Schoen, S.C. Schoenbaum, M.M. Doty, A.L. Holmgren, J.L. Kriss, and K.K. Shea. 2007. *Mirror, mirror on the wall: An international update on the comparative performance of American health care*. Commonwealth Fund.

Durand-Zaleski, I., and K. Chevreul. 2011. The French health care system, 2011. In S. Thomson, R. Osborn, D. Squires, and S.J. Reed, eds., *International profiles of health care systems, 2011* (45–56). The Commonwealth Fund. Pub. No. 1562

Foubister, T., S. Thomson, E. Mossialos, and A. McGuire. 2006. *Private medical insurance in the United Kingdom*. Great Britain: The Cromwell Press.

Harrison, A., S. Gregory, C. Mundle, and S. Boyle. 2011. The English health care system, 2011. In S. Thomson, R. Osborn, D. Squires, and S.J. Reed, eds., *International profiles of health care systems, 2011*.The Commonwealth Fund. Pub. No. 1562.

HealthlyPeople.gov. n.d. http://healthypeople.gov/2020/LHI/2020indicators.aspx (accessed August 2012).

Iglehart, J.K. 1991. Germany's health care sytem. *New Engl J Med* 324: 503.

Kindig, D. 2007. Understanding population health terminology. *Milbank Q* 85(1): 139–61.

_____, and G. Stoddart. 2003. What is population health? *Am Pub Health* 93: 380–83 .

Maciosek, M.V., A.B. Coffield, N.M. Edwards, T.J. Flottemesch, M.J. Goodman, and L.I. Solberg. 2006. Priorities among effective clinical preventive services: Results of a systematic review and analysis. *Am J Prev Med* 31:52–61.

McClellan, M., A.N. McKethan, J.L. Lewis, J. Roski, and E.S. Fisher. 2010. A national strategy to put accountable care into practice. *Health Affairs* (*Millwood*) 29(5): 982–90.

Mokdad, A.H., J.S. Marks, D.F. Stroup, and J.L. Gerberding. 2004. Actual causes of death in the United States, 2000. *JAMA* 291:1238–45.

Nash, D.B. 2012, Spring. Population health and health reform: Inseparable concepts. *Prescriptions for Excellence in Health Care* 16: 1–2.

O'Neill, J.E., and D.M. O'Neill. 2007. Health status, health care, and inequality: Canada vs. the U.S. Cambridge MA: National Bureau of Economic Research (Working Paper 13429). Retrieved from http://www.nber.org/papers/w13429.

Public Health Functions Steering Committee. 1994. Public health in America, 1994. Retrieved from www.health.gov/phfunctions/public.htm (accessed July 12, 2000).

Sidel, V.W., and R. Sidel. 1983. *A healthy state*. New York: Pantheon Books.

Taylor, M.G. 1990. *Insuring national health care: The Canadian experience*. Chapel Hill: University of North Carolina Press.

World Health Organization. 2007. History of WHO. Retrieved from http://www.who.int/about/history/en/index.html (accessed June 13, 2007).

Zell, B.E. 2012, Spring. For health reform success, context matters. *Prescriptions for Excellence in Health Care* 15: 8–10.

Appendix A Resources on Policies Addressing Social Disablement

General Resources

A Guide to Disability Laws: http://www.ada.gov/cguide .htm#anchor62335.

American Occupational Therapy Association: http:// www.aota.org. Provides information about bills and advocacy resources.

American Physical Therapy Association: http://www.apta .org. Provides information about bills and advocacy resources.

National Disability Rehabilitation Center: http://naric .com. Contains resources about disability and rehabilitation.

Thomas.gov: http://thomas.loc.gov/home/thomas.php#. Library of Congress site for information on current and past legislation.

USA.gov: http://www.usa.gov/Topics/Reference_Shelf .shtml#Laws. Contains many resources about the federal government, including disability laws.

Americans with Disabilities Act (ADA)

ADA Accessibility Guidelines for Buildings and Facilities: http://www.access-board.gov/adaag/html/adaag.htm. "Contains very specific guidelines for "scoping and technical requirements for accessibility to buildings and facilities by individuals with disabilities under the Americans with Disabilities Act (ADA) of 1990."

ADA National Network: **ada**ta.org. "The ADA National Network provides information, guidance, and training on the Americans with Disabilities Act (ADA), tailored to meet the needs of business, government, and individuals at local, regional, and national levels."

U.S. Department of Justice: ADA Homepage: http://www.ada .gov. Contains many resources with the latest information about the ADA.

Assistive Technology Act (ATA)

Association of Assistive Technology Programs: http://www .ataporg.org. "Provides support to state AT Program members to enhance the effectiveness of AT Programs on the state and local level, and promote the national network of AT Programs."

Rehabilitation Engineering and Assistive Technology Society of America: http://www.resna.org. "RESNA is a professional society for individuals and organizations interested in technology and disability."

Developmental Disability Act (DDA)

The Arc: http://www.thearc.org. Resource for people with developmental and intellectual disabilities.

Association of University Centers on Disability: http://www.aucd.org/template/page.cfm?id=272. "A network of interdisciplinary centers advancing policy and practice for and with individuals with developmental and other disabilities, their families, and communities."

The National Disability Rights Network: http://www.napas.org. Provides information about Protection and Advocacy (P&A) and Client Assistance Programs (CAP).

Fair Housing Act (FHA)

U.S. Department of Housing and Urban Development: http://portal.hud.gov/hudportal/HUD?src=/program _offices/fair_;housing_;equal_;opp/FHLaws.

Individuals with Disabilities Education Improvement Act (IDEA)

U.S. Department of Education: http://idea.ed.gov.

Appendix B   Advocacy Resources

General Internet Sites Related to Health Care Public Policy

Duke University: Center for Health Policy and Inequalities Research: http://chpir.org. This site addresses research about health policy and health disparities.

FamiliesUSA: http://www.familiesusa.org. This national nonprofit organization advocates for "high-quality affordable health care for all Americans". It focuses on the following health care policies: Medicaid, managed care, Medicare, children's health, and the uninsured. The site contains links to information about advocacy.

Heritage Foundation: http://www.heritage.org. "The Heritage Foundation is a research and educational institution— a think tank—whose mission is to formulate and promote conservative public policies based on the principles of free enterprise, limited government, individual freedom, traditional American values, and a strong national defense."

Kaiser.edu: http://www.kaiseredu.org. This site has educational resources, including tutorials and presentations, issue modules, videos and research tools, about health care public policy.

Kaiser Family Foundation: http://www.kaisernetwork.org. This nonprofit foundation addresses health-related policies and trends through examining health policies, journalism, and communication. The site is a source for health policy information about current issues, and one can get on their e-mail list to receive health care policy updates.

Government Public Policy Resources and Bill Language

Congress Website: http://www.congress.org. Provides information about what is happening in Congress.

The Dirksen Congressional Center: http://www.congresslink .org. An educational site that provides information about Congress and public policies.

Federal Disability Laws: http://www.usa.gov/Topics/Reference _Shelf.shtml. This site contains the full text of the federal disability laws.

House Website: http://www.house.gov. This site contains resources pertaining to the U.S. Congress. For example, one can find out who is on committees and what the different committees address. Representatives specifically involved with health policy often have statements on their own sites.

Senate Website: http://www.senate.gov. This site contains many resources pertaining to the U.S. Senate. Senators specifically involved with health or disability public policy often have statements on their own sites.

Thomas: http://thomas.loc.gov. This site has all the current bills listed in abbreviated and completed forms. From this site, one can identify the status of different bills, such as where they are in the legislative process. Older bills from previous Congresses can be accessed. Site includes educational information, such as information about the legislative process.

Centers for Medicare and Medicaid: http://www.cms.gov. This is the site for the Centers for Medicare and Medicaid Services, the agency that governs Medicare, Medicaid, and child health insurance programs. There is a plethora of resources on the site about these government programs and how they are regulated. The most current guidelines for Medicare can be located in the web-based manuals.

Professional Organizations with Public Policy Resources

Agency for Health Care Policy and Research: http://www.ahrq .gov. Part of the Public Health Service in the U.S. Department of Health and Human Services, this agency supports efficacy and cost research. Specific information is provided for policymakers.

American Association of Retired Persons: www.aarp.org. This site has many resources for Americans age 50 and older and is strongly involved in policymaking.

American Chiropractic Association: http://www.acatoday.org.

American Health Care Association: http://www.ahca.org. This association addresses concerns of people in the long-term care community.

American Medical Association: www.ama-assn.org.

American Medical Student Association: http://www.amsa.org.

American Occupational Therapy Association: http://www.aota.org.

American Physical Therapy Association: http://www.apta.org.

American Psychological Association: http://www.apa.org.

American Public Health Association: http://www.apha.org .

Center for Medicare Advocacy: http://www.harp.org. This private nonprofit organization focuses on Medicare and issues for those with chronic conditions.

Joint Commission on Accreditation of Healthcare Organizations: http://www.jcaho.org. This agency evaluates and accredits health care organizations.

National Information Center for Children and Youth with Disabilities: http://www.nichcy.org.

National Rehabilitation Organization: http://nationalrehab.org.

National Senior Citizens' Law Center: www.nsclc.org. The center helps with advocacy for older adults with low incomes.

Quackwatch, Inc.: http://www.quackwatch.com. This site provides resources for dealing with medical quackery.

National Organizations for Disease and Disability Conditions

Most of these organizations have policy sections. Consider networking with them about mutual concerns.

Alzheimer's Disease

Alzheimer's Association: http://www.alz.org.

Arthritis

Arthritis Foundation: www.arthritis.org.

Autism

National Autism Association: http://www.nationalautismassociation.org.

Family Caregiver Alliance: http://www.caregiver.org.

Brain Injury Association: http://www.biausa.org.

Cerebral Palsy

United Cerebral Palsy: http://www.ucp.org.

Diabetes

American Diabetic Association: http://www.diabetes.org.

Emphysema

National Emphysema Foundation: http://www.emphysemafoundation.org.

Epilepsy

Epilepsy Foundation: http://www.efa.org.

Heart/Stroke

American Heart Association: http://www.americanheart.org.

American Stroke Association: http://www.strokeassociation.org.

Hospice

Hospice Foundation of America: http://www.hospicefoundation.org.

National Hospice and Palliative Care Organization: http://www.nho.org.

Mental Illness

National Alliance for the Mentally Ill: http://www.nami.org.

National Mental Health Association: http://www.nmha.org.

Muscular Dystrophy

Muscular Dystrophy Association: http://www.mdausa.org.

Multiple Sclerosis

Multiple Sclerosis: http://www.msfacts.org.

Osteoporosis

National Osteoporosis Foundation: http://www.nof.org.

Parkinson's Disease

American Parkinson Disease Association: http://apdaparkinson.org.

Spinal Cord

National Spinal Cord Injury Association: http://www.spinalcord.org.

Vision

Glaucoma Research Foundation: http://www.glaucoma.org.

Macular Degeneration International: http://www.maculardegeneration.org.

NEWS SITES

Congressional Quarterly: http://www.cq.com. This subscription site provides specific information about what is happening in Washington, DC, with bills.

C-span: http://c-span.org. This is an excellent resource for more current bills.

New York Times: http://www.nytimes.com. The *New York Times* provides information about political issues.

Washington Post: http://www.washpost.com. The *Washington Post* provides information about political issues.

Yahoo: http://www.Yahoo.com. The news section provides policy information, particularly about recent bills.

Glossary

Acceptability is a component of access related to the degree of congruence of cultural values between provider and patient.

Access The ability to obtain a health care service when you need it.

Accessibility is a component of access related to congruence of location and transportation resources of provider and patient.

Accommodation is the organization and appropriateness of health care services.

Accountable Care Organizations are integrated health systems established by the PPACA to contract with the Medicare program to provide services with an incentive for shared savings of any efficiencies.

Accreditation A voluntary quality-assurance and improvement process whereby an organization is rated against accepted standards of performance.

Actuarial Analysis The insurance process that predicts the risk of covered events in the risk pool and calculates a premium for pool members called actuarial adjustment.

Actuarial Value The percentage of average costs that a health insurance plan will cover.

Adverse Selection A form of moral hazard resulting in a high-risk, high-cost insurance pool.

Advocacy The process of identifying issues and participating in policymaking and policy change.

Affordability is the price of health care related to the population's ability to pay.

Aggregation The degree or extent of integration of financing and delivery of health care in a managed care plan.

Alternative Medicine A form of health care that has emerged in contrast to the bioscientific, allopathic model of care that dominates in the United States; examples of alternative medicine include naturopathy, homeopathy, and chiropractic.

American Health Benefit Exchanges State-based insurance marketplaces established by the PPACA to improve access to private health insurance.

Assignment of Benefits The process whereby a patient transfers insurance benefits directly to the provider from the insurer.

Assistive Technology Equipment, software, and devices that enable persons with disabling conditions to access and become more independent in their environments.

Barriers Physical, social, and attitudinal obstructions to full participation in society for persons with disabling conditions.

Benchmarking The measurement and comparison of performance over time or against a known standard.

Beneficiary The recipient of the benefits from an insurance contract.

Benefit Period The length of time from day of admission to the hospital to 60 days post-hospital or SNF discharge. Used in determining deductible and co-insurance payments for the Medicare program.

Biomedical Model A perspective on disablement that locates the problem in the person with the disabling condition and the solution in medical care services.

Bundled A term for the collation of fees for individual but related services into one new fee category.

Capitation Payment mechanism for health care whereby a provider is paid a flat fee for each covered member in a health plan per month.

Case Management The process of eligibility determination and coordination of services for a person receiving multiple health care services.

Case Mix Adjustment A system of classifying patients for payment purposes by clinical characteristics and anticipated resource utilization.

Case Rate A negotiated payment based on a visit, day, or episode of care.

Categorical Eligibility One of the methods to qualify for Medicaid; mandated in all states. Includes low-income women and children, wards of the state, and persons with disabilities (receiving SSI payments).

Certification Approval by a physician of a therapy plan of care for a Medicare beneficiary.

Children's Health Insurance Program Enacted by Congress in 1997, this state program expands insurance coverage to low-income, uninsured children.

Clinical Pathway A statement of the process of care based on the best available evidence of the effectiveness and efficiency of care.

Coalition A group of individuals or organizations that come together to participate in advocacy; a prerequisite for effective advocacy.

Co-Insurance A share of health care costs owed by the beneficiary in an insurance contract; typically expressed as a percentage of the approved cost.

Community Rating A process of actuarial adjustment that assigns a premium rate based on people living in a geographic region.

Complementary Medicine Alternative medicine procedures that are used as an adjunct or in addition to allopathic medical care.

Consolidated Billing The requirement for SNF to bill for all Medicare Part A services that prevents contractual providers (e.g., therapists) from independently billing for their care.

Consumer-Directed Health Care   A health insurance product that consists of a high deductible form of health insurance and a health savings account.

Conventional Medicine   Another term for the bioscientific, allopathic medical care model that is dominant in the United States.

Co-Payment   A flat fee owed for a service by a beneficiary covered by an insurance contract.

Core Functions   are defined roles and purposes for public health agencies in addressing population health concerns.

Cost-Based Reimbursement   A retrospective method of health care financing whereby a provider reports costs of providing care and is paid by an insurer.

Cost Containment   is a set of policies aimed to control the growth in health care expenditures.

Cost Limits   Payment mechanisms utilized in insurance contracts to share/limit costs of health care. Includes plan limit, first-dollar coverage, co-insurance, co-payment, and deductible.

Cost Shifting   Associated with underpayment of the true costs of caring for Medicare beneficiaries, which are then paid by private insurers who pay artificially high prices for care.

Coverage Determinations   A process used by insurance companies to analyze and decide whether or not to pay for a claim.

Credentialing   A process used by insurers and some health care organizations to ensure that providers achieve minimum standards of education and experience.

Custodial Care   A facility that provides long-term residential and skilled health care services.

D

Deductible   First-dollar expense owed by the beneficiary to pay for a health care cost prior to any payment by the insurer.

Defined Benefit Plan   The sponsor of the insurance plan predetermines the benefits for a health insurance plan. Typical of most forms of health insurance today.

Defined Contribution Plan   The sponsor of the insurance plan (e.g., business or government) predetermines the level of funding for a health insurance plan offered to eligible beneficiaries. Benefits are provided based on this funding and excess beneficiary contributions.

Determinants   are social, economic, and environmental factors that influence the health status of a population.

Direct Access   The ability of a patient to obtain physical therapy and occupational therapy services without requiring referral from another provider.

Disablement   A process whereby a person who experiences an illness or injury develops a set of impairments, activity limitations, and participation restrictions.

Distributive Justice   An ethics of social policy that advocates for a just distribution of resources and benefits in a society.

Dual Eligibility   Persons who qualify for both Medicare and Medicaid coverage. Typically low-income elderly or persons with disabilities.

Dualism   Two sources of health policymaking in the United States: government and private enterprise. A unique feature of the U.S. health care system.

E

Early Intervention   is a set of special education services, including therapy, provided to children, ages birth to three, typically in the home setting.

Effectiveness   is the best care provided under ordinary, everyday circumstances.

Efficacy   is the best care provided under ideal circumstances.

Efficiency   is care that considers the relationship of cost to the amount of improvement in health.

Empowerment   A social attitude and philosophy that provides an environment and skills that enable people with disabling conditions to make and act upon individual choices.

Enabling Factors   System characteristics that predispose a person to be able to access health care services (e.g., availability of insurance, provider location).

Entitlement   A statutory guarantee to a set of benefits for eligible persons.

Epidemiology   The science of public health; the systematic monitoring and investigation of disease and injury.

Equity   is care that meets societal expectations for fairness and justice.

Essential Health Benefits   A list of health care services mandated to be covered in insurance plans offered by American Health Benefit Exchanges.

Evidence-Based Practice   A process of delivering health care based upon the best available evidence of effectiveness and efficiency.

Expenses   are the amount of money spent on health care services in a specified time frame. Expenses to a health care provider would be revenue.

F

Favorable Selection   A form of moral hazard resulting in the selection of a low-cost, low-risk insurance risk pool; the opposite of adverse selection.

Federal Poverty Level   An annual income based on family size to determine a minimum, subsistence income; used for means-testing for several government insurance programs.

Fee for Service   Payment mechanism for health care whereby a provider is paid an amount of money for each procedure performed.

Fee Schedule   A list of procedures with an associated payment amount for each service.

Financing   The methods of paying for health care. Broadly speaking, includes private insurance, out-of-pocket payments, and government insurance programs.

Formal Care   The personal health care system consisting of a mix of acute, subacute, and long-term care facilities and related health care personnel.

G

Gatekeeper   A primary care provider in a health maintenance organization, usually a physician, who provides primary care and coordinates/controls access to the rest of the health care system.

Global Budgeting   Payment mechanism for health care whereby a provider is given a lump sum of money to care for a population for a period of time, usually a year.

Gross Domestic Product   Total output of goods and services in the United States in a year.

Guaranteed Issue   A requirement that health insurance be offered regardless of proof of insurability, (e.g., preexisting conditions exclusion).

H

Health Disparities   Differences in health status or health care based upon geographic or demographic characteristics of a population.

Health Maintenance Organization   is a form of managed care that demonstrates a strong integration of financing and delivery of care such as gatekeeper physicians, extensive utilization review, capitated financing.

Health Savings Account   A tax-protected pool of money set aside by a person to pay for out-of-pocket health care costs; usually associated with a high deductible form of health insurance.

Health Services   Related policy and systems that organize, finance, and deliver health care.

High Deductible Health Plan   A form of private health insurance, usually a PPO, that has a high annual deductible and is usually offered with a health savings account.

Home and Community-Based Waiver   An option for state Medicaid plans that will allow for coverage of noninstitutional health care services for eligible beneficiaries.

Hospitals   The institutional core of the acute medical care system; site of most tertiary and quaternary care in the United States.

I

Inclusion   A social philosophy that minimizes barriers and empowers persons with disabling conditions to achieve full participation in society.

Independent Living   A social movement that promotes employment, access to adequate housing, education, and employment, and acts against discrimination for persons with disabling conditions.

Individual Mandate   A requirement in the PPACA that all Americans purchase health insurance or pay a tax.

Informal Care   Personal health care that is provided by nonprofessional workers, primarily family and friends.

Integrated Health Care System   A combination of primary care, secondary care, tertiary care, and quaternary care providers through a process of vertical or horizontal integration.

Intermediate Care   A facility that provides residential services and a minimum level of professional care focusing on periodic monitoring and basic personal care.

Interpersonal Excellence   A component of health care quality that includes the caring and affective elements of patient care.

L

Legitimate   health care is care that meets societal expectations for optimal health care.

Level of Care   A stage of the informal or formal care system; often considered to be part of a "continuum of services."

Leverage   A position of dominance in an economic market that forces other players to negotiate on terms favorable to the person in the dominant position.

Lobbying   The process of redressing grievances to elected representatives; a First Amendment right in the United States.

M

Managed Care   is the integration of financing and delivery of health care services.

Managed Indemnity   is the least aggregated form of managed care characterized by fee-for-service reimbursement with preauthorization and utilization review for high-cost services.

Marginalization   A social process that isolates and stigmatizes persons with disabling conditions from the general population.

Matrix System   An organizational structure in a hospital that matches a product line team to a discipline-specific management structure.

Markets   An interaction between buyers and sellers involved in the exchange of economic resources (i.e., money, goods, and services).

Means-Tested   Prequalification process for Medicaid and SCHIP that requires eligible beneficiaries to meet certain income and asset requirements.

Medicaid   is a state-federal insurance program targeted to provide health insurance for low-income children, mothers, persons with disabilities, and elderly persons.

Medical Negligence   An act (or failure to act) by a health care professional that causes an injury or other adverse event to a patient.

Medically Necessary   Sometimes termed medical "necessity." The determination by a provider with physician status that a health care intervention is required. A prerequisite for all forms of health care insurance reimbursement. Associated with the certification and recertification process in Medicare.

Medically Needy Eligibility   A state-option qualification for Medicaid based on demonstrated medical need and, in some cases, income/asset level.

Medicare Administrative Contractor   A nongovernment entity, typically an insurer, that receives, reviews, and determines coverage for the Medicare program.

Medicare Assignment   An agreement between a provider and Medicare to accept (participate) the fee schedule as payment in full for services (minus the appropriate deductible and co-insurance).

Medicare Physician Fee Schedule   is the list of procedures and prices for outpatient therapy services for the Medicare program; updated annually and regionally adjusted.

Medicare-Medicaid Dual Eligibility   A classification of Medicaid eligibility that pays out-of-pocket Medicare expenses for low-income beneficiaries.

Medigap   A term for private supplemental insurance plans that provide benefits for services not covered by traditional Medicare.

Mental Health Policy   is the set of private and public statements, statutes, and regulations that address the needs of persons with mental illness.

Mental Health Settings   are sites of delivery of health care services to persons with mental illness such as hospitals, community mental health centers, day rehabilitation programs.

Moral Hazard Financially irresponsible behavior regarding insurance experienced as favorable selection and adverse selection.

Multiple Procedure Payment Reduction is a Medicare cost containment strategy that reduces the practice expense portion of the fee schedule amount for multiple procedure codes when used in the same visit.

N

Need Factors The presence of a medical condition that predisposes a person to access health care services.

O

Olmstead **Decision** is a legal ruling by the United States Supreme Court that established a legal right to integrated, community-based services for persons with disabilities.

Optimal health care maximizes the efficiency of health care delivery (i.e., the best value).

Outcome The results of a health care intervention.

P

Panel A group of providers selected by a managed care organization to provide services to plan members. May be open or closed.

Patient-Centered Medical Home is an integrated outpatient care system designed to increase the efficiency of ambulatory health care.

Patient-Focused Care Developed initially in hospitals, a redesign process of health care services from the perspective of the patient.

Patient Privacy A basic expectation of health care quality is that the patient's identity and records are kept confidential from the general public.

Patient Protection and Affordable Care Act of 2010 Landmark federal legislation that reforms the United States health care system.

Patient Safety A basic expectation of health care quality is that the patient is protected from unnecessary harm or from harm that can be anticipated.

Pay for Performance Incentive payment systems that reward high-quality care or penalize poor-quality health care.

Peer Review A process whereby therapist activity is examined and compared to accepted standards of practice.

Peer Review Organizations Medicare-sponsored organizations that perform quality-control, investigatory, and patient-education functions.

Penetration The percentage of the insurance market that is controlled by managed care.

Personal Care Services Home-based attendant care for persons with disabilities. Care assists with community integration (e.g. bathing, dressing).

Physician-Hospital Organization An integration of physician practices and the hospital to create leverage and compete with managed care organizations.

Physician Quality Reporting System is a quality reporting mechanism for Medicare. Currently voluntary, the program will soon be mandatory for outpatient therapy services.

Point of Service plan is a hybrid form of managed care typically combining a health maintenance organization and preferred provider organization form of insurance into one product.

Population Health is the assessment of health status and focused interventions for groups of people, communities, nations, or the world.

Preferred Provider Organization is a form of managed care with a discounted fee-for-service model, pre-authorization, utilization review, and reduced payment for out-of-network services.

Premium An amount of money paid by a beneficiary each period into a risk pool in order to qualify and pay for insurance benefits.

Presumptive Eligibility Used in the Medicaid program to provide temporary benefits until permanent eligibility can be determined.

Primary Care The most common form of health care in the United States. Care for common, episodic illnesses. Occurs primarily in outpatient settings.

Process The delivery of health care services, including physical therapy and occupational therapy. It has two components: technical excellence and interpersonal excellence.

Product-Line Teams The reorganization of patient care services away from traditional discipline-specific services to patient-focused teams (e.g., a joint-replacement team).

Professional Regulation A voluntary or mandatory process of ensuring the competence of health care providers. It has three levels: registration, certification, and licensure.

Prospective Payment A form of health care payment whereby providers are paid a set fee or rate prior to the delivery of services. Case-based payment, capitation, and Medicare Part A payment mechanisms are examples of prospective payment schemes.

Public Health Health care for populations that focuses on identification and intervention for the agent, host, and environment of disease and injury.

Q

Quality Improvement A process that identifies quality issues, sets goals to improve performance, and measures progress towards those goals.

Quaternary Care High-technology health care for uncommon, acute, and chronic disorders (e.g., organ transplantation). Associated with academic medical centers.

R

Reasonable Accommodations Legal language in the Americans with Disabilities Act requiring employers to address barriers experienced by persons with disabilities seeking employment.

Reflection A process of self-examination that is critical in understanding the personal motivations that affect the advocacy process.

Related Services Services for students defined in the Individuals with Disabilities Education Act that are mandated to assist students to access a public education; includes occupational therapy and physical therapy.

Rescission An insurance process outlawed by the PPACA (except for fraud) that prevents insurance companies from cancelling existing insurance contracts.

Revenue is the source of money to pay for health care services such as health insurance premiums or taxes.

Risk An insurance term that identifies the likelihood of a person or group incurring a loss, i.e., need for benefits.

S

Safety-Net Provider A health care provider that provides care to a large or predominantly uninsured or underinsured population.

School-Based Practice The site of delivery of therapy services as a component of special education; different goals and expectations from medically-based practice.

Scope of Practice is a legal definition of the procedures and level of decision making that can be performed by a profession.

Secondary Care Care for common, chronic-type disorders (e.g., diabetes mellitus, hypertension).

Social Disability A perspective on disablement that locates the problem in the policies, systems, and attitudes of those who are not experiencing disablement.

Social Insurance A form of government-sponsored health insurance whereby people paying premiums (taxes) are not eligible for benefits. Benefits are paid to those who have a defined social need. Examples are Medicare and Medicaid.

Social Media Technology-based communication methods, such as Twitter, increasingly used in political advocacy.

Special Education Services Primary and secondary education for children from birth to age 21 who have disabilities; includes related services (i.e., occupational therapy and physical therapy).

Spend-Down A process whereby a person with potential Medicaid eligibility "spends down" his or her assets to a certain level in order to gain eligibility for the program.

Spousal Impoverishment Associated with the spend-down program in Medicaid, this provision allows the spouses of Medicaid beneficiaries to remain in the community.

Standard An accepted or, in some cases, optimal level of practice or performance.

State Option Eligibility criteria for Medicaid that can be included or excluded by the states (e.g., medically needy eligibility).

Structure The stable elements of the health care system (e.g., physical structures, human resources).

Sustainable Growth Rate is a Medicare cost containment strategy to limit the growth in the Medicare Part B program by reducing the standardized conversion factor.

Swing Bed Unit A subacute care ward, typically in a hospital, for patients recovering from an acute illness or injury.

T

Technical Excellence A component of health care quality that considers the knowledge and expertise of the provider in the health care encounter.

Tertiary Care A technologically sophisticated level of care associated with inpatient hospital stays.

Testimony Providing information to public policymakers in verbal and written form as well as in response to questions.

Therapy Benefit Manager A contractor used by an insurance company to analyze and advise on the appropriateness of therapy claims.

Therapy Cap is the annual financial limit placed on outpatient occupational therapy and physical therapy. For physical therapy, the limit is combined with speech therapy.

TRICARE is the civilian health insurance program for active military, certain retirees, and their beneficiaries.

Tribal Self-Determination An option for American Indian/Alaska Native tribes to organize their health care system vs. direct delivery by the Indian Health Service.

U

Underinsured People with health insurance but who have impaired access to health care due to fewer plan benefits.

Underwriting The insurance process that examines individual characteristics to determine eligibility and cost of insurance.

Uninsured People who have impaired access to health care due to lack of health insurance.

Universalism A philosophy on disablement that emphasizes the common experience of disability and advocates policies that reduce barriers and reinforce inclusion for all persons.

Utilization Review is a process of review of patient records and the process of care for individuals to determine the appropriateness of services.

V

Vested After payment of taxes into the Medicare trust fund for 40 quarters, a person is eligible for Part A benefits upon reaching retirement age, experiencing permanent disability, or developing end-stage renal disease.

Vocational Rehabilitation A process of assessment, education, training, and support for persons with disabling conditions to prepare them for the workforce.

Voluntary Agency Not-for-profit organization that provides advocacy, education, and limited personal health care for persons with illness or disease (e.g., the National Multiple Sclerosis Society).

Index